Detection of Malingering during Head Injury Litigation

CRITICAL ISSUES IN NEUROPSYCHOLOGY

Series Editors

Antonio E. Puente
University of North Carolina, Wilmington

Cecil R. Reynolds
Texas A&M University
and Bastrop Mental Health Associates

Current Volumes in this Series

CONTEMPORARY APPROACHES TO NEUROPSYCHOLOGICAL ASSESSMENT
Edited by Gerald Goldstein and Theresa M. Incagnoli

DETECTION OF MALINGERING DURING HEAD INJURY LITIGATION
Edited by Cecil R. Reynolds

FAMILY SUPPORT PROGRAMS AND REHABILITATION:
A Cognitive–Behavioral Approach to Traumatic Brain Injury
Louise Margaret Smith and Hamish P. D. Godfrey

HANDBOOK OF CLINICAL CHILD NEUROPSYCHOLOGY, Second Edition
Edited by Cecil R. Reynolds and Elaine Fletcher-Janzen

HANDBOOK OF NEUROPSYCHOLOGY AND AGING
Edited by Paul David Nussbaum

NEUROPSYCHOLOGICAL EXPLORATIONS OF MEMORY AND COGNITION:
Essays in Honor of Nelson Butters
Edited by Laird S. Cermak

NEUROPSYCHOLOGICAL TOXICOLOGY:
Identification and Assessment of Human Neurotoxic Syndromes, Second Edition
David E. Hartman

THE PRACTICE OF FORENSIC NEUROPSYCHOLOGY:
Meeting Challenges in the Courtroom
Edited by Robert J. McCaffrey, Arthur D. Williams, Jerid M. Fisher, and Linda C. Laing

---

A Continuation Order Plan is available for this series. A continuation order will bring delivery of each new volume immediately upon publication. Volumes are billed only upon actual shipment. For further information please contact the publisher.

Detection of Malingering during Head Injury Litigation

Edited by

Cecil R. Reynolds

Texas A&M University
College Station, Texas, and
Bastrop Mental Health Associates
Bastrop, Texas

Plenum Press • New York and London

Library of Congress Cataloging-in-Publication Data

Detection of malingering during head injury litigation / edited by
Cecil R. Reynolds.
p. cm. -- (Critical issues in neuropsychology)
Includes bibliographical references and index.
ISBN 0-306-45655-9
1. Forensic neuropsychology. 2. Malingering--Diagnosis. 3. Head--Wounds and injuries--Complications. I. Reynolds, Cecil R., 1952- . II. Series.
[DNLM: 1. Head Injuries--complications. 2. Malingering--diagnosis. 3. Jurisprudence. WE 706 D479 1997]
RA1147.5.D48 1997
614'.1--dc21
DNLM/DLC
for Library of Congress

97-34812
CIP

ISBN 0-306-45655-9

A Division of Plenum Publishing Corporation
233 Spring Street, New York, N.Y. 10013

http://www.plenum.com

10 9 8 7 6 5 4 3 2 1

Printed in the United States of America

Contributors

Margaret A. Ackley • Department of Psychology, University of Rhode Island, Kingston, Rhode Island 03881

David T. R. Berry • Department of Psychology, University of Kentucky, Lexington, Kentucky 40506

James N. Butcher • Department of Psychology, University of Minnesota, Minneapolis, Minnesota 55415

David Faust • Department of Psychology, University of Rhode Island, Kingston, Rhode Island 03881

Charles J. Golden • Center for Psychological Services, Nova Southeastern University, Fort Lauderdale, Florida 33314

Wm. Drew Gouvier • Department of Psychology, Louisiana State University, Baton Rouge, Louisiana 70803

Christine A. Grier • Center for Psychological Services, Nova Southeastern University, Fort Lauderdale, Florida 33314

Ruben C. Gur • Brain Behavior Laboratory and the Neuropsychiatry Section, Department of Psychiatry, University of Pennsylvania, Philadelphia, Pennsylvania 19104

Juan Manuel Gutiérrez • Brain Behavior Laboratory and the Neuropsychiatry Section, Department of Psychiatry, University of Pennsylvania, Philadelphia, Pennsylvania 19104

Lawrence C. Hartlage • Augusta Neuropsychology Center, Augusta, Georgia 30809

Jill S. Hayes • Department of Psychology, Louisiana State University, Baton Rouge, Louisiana 70803

Ralph M. Reitan • Reitan Neuropsychology Laboratory, Tucson, Arizona 85713

Cecil R. Reynolds • Department of Educational Psychology, Texas A&M University, College Station, Texas 77843

Brandi B. Smiroldo • Department of Psychology, Louisiana State University, Baton Rouge, Louisiana 70803

J. Michael Williams • Department of Clinical and Health Psychology, Allegheny University of the Health Sciences, Philadelphia, Pennsylvania 19102

Deborah Wolfson • Reitan Neuropsychology Laboratory, Tucson, Arizona 85713

Preface

The issue of potential malingering in the context of head injury litigation has seen an explosion of research and commentary in recent years. In reviewing various journals devoted to clinical practice of the 1950s, 1960s, and even into the 1970s, one rarely sees a paper focused on the issue of malingering in civil litigation; occasional papers deal with malingering with regard to military service and criminal prosecution, but even in these areas there is relatively scant work. During this time period, neuropsychology was principally an academic endeavor with few clinical practitioners. Largely through the efforts of Ralph Reitan, Oscar Parsons, Art Benton, and a bevy of their former students (Lawrence Hartlage and Charles Mathews, among others), clinical practice in neuropsychology became the norm. With this growth of practitioners and the founding of journals to support scholarly inquiry and clinical practice in the field came many revelations about the effects of closed head injury, an injury for many years believed to be of little consequence and one known at times as a silent epidemic. Coupled with the growth of knowledge about the potential deleterious effects of closed head injury has been growth in personal injury litigation and product liability suits. As more and more injuries have come to be litigated and the potential sums of money involved have become enormous (a jury in Dallas in 1996 awarded $25 million to a man in his 50s in a closed head injury claim involving a motor vehicle accident), issues and concerns about malingering have grown substantially. By the mid-1980s, malingering and its evaluation and detection had found a routine place in the primary journals of neuropsychology. Seldom does a month go by that I do not find at least one thoughtful study of this problem.

The rapidity and need for this research has prompted many strong ideas and creative approaches to the detection of malingering but has likewise spawned a considerable tautology and clinical mythology. The diagnosis of malingering is not just a scientific controversy but has become an emotional one as well. As editor-in-chief of *Archives of Clinical Neuropsychology*, I have received letters of complaint about the "defense posture" of the journal while receiving letters complaining about the journal favoring plaintiffs' allegations of injury, only to find the neuropsychologists writing to me were complaining about the same papers. As health care providers it is, and should be, difficult from a personal perspective to designate a patient a malingerer. It is a diagnosis with clear negative implications and is tantamount to calling a potentially injured patient a liar, something we are loathe to do. Therefore, we tend to seek stronger, more convincing evidence for such a diagnosis than is the case for many clinical diagnoses we make on a routine basis.

The diagnosis of malingering is fraught with conceptual, philosophical, and logistical potholes. Although some may think it more fitting as a closing chapter, Faust and Ackley have been given the opening chapter of this volume to disclose the methodological and conceptual problems in the diagnosis of malingering to establish clearly a mind-set of critical analysis before reading about methods proposed by other authors. The chapters that follow provide current methods and thinking on multiple approaches to the detection of malingering during head injury litigation, including specific symptoms such as memory loss to more global claims of diffuse loss of function to cognitive and psychomotor arenas. The various presentations range from the strong actuarial methods of Reitan and Wolfson, which have a false-positive rate of nearly zero (but at what sacrifice to false-negative rates we are uncertain), to the careful, consummate clinical reasoning of Hartlage, known as a gifted clinician in addition to a leader in professional activities in the profession. This book has been developed for the thoughtful, serious clinician who may be involved in evaluating patients with head injury who often become involved in litigation with regard to these injuries. The book contains many "how-to" sections, but just as many cautions and concerns are expressed about how we approach the problem of malingering.

Several things are clear at this stage. The first is that malingering is a substantial problem in head injury litigation; reasonable and thorough research indicates that at least 25% of cases of head injury in litigation involve malingering. Secondly, we must consider the possibility of malingering in all cases and be prepared to make the diagnosis when it is the most probable diagnosis despite our reluctance to make the call of malingering and despite the many methodological, conceptual, and logistical caveats expressed so eloquently in the opening chapter. Hopefully, this work will demonstrate the utility and the pitfalls of various actuarial and clinical approaches to the diagnosis of malingering and equip the clinician with the necessary tools, knowledge, and logic to consider malingering and its alternative diagnoses intelligently. As with much of what we do, the evaluation of malingering cries out for intelligent testing.

I must express my appreciation to the chapter authors, who have laid bare their own methods and reasoning in the evaluation of malingering. Each has provided original insights, methods, and commentary on the issues that go beyond what any one of us could conceptualize. Their willingness to share in the movement toward advancement in the diagnosis of malingering is much appreciated. A special thanks also goes to Jean Whitaker, for her hard work in preparing such a thorough index. To my editor at Plenum, Mariclaire Cloutier, I would like to express my appreciation for her continuing faith in my efforts to produce works that contribute to the growth of neuropsychology and in particular for her affable nature in both pulling and prodding work that is so often delayed. To the Plenum production editor, Michele Fetterolf, thank you for your tenacity in chasing author queries and in bringing the manuscript to its published conclusion with such promptness and with such style and for putting up with me in the process. To my wife, Dr. Julia A. Hickman, goes my continuing and unfaltering appreciation for her support and understanding during those times devoted to manuscripts such as this that pull from time otherwise spent together. Thank you.

Cecil R. Reynolds
Bastrop, Texas

Contents

1

Did You Think It Was Going to Be Easy?

Some Methodological Suggestions for the Investigation and Development of Malingering Detection Techniques

DAVID FAUST AND MARGARET A. ACKLEY

One disadvantage of no longer taking a problem for granted is that one may begin to appreciate just how difficult the problem is. In a 1992 address to the American Psychological Association, Ralph Reitan indicated that the development of methods for the detection of malingering might require an effort not that different in scope from that required to derive neuropsychological methods for the detection of brain dysfunction. That distressing thought could certainly be viewed as a constructive call to action.

Indeed, over the last decade, and particularly in the last few years, psychologists and neuropsychologists have mounted a major research campaign in the area of malingering detection, perhaps motivated in part by the increasing recognition of the importance and potential difficulty of the problem. Unlike a decade ago, there is now a sizable body of research to consider that extends well beyond the Minnesota Multiphasic Personality Inventory (MMPI) (Butcher, Dahlstrom, Graham, Tellegen, & Kaemmer, 1989; Hathaway & McKinley, 1983) and anec-

DAVID FAUST AND MARGARET A. ACKLEY • Department of Psychology, University of Rhode Island, Kingston, Rhode Island 02881.

Detection of Malingering during Head Injury Litigation, edited by Reynolds. Plenum Press, New York, 1998.

dotal reports, and various scientific advances to point to as indications of real progress.

Our aim in this chapter is not to critique this now considerable body of literature study-by-study, nor to address basic methodological points that competent researchers fully recognize and that seem to emerge in cookie-cutter fashion in almost every review of difficult areas of applied clinical research. Readers do not need yet another article telling them to watch their subject-to-variable ratios, be alert for Type I and Type II errors, and exercise caution when combining results across studies using different measurement techniques. Rather, our main intent is conceptual and prospective, that is, to reflect on our current state of knowledge and methodology, propose some directions we might think of heading next, try to frame what we believe are key issues and problems in the area, and offer suggestions that might aid progress on some of the most difficult methodological problems we face. Accordingly, in order, we will address a series of major conceptual and methodological concerns, discuss malingering indices present and future, and finally expand on the suggestions for research described throughout the chapter.

LEARNING TO DETECT MALINGERING VIA EXPERIENCE

Meta-analysis of MMPI malingering indices shows impressive effect sizes, usually surpassing one standard deviation and sometimes two standard deviations. (Issues about the fidelity of MMPI malingering studies, which we discuss later, are of little relevance to the immediate discussion.) This impressive achievement is a product of gifted individuals applying the best epistemic game in town—science—to a difficult problem.

It is instructive to contrast studies examining the success with which MMPI malingering indices versus laypersons and professionals detect falsification. Considerable literature suggests that laypersons and professionals from various walks of life (e.g., psychologists, psychiatrists, lawyers, judges) have considerable difficulty detecting lies (DePaulo, 1994; Ekman & O'Sullivan, 1991). Further, research that has directly examined the capacity of clinicians to detect malingering has provided little basis for confidence in their success. For example, in Heaton, Smith, Lehman, and Vogt's (1978) study, clinicians performed at chance level to 20% above chance level in separating the testing results of individuals with serious brain injuries versus those faking brain injury. Frederick, Sarfaty, Johnson, and Powell's (1994) study also suggested problems detecting malingering, even among neuropsychologists who performed comprehensive assessments and had face-to-face contacts with examinees. The clinicians in Faust and colleagues' studies (Faust, Hart & Guilmette, 1988; Faust, Hart, Guilmette, & Arkes, 1988) showed similar difficulties detecting malingering.

Various methodological criticisms have been raised about these types of studies (e.g., Bigler, 1990), a number of which certainly merit attention and further study but others of which sometimes seem weak or raise straw-man arguments. For example, in contrast to the idea that these studies must have included hacks, the list of clinicians in the Heaton et al. (1978) study is rather impressive, including such individuals as Igor Grant and Charles Matthews. The Faust et al. studies included both clinicians with limited and extensive experience and found no difference in outcome. The idea that clinicians would have done better had they had a chance to observe patients may be correct, but studies examining the accuracy of judgments about falsification based on personal contact are not at all encouraging on this score, and Frederick and colleagues' (1994) results run counter to the conjecture.

Additionally, these studies on malingering detection and the relative success of subjective versus empirically validated and objective decision methods do not exist in a vacuum. Studies in other areas demonstrate the same types of difficulties identifying malingering or exaggeration (e.g., Albert, Fox, & Kahn, 1980; Rogers, 1988). There is also a massive body of literature demonstrating the relative superiority of empirically based, systematic, and formally validated decision procedures over subjective methods (Dawes, Faust, & Meehl, 1989; Grove & Meehl, 1996). In contrast, there is a relative paucity of evidence suggesting that clinicians do particularly well identifying malingering using subjective judgment methods. Finally, researchers who have directly examined the capacity of clinicians to detect malingering, such as Heaton, Frederick, and Faust, have never claimed that their studies can be safely and directly generalized to everyday clinical practice, but rather that their results raise concerns or questions about clinicians' capacity to detect malingering.

Whatever one's exact views on the methodology of malingering detection studies, the current box score strongly favors indices and procedures derived through formal scientific study over subjective or clinical judgment. Such differential success suggests at least two points. First, it is likely that subjective clinical judgment often does not make optimal or near-optimal use of information bearing on malingering when evaluating cases, for if that were so, clinicians in the studies would at least be matching, if not outperforming, formal decision rules and procedures, which they are not doing. The relative success, and relatively greater success, that formal decision procedures achieve in malingering detection indicates that the available information frequently is sufficient to make accurate identifications, but that too often this information is being overlooked or countervailed or combined improperly. Second, the studies do not support the idea, often taken for granted, that experience provides a major assist in learning to detect malingering.

It is precisely this difficulty in learning to detect malingering via experience that provides the major rationale and impetus for research on malingering detection. A recognition of the factors that impede experiential learning is essential in practice and research. In practice, a healthy respect for the benefits and limits of experiential learning alerts us to the need to use helpful decision aids. In research, this same understanding helps to set the research agenda, provides insight into the tasks that clinicians face, and can alert us to potential methodological boondoggles that compromise the value of investigations.

Let us consider the conditions that promote or inhibit experiential learning (Dawes, 1989; Faust, 1989). Experiential learning tends to be most successful when feedback is immediate, clear, and deterministic. By *deterministic*, we mean that the feedback is unfailingly or perfectly related to its antecedent, in particular the accuracy of judgments or conclusions. Thus, each time we are right we are told we are right, and each time we are wrong we are informed so. At the other end of the spectrum, learning can become difficult or impossible when no feedback is received. In between, as the error term in feedback increases, that is, as the level of noise and inaccuracy in feedback grows, the more difficult learning tends to become.

The Category Test (Reitan & Wolfson, 1993) can serve to illustrate these points. Following the examinee's response, he is immediately informed whether he is right or wrong in no uncertain terms. The feedback is deterministic, for each time he is right he is told he is right, and vice versa. These are excellent conditions for learning from experience, and most examinees benefit greatly from the feedback, performing well above chance level. Further, if normals were given the chance to take the Category Test again and again within a brief period of time, many would rapidly move toward very high levels of accuracy.

Imagine, however, if conditions were changed so that in many instances, the feedback that was received was no longer an easily distinguished bell or buzzer but something that perhaps sounded a little more like a bell than a buzzer or a little more like a buzzer than a bell. Imagine further that in many instances, feedback was delayed, perhaps by minutes or hours or days, and that in the interim intervening events might occur that could alter the seemingly simple association between response accuracy and feedback. For example, in some instances some event might occur that distorted the initial response such that 2 was misrepresented as 3, with feedback given accordingly. Imagine if, in addition, the feedback was systematically skewed in some fashion, for example, if the examinee were repeatedly informed that a certain type of misconception was instead correct. Imagine further that at times, perhaps more often than not, no feedback was given at all. It is obvious from this example that learning via experience would become much more difficult, and that one might welcome a community of scientists mounting a concentrated effort to unlock the keys to the Category Test.

We do not think it is at all exaggerating to say that a clinician who depended solely on experience to learn malingering detection would be faced with much the same conditions as an examinee trying to learn under conditions of sporadic, skewed, delayed, noisy, and all too often misleading feedback. In many, if not most, instances, the clinician does not receive feedback on the accuracy of positive or negative identifications of malingering. When feedback is obtained it is often delayed, ambiguous, and skewed or distorted. For example, if the clinician falsely diagnoses genuine disorder, it would be the rare event for the malingerer to correct the misimpression. If the clinician falsely diagnoses malingering, then the plaintiff's sincere claims of disorder have not been believed in the first place, and subsequent sincere disagreement, should the plaintiff learn of the conclusion and have a chance to dispute it, are likely to be similarly rejected. The outcome of a trial, should the case be one of the small percentage that ever get that far, does not necessarily indicate the true answer and can be contaminated by the clinician's own input. Although it is true that the clinician who believed the claimant was sincere might be confronted at trial with a videotape that provides convincing evidence that the practitioner was fooled, she has learned little else than that she is not right all of the time, something that all but the most foolishly arrogant already know.

There is another, perhaps more subtle, but no less important facet of this problem of learning from experience. In malingering detection, as is true with most diagnostic and predictive tasks in psychology, conditions or states are inferred from probabilistic indicators, rather than directly observed. Further, these probabilistic indicators are usually found in both the target and nontarget populations. For such indicators to be effective, they of course must occur with different frequency across the target and nontarget populations. If they are more frequent in the target population, they can be viewed as positive indicators, and if they are less frequent, they can be viewed as negative indicators. One hopes for markedly different frequencies across the target and nontarget populations, but sometimes separations are not that great. For example, both brain-damaged patients and normals report interpersonal conflicts. Even when separations along particular characteristics or on particular items are not that great, the proper combination of multiple, nonredundant indicators of modest validity can sometimes achieve respectable or high accuracy rates. In other instances we settle for indicators of modest accuracy because they allow us to do better than we could otherwise do without them, and they do not shift the balance of false-negative and false-positive error in an unacceptable direction.

The clinician who attempts to identify and apply malingering indicators via experience, or perhaps to modify empirically validated procedures on this same basis, is operating under terrible disadvantages. If one does not consistently know who are and are not the malingerers among those one evaluates, how can one determine the relative frequency of potential indicators across the target and nontarget groups? Even if such identifications are possible in some cases, absent a representative sample of cases, as opposed to the sample and distribution of cases the clinician happens to see in his setting, differential frequencies may be substantially misrepresented. An accurate appraisal of these differential frequencies is necessary to determine whether a sign is useful, just how useful it might be, how it compares with other signs, whether it should be added to other available predictors, and how it is to be combined with other predictors. For example, the clinician may observe that almost all malingerers she feels confident she has correctly identified show grossly implausible results on forced-choice methods. However, the majority of malingerers may not show such results, and thus the absence of such an indicator may be of little differential value. As the Chapmans' original research (1967, 1969) and much work thereafter has shown (Wedding & Faust, 1989), it can be very difficult to determine the association between variables, such as potential signs and disorder, in the course of clinical practice and observation. We are prone to forming false associations between signs and disorder and overestimating the strength of associations.

When attempting to determine the potential utility of diagnostic signs, we are helped greatly if we can obtain a representative sample of the target and nontarget populations. We are not so interested in subgroups of the nontarget population that we can easily distinguish from the target group (the malingerers) in the first place, such as patients with severe strokes or advanced dementias. Rather, we are interested in the nonmalingerers that might be, or particularly that are most likely to be, misidentified as malingerers, that is, those individuals the clinician needs to distinguish from malingerers. For example, the clinician almost never needs to discriminate between those who appear to be injured but are malingering and those who do not appear to be injured and are responding to the best of their capability. One needs an appropriate contrast group, or what might be conceptualized as the proper counterfactual.

If and when valid signs are identified, one then wishes to adjust, as needed, the manner in which they are used or the cutting scores that are applied in accord with the relative frequencies of the target and nontarget populations in the setting of utilization. A decision rule that is effective in a setting with a very high rate of malingering will probably lead to far too many false-positive identifications if applied unchanged within a setting with a much lower frequency. Decision rules should be adjusted in accord with frequencies or base rates in the setting of application (Meehl & Rosen, 1955). Optimum cutting points shift depending on the frequency of conditions.

The task that faces the clinician who tries to learn malingering detection via experience is thus as follows. The clinician needs a way to determine true status, determine the differential frequency of the target and relevant nontarget groups in the setting of interest, obtain representative samples of these groups, separate the valid and invalid signs through adequate testing in these groups, and then devise a proper means for combining the range of valid predictors that have been uncovered, preferably by considering such matters as their nonredundant contribution to predictive accuracy and the extent to which predictions should be regressed. To say the least, this is a formidable task. It is also one that lays out a blueprint for researchers.

The same types of conditions required for learning through clinical experience need to be met for learning through research, and to the extent that studies fall short, the pragmatic help they can provide to clinicians will be compromised. Of course, this does not justify the stance that because such conditions are imperfectly met by one or another investigation, one can then resort to experiential learning in which one usually violates, to a far greater extent, the epistemic shortcomings of research studies.

THE VALUE OF EXPERIENCE AND CASE STUDY

The preceding statements should not be confused with the view that clinical experience and impressions are of no use. Rather, it is important to recognize the strengths and limitations of this type of evidence. Clinical observation has led to brilliant insights, and it is sometimes hard to imagine how such ideas could have evolved in any other context. It seems almost pedantic to say that all forms of evidence do not serve all masters equally well. Those evaluating malingering research sometimes apply criteria rigidly across too diverse a set of contexts, or in situations in which they are not fully or at all appropriate. It is a related mistake to assume that if information meets evaluative criteria in one context it will do so across other contexts, without considering the shift in epistemic standards that may be necessitated by context and intended use.

Much of the work on malingering is based exclusively or primarily on clinical impressions or anecdotal evidence (although terminology or descriptions of methodology sometimes make it sound as if the data were something more than this). An article that offers opinion or conjecture on malingering based on clinical experience provides an example. Other works consist of case studies, or descriptions of a series of cases. A close cousin is the work that reports on a series ("group") of malingerers who have been detected, or presumably detected. Unfortunately, in some of these articles, the authors are too quick to attempt broad generalizations, or to claim that the evidence they obtained helps to validate (or invalidate) certain potential indicators of malingering. In contrast, other reviewers may immediately dismiss such studies as useless, arguing that they do not provide an appropriate means for testing malingering indicators.

One problem with these case study methods is that the researcher may not have that strong a basis for determining whether those who were "caught" were truly malingerers. Further, one does not know how many malingerers escaped detection. Consequently, at least based on current methods, it can be very difficult to determine the representativeness of the investigator's sample (we discuss below a possible method for dealing with this problem). Additionally, there are strong armchair reasons to doubt that the obtained sample is representative of the target population. The researcher is studying the malingerers who were caught, or in essence the characteristics that led them to be caught, so as to devise means to catch the malingerers who were not caught, or to uncover the discriminating features of this latter group. However, one might well expect a negative correlation between the characteristics that led an individual to be caught and thereby included in the sample and the characteristics that led an individual not to be caught and thereby excluded from the sample; and yet it is exactly the excluded sample about which we most want to learn. After all, we are not interested in the malingerers we already know how to detect, and who likely on average fall toward the lower end of the malingering-skills continuum, but more so in learning how to detect the malingerers who we do not know how to detect or who we have trouble detecting.

Whether or not these armchair speculations about negative relations between the caught and the not-caught seem reasonable, the key point is that we presently lack a method to gauge the representativeness of samples obtained in these catch-as-catch-can studies. Thus, even if a particular sample happens to be representative, it does us little good because we have no way of knowing that it is the case, and at the same time we know that samples may well be non-representative. As such, these studies by themselves do not offer a means to determine whether the signs and indicators found in the sample have diagnostic utility. They may or may not have utility, but unless one can make that determination the information by itself is close to useless in the clinical setting. For these reasons, a researcher who cites such evidence to make anything approaching strong claims about validity or invalidity is probably committing a serious methodological error.

Although the distinction is somewhat artificial and the boundaries not nearly as clear as one might think, it is still helpful to distinguish the context of discovery and what Reichenbach (1938) referred to as the context of justification. To aid in detecting malingering, one ultimately strives to provide the clinician with potent predictors. Of course, one cannot validate or apply predictors that no one has ever thought of, and surely no philosopher of science would suggest that the researcher "only identify potential predictors that are known in advance to be highly valid," because we are aware of no method for doing so and such a prescription would impossibly hinder investigation. More reasonable epistemic advice might be something like, "Test your best ideas or conjectures about potential predictors, and try to avoid potential predictors that have very little chance of success, unless you are totally stuck, or unless improbable indicators, should they pan out, are likely to be very powerful; but don't inhibit yourself too much because it's hard to anticipate nature and occasionally a seemingly outlandish idea turns out to be highly progressive." In the context of discovery, one exercises considerably greater leniency when evaluating ideas.

One of course prefers ideas that are more likely to be correct because it is the correct answer we are seeking and because economy of research effort is extremely important (there are only so many scientific hours and tax dollars to be spent on any particular problem). However, it is often very difficult to make such judgments at the outset and, again, our ultimate methods and ideas will be no better than the ideas we think of and test. In the context of discovery, one might say that the only requirement is that the idea or method or sign might work, not that it will or does work, and at least for now the scientist has few or no formal methods for deriving probabilities (although Faust & Meehl [1992] are working on these and related metascience problems).

If anecdotal evidence, case studies, and naturalistic studies of "caught" malingerers are viewed mainly within the context of discovery and not verification, we can readily acknowledge their value in uncovering variables or indicators that may prove discriminatory, or in providing the needed grist for the verification mill. However, when the value of evidence is mainly limited to the domain of discovery, it is helpful to recognize and acknowledge these limitations, just as it is unfair to criticize a researcher whose intent is discovery for failing to meet stringent tests of verification. More generally, to the extent that a study lacks external validity, one might think of it more as an exercise in the context of discovery versus verification.

Having said all this, there are still some situations in which the problems with representativeness that typically plague case study methods are not of much concern. For example, if we can identify clinicians who are highly skilled in detecting malingering, and if our hope is to learn how they achieve this success so that others can benefit from it, we do not really care if their abilities and methods are atypical. Also, occasionally, such extreme claims are made that single clear counterinstances provide powerful disconfirming evidence. For example, suppose someone claims that the only explanation for a very low score on a forced-choice method is malingering. A single solid counter-example can offer a powerful form of disproof, as might occur were the technician to mangle the instructions and tell the examinee to select the number that was not presented before.

CLINICALLY RELEVANT DISTINCTIONS

Dimensions of Malingering

One of the most common types of malingering study involves the sort of discrimination that clinicians or forensic evaluators are almost never called on to make: the distinction between normal individuals performing to the best of their abilities and normal individuals faking bad. Rather, ignoring complexities and mixed presentations for the moment, the examiner is almost always trying to separate individuals who have some form of disorder from those purposely falsifying information about disorder. The clinician's typical task is far more difficult than separating normals doing their best from those faking bad, and can certainly involve different qualitative elements.

It is not an academic exercise to ask, "What is the nature of the thing we are addressing when we refer to malingering or falsification?" This is not a question of definition, which is not too difficult. Instead it is a question of proper conceptualization of external (real-world) correlates, and in particular whether we are referring to an artificial conglomeration of attributes and behaviors as opposed to something with taxonicity or internal coherence, a type or types of some sort. How are we to think about the clinician's task if we do not have a reasonably clear idea about just what it is we are trying to identify? For example, the inferences or conclusions we should draw from data can differ greatly depending on whether malingering or falsification represents a continuum, or if falsification in one domain bears a high versus negligible correlation with falsification in other domains. If plaintiff Jones falsifies an early history of alcohol abuse, how much does this tell us about the likelihood that he is also lying about his fall down the stairs? If falsification is minimally related across domains, it tells us little; but if it is highly interrelated, then knowing that Jones underestimates his drinking by 50% could practically tell us that he fell down three steps, not the six he reported.

In conceptualizing what malingering might be, at least two dimensions seem to be required. One dimension involves misrepresentation of one's own health status (defined broadly) and the other intentionality. Whether the clinician wants to become involved in examining both dimensions, and whether or not the practitioner thinks that intention can be evaluated, are separate considerations from whether or not intentionality is needed in a conceptualization of malingering, which it is. For example, we would not want to identify a horribly depressed patient who misperceives his functioning in an overly negative way, or a patient with a right parietal tumor who claims her right hand is not her own, as malingerers.

It could easily be argued that a definition of malingering should also include the aim or hoped for goals of the intentional misrepresentation. Surely there would seem to be a difference between an individual who fabricates a disorder in an effort to avoid responsibility for a vicious crime and a crime victim who feigns death to save his life. One of the difficulties here is unpacking the ontologic and moral issues. On the one hand, there might well be differences between individuals who fake illness for altruistic or at least neutral reasons and those who do so for self-gain, even when it harms innocent individuals. On the other hand, these types of distinctions between honorable and dishonorable reasons for malingering may lack objective grounding and can become rather arbitrary or almost purely subjective. For example, the same hockey player who fakes injury to draw a major penalty may be a villain in the visiting arena and a hero in the home arena, and it does not make much sense to say the justifications for his actions change when he lands in Montreal. Contrast this to a situation in which an individual plans and carries out a brutal murder for monetary gain and then feigns insanity.

Some social scientists think that these types of value judgments are arbitrary or irrelevant, but assuredly the courts do not share their views. The stated purpose of the legal system is to resolve disputes in a fair manner, and this indeed often involves moral judgments and questions of culpability. A person's intended goals or reasons for doing something and their legal/moral correctness frequently decide the outcome of cases. An abused woman who feigns unconsciousness to avoid physical injury is likely to be judged quite differently than an abusing husband who fakes incapacitation so as to lure his spouse into a trap and harm her, even though both are intentionally faking disorder.

These value issues involve such considerations as whether there would seem to be a morally just versus immoral reason to malinger; whether the malingerer's motives are altruistic, neutral, or self-interested; and whether the act of deception comes at cost to others or victimizes them. Hence, in considering the dimensions of malingering, one might need to ask not only whether the act of providing false information is intended, but also what the individual intends to accomplish and is willing to do given an awareness of the possible consequences for others. Such judgments may reflect societal perceptions for the most part and in some instances are arguably relativistic. Nevertheless, there may well be an intrinsic, qualitatively different dimension one taps beyond falsification and intention when one looks for differences between individuals who will and will not violate major societal norms or engage in deceit for moral versus immoral reasons. Whatever the case, we will mainly limit our focus here to the first two dimensions of intent and misrepresentation. It seems likely that in most clinical and legal cases, more serious forms of intended misrepresentation are not altruistic.

In legal cases, there is another element that must be considered, although it does not belong on a list of candidate dimensions for malingering. In tort law, a determination of culpability, and the assignment of damages, often depend not only on the presence and extent of harm, but also on cause. Smith may be terribly damaged, but if it is not the car accident but the 20-year addictive history that accounts for lowered scores on neuropsychological testing, then the driver who carelessly hit him may owe nothing for neurocognitive maladies.

A plaintiff who is claiming brain damage may not need to fake or exaggerate disorder at all to mislead the clinician into adopting a conclusion favorable to her case. For example, the plaintiff can simply try to mislead the clinician about cause by hiding or covering up alternative factors that explain her difficulties. Plaintiffs may also overstate prior functioning so as to create a false impression about loss of functioning. Whether these alternative forms of deceit represent another separate qualitative dimension or just another phenotypic variation of a genotype is difficult to say, but there is no question that clinicians desire methods for identifying these types of deception as well. In fact, attempts to lead clinicians down the wrong causal path may be one, if not the most, common form of falsification in legal settings and deserves the careful attention of researchers.

Qualitative and Quantitative Differences in Presentation and Interrelation with Clinical Distinctions

If we momentarily limit ourselves to the dimensions of intention and falsification, and if we avoid seeing these variables as dichotomous or all or none, which almost certainly they are not, the number and types of distinctions the clinician must make become apparent. As illustrated in Figure 1, suppose we arrange the accuracy of information that is available to the clinician about the examinee's

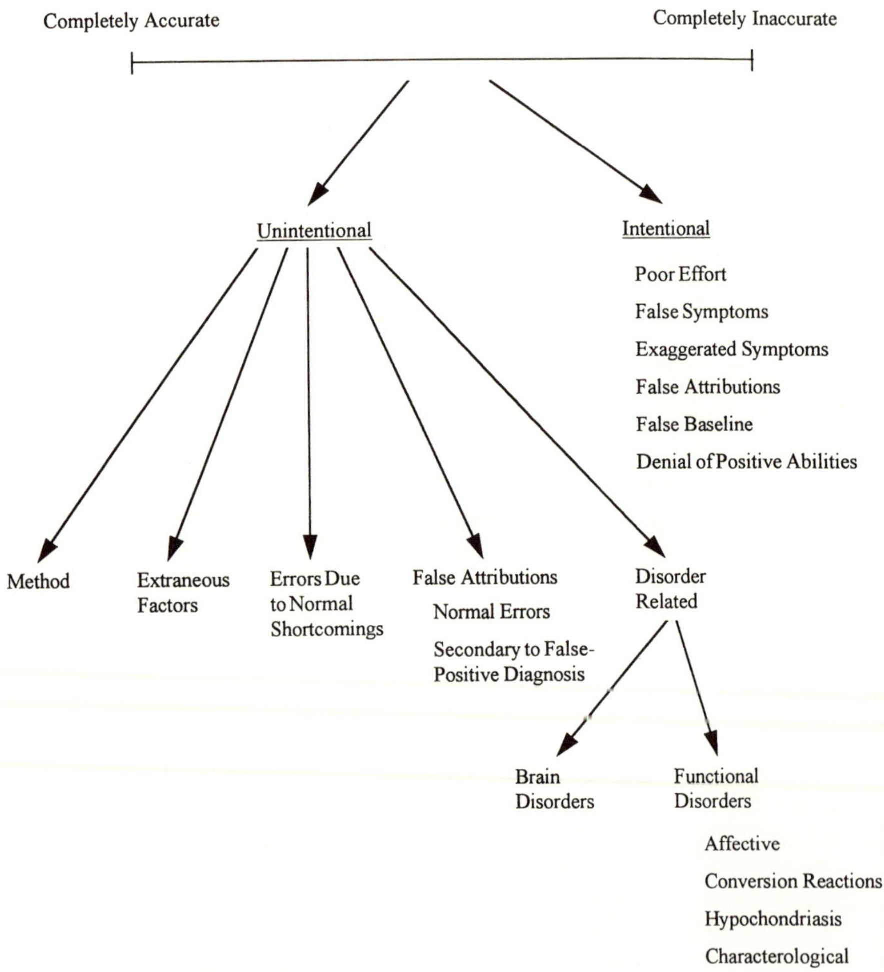

FIGURE 1. Sources of inaccuracy in assessment data.

condition along a continuum, ranging from completely accurate to completely inaccurate. Inaccuracies can arise from various factors, including not only misrepresentations stemming from an individual but also from such sources as measurement error. It would immediately seem clear that we are almost never, or never, at either end point of the continuum, but rather some place in between, that is, we have some balance of accurate and inaccurate information.

Types of inaccuracy can then be divided into two subtypes, intentional and unintentional (although we realize that some individuals would place this dimension on a continuum as well). Note again that in this context we are not using the term *unintentional* to refer exclusively to a mental state, but rather in a more general sense to encompass various sources of inaccuracy in neuropsychological data, none of which anyone sets out to find or create. For example, inaccurate information can stem from problems in method (e.g., measurement error, misadministration of tests). Inaccuracy can also result from the operation of various extraneous factors that contaminate the data or lead to results that misrepresent the patient's more typical or characteristic state, such as a very poor night of sleep before the day of the evaluation, a flare-up in medication side effects, or a transient poor mood that impedes the examinee's efforts.

Other unintentional forms of inaccuracy originate from the patient. Some are disorder related. For example, brain damage may impair insight, and a grievously injured patient may report minimal difficulties in everyday functioning. Functional or personality factors and disorders, including normal human shortcomings, can also lead to misreporting. After all, who has perfect insight into their own strengths, weaknesses, and personal characteristics? Some individuals characteristically or stylistically under- or overperceive their capacities. Individuals with affective disorders may underestimate their behavioral and cognitive capabilities and overperceive their functional difficulties. Individuals with conversion or somaticizing disorders may believe they are brain impaired when they are not, or that they are more incapable or impaired than they are, and they may misperceive normal behavior as indicative of disorder, skewing their self-reports.

False-positive diagnoses may lead examinees to mistakenly believe that they are brain-damaged and to greatly overestimate the frequency of neuropsychological difficulties. On the opposite end of the spectrum, false-negative diagnoses may lead to the opposing error type in self-perceptions and self-reporting. Alternatively, as Mittenberg, DiGiulio, Perrin, and Bass (1992) pointed out, individuals may reconstruct an overly positive image of preaccident functioning and may misperceive their present normal shortcomings as pathologic, or as representing a change in their status. In turn, they may describe a long list of "symptoms" secondary to their injury.

Individuals can easily form false attributions about the causes of their problems (for if these judgments were always so easy there would be little need to consult highly trained specialists to determine etiology). The dementing patient who has been slowly declining may suddenly come to attention after a mild head injury causes a temporary diminution in cognitive functioning, with subsequent problems blamed entirely on the car accident. The patient who shows persisting symptoms may attribute them to medication side effects rather than the head trauma, the patient who can't concentrate on work may blame the problem on exposure to toxins rather than her sleep disorder, and so on. Clinicians usually ask patients to discuss possible precipitating factors and may give great weight to their reports, sometimes above all other information. (It would be fascinating to study, absent any incentive to mislead and, instead, quite the opposite, the frequency with which patients draw correct conclusions about the causes of their conditions.) Considering the many ways examinees can inadvertently mislead themselves and others, it would be outrageous to assume that any type of misrepresentation provides strong evidence of malingering; this is exactly why we cannot overlook the element of intentionality.

Intentional inaccuracy or misrepresentation can take various forms. For example, the examinee may make a poor effort on testing, may make up symptoms, may overstate symptoms, may purposely cover up or mislead about causality, may present a false baseline, or may fail to acknowledge strengths, positive abilities, or positive areas of functioning.

The pragmatic task facing the clinician (and the researcher) would not be nearly as hard if the array of information that was available on examinees tended to show powerful intercorrelations. Were this the case, then if one could identify a few pieces of information or variables that could be accurately sorted into one or another class, the overall class could probably be determined with a high degree of accuracy, that is, one would usually be able to predict or determine the class within which much of the remaining data would fall. For example, were malingering on the Dr. Soothsayer Inventory strongly predictive of malingering on all other tests, clinical life would be relatively easy. However, it is exactly because intercorrelations are so imperfect that we are usually surprised when virtually everything in an assessment lines up in just the same direction and the case becomes as trivially obvious as it is atypical. There would be no need to calculate the F-back on the MMPI if there were a very high correlation between responses on F items across the entire MMPI, but this is not the case even for these very closely aligned items (Butcher et al., 1989).

In one forensic case in which one of the authors consulted, almost half of the plaintiffs were captured on videotape engaging in some sort of physical activity that they had unequivocally denied the capacity to perform. Most of these same plaintiffs obtained unremarkable scores on symptom validity testing and the MMPI. It was because the intercorrelations were limited across these various techniques that one could not have predicted, based on one plaintiff's normal MMPI findings and symptom validity testing, that despite his claims of physical infirmity and severe vertigo he would be caught on a 40-foot-high barn roof directing a demolition crew and using a chain saw.

We do not intend to review factors that often produce low intercorrelations among various measures of accuracy in self-report and test behavior (e.g., measurement error, variable levels of validity, selectivity in what is falsified), but the point remains that it is there. Consequently, being able to accurately classify results on one particular score or variable frequently does not allow one to predict the classification (or determine the underlying explanation) of other data points.

Even if we cannot necessarily obtain high or consistently high intercorrelations, in part perhaps because we are measuring different dimensions, we still want to know the strength of relations between variables. At least then we would be able to intelligently address the question, "Knowing the correct classification on Variable(s) A (B, C, and D), what can I predict about classification on other variables or groups of variables?" Further, knowledge of the intercorrelation matrix can help direct our attention toward variables or combinations of variables that show the broadest predictive power or the strongest loadings on the dimensions or qualities that comprise malingering.

Some clinicians, having obtained powerful evidence for suboptimal performance on one or another test or subtest or set of items, may select the default option and indicate that the result raises so much doubt about the validity of the entire assessment that they can go no further. Absent good knowledge of interrelations among variables and measures at the present time, it is difficult to criticize such an approach. Of course, if we had such knowledge, we would know just how much more we were and were not justified in indicating.

Similarly, having obtained unremarkable results on one or a few "malingering" tests (which are often structurally similar to other tests in a battery on which an individual may have performed very poorly), another clinician might conclude that good effort has been exerted across the entire battery. Structurally, it would seem as if this type of generalization is usually just as risky as those involving inadequate effort, if not more so, because the sensitivity of malingering tests is often poor (e.g., see Rogers, Harrell, & Liff, 1993; Wiggins & Brandt, 1988). In either case, the clinician is moving from one or a few samples of good or poor effort to generalizations about level of effort or cooperation across the entire battery. What does not seem justified, at least in the forensic arena, and absent a good knowledge of base rates, is altering standards of evidence such that the same clinician is much slower to generalize from suboptimal effort on measures than she is to generalize from satisfactory effort, or vice versa. Given these considerations, it seems apparent that a far better understanding of the interrelations between results on measures of malingering and effort, as well as the various measures of neuropsychological functioning included in neuropsychological batteries, would be very helpful in applied clinical and forensic work.

This question of interrelationships should not be viewed too simplistically. The question is not so much, "If Smith intentionally performs below her capability on one measure, can we predict suboptimal effort and false reporting on all other measures?" but rather, "If we know Smith has intentionally produced misleading results on one or another variable, to what extent can I explain the other things that seem to trouble her on this same basis?" The latter question can also be framed obversely: "If I know that Smith's effort or the accuracy of her report has been satisfactory in one area, to what extent can we trust that the things that seem to trouble her are genuine?" Within this framework, if Smith's far-below-chance performance on a multiple-choice measure of anosmia *required* intact smell, and if this were the only deficit Smith was claiming, the clinician should not be too troubled about the issue of generalization, nor should we expect a high association between performance on this anosmia measure and other measures. In contrast, if Smith has decided to portray global impairment, then there should be a high intercorrelation between the malingered result on the anosmia measure and level of performance across the battery, or more precisely, across measures that are sensitive to fake-bad response sets.

Studies of intercorrelations will therefore ultimately need to take into account discrepancy from true status and the scope of the problem the subject is attempting to malinger. In turn, accounting for true status will often require something different from, or more than, a standard of normality, and rather a determination of the subject's true baseline. Many of the types of studies that need to be done on malingering detection will involve subjects whose true baseline or starting point is *not* normal functioning across all domains or some variation of normal overall functioning, but rather some combination of normal and abnormal functioning. For example, not all malingerers are perfectly normal individuals faking bad; rather, some are injured individuals who are exaggerating or also fabricating. This is why it is so encouraging to see an increasing number of studies in which individuals are instructed to fake a particular type of disorder or target symptoms and in which simulators include patient groups that are instructed to exaggerate (e.g., Rogers, Bagby, & Dickens, 1992; Rogers, Sewell, & Ustad, 1995). Such research will help create a basis for relating negative or positive performance on measures sensitive to malingering to performance on tests that are not sensitive to malingering. This will help avoid mistakes in both directions, for example, a false conclusion that suboptimal performance on one measure explains away all deficits in an individual who has genuine, serious symptoms from a major head injury, or the mistaken belief that unremarkable performance on a malingering measure more or less rules out the possibility that a person displaying terrible performance across a range of measures following a very mild head injury really has grievous losses.

The practitioner's world, and hence the world of the investigator who is trying to address the practitioner's applied problem, is not a simple one. The clinician, especially in the forensic context, rarely worries about confusing a normal person doing his best and one faking bad. Thus, although the typical simulation study can serve as a very helpful beginning in evaluating malingering measures or in the context of discovery, it will rarely yield findings that, by themselves, can be safely applied to clinical practice. In fact, one usually has little basis for determining how well such methods will work in practice. Further, the clinician's fundamental task is to separate signal from noise, and there are multiple sources of potential inaccuracy in assessment data, intentional misrepresentation being just one of them. A range of conditions, alone or in combination, can lead to nonrepresentative or lowered test performance and to misreporting of symptoms and history.

Some clinicians will decide to stop (at least temporarily) when they find that some major source of inaccuracy has entered into the evaluation. Others will attempt to distinguish between potential sources of inaccuracy and may try to determine whether intentional misrepresentation occurred. In this effort, the clinician must consider such sources of inaccuracy as methodological ones (e.g., measurement error), transient factors, individual and personality factors, forms of pathology that can lead to misrepresentation, inadvertent false attributions, and the various forms of intentional falsification that might occur. Some of these possibilities are likely to influence performance or reporting in select domains, and others are likely to have a wider impact. For example, an inadvertent causal misattribution is unlikely to impact very much on test performance, whereas the intentional effort to portray memory deficit is likely to affect the patient's self-report, the history he provides, and test performance. Furthermore, the clinician would like to know, should she obtain definite or strong evidence about level of effort or accuracy on one or a few variables, whether, and to what extent, generalizations can be made about the genuineness of the dysfunctions that have been reported or observed in other areas and about information pertaining to cause.

In the planning and design of malingering research, it is helpful to maintain a broad appreciation of the clinician's task and the types of distinctions that need to be made, such as those outlined above. The practitioner wants to be able to separate an individual with a conversion reaction who has experienced a mild head injury and who genuinely believes she has memory difficulty but does not, from one who has experienced a mild head injury and who had memory problems but now does not and is faking deficit. Or the clinician may be trying to differentiate between a moderately head-injured individual who has serious memory difficulties, has organically based motivational problems, and, because of affective disorder, tends to overperceive his level of difficulty, and a moderately head-injured individual who does have mild memory difficulties but is portraying moderate to severe memory problems. If the practitioner is not enthusiastic about an MMPI study involving distinctions he is almost never required to make, it may reflect an appropriate recognition of the gap between such research and clinical needs (which, at the same time, certainly does not justify or bolster the use of methods with even weaker evidentiary bases).

It is understandable that many malingering studies have examined simple distinctions as a way of getting started. However, as an increasing number of researchers are now doing, it is time to begin focusing on the more complex and difficult distinctions that commonly need to be made in clinical and forensic practice. In our opinion, such research will take into account variables of the type we have outlined above. One can thus see why a person of Ralph Reitan's acumen might describe the task as difficult. As we imagine he would agree, given the progress that is being made, there is good cause for optimism. In the remainder of this chapter, we will suggest some directions that we hope will contribute to the effort.

RELATION BETWEEN THE NATURE OF THE BEAST AND MEASUREMENT

If we were to move 20 to 40 years forward in time, what type of malingering assessment devices would we find? Would we find a single falsification index, would we see MMPI-like profiles that provided results on multiple scales, or would we find some complex multidimensional space within which the examinee was located? Would we uncover neuropsychological profiles with differentially weighted malingering corrections on certain scales or measures?

Anyone with a little scientific realism in the blood would likely say that measurement should eventually be dictated by external reality, that is, measurement is intended not to construct but rather to reflect what is out there. Therefore, to a large extent, the "shape" of malingering measures should be dictated by the shape of malingering. If malingering is a true category or class that is captured for the most part by two dimensions, measurement devices might in turn be limited to scores on two scales, but if malingering has a more complex structure, measurement approaches will need to change accordingly. Similarly, measurement approaches will also need to differ if malingering is or is not a taxon.

It would seem that we encounter an obvious circularity at this point. Measuring devices should fit the shape of malingering, but we do not yet know the shape of malingering and need good measurement so as to obtain this knowledge. Hence, it would appear that we need to know more than we know if we are to learn what we need to learn. Under such conditions, how can we proceed? Psychology's response to such dilemmas has often been to adopt some form of pseudopositivism or operationalism (e.g., "Malingering is defined as performance above a certain level on some measure," or, "We will avoid mentalistic terms") that compounds the problem or tries to bypass the very conceptual issues that need our attention.

Ironically, it is commonplace within science (and within the course of human development for that matter) to need to know more than we know if we are to learn what we need to learn, and yet to find some way to do it. In science, this often involves some fairly crude groping around in the dark and a good deal of trial and error (Faust, 1984). We can usually determine whether we are getting somewhere by examining classic criteria for scientific ideas, such as the power to predict, and, most importantly and globally, the orderliness of the data revealed (Faust & Meehl, 1992; Meehl, 1991). A phrase like "orderliness of the data" might seem vague and circular, but it has clear conceptual implications among philosophers of science and is probably the most generally accepted criterion for evaluating theories. Circularity, although indeed present, is not that problematical (see Meehl, 1991, 1992). The relation between knowing (malingering) and measurement is dialectical—the development, ongoing evaluation, and modification of malingering detection devices ought to be based on what we come to know about malingering (our ontological knowledge), whereas our capacity to learn about malingering depends on the state of our measurement tools (our methodological or epistemological competence). Hence, knowing or attempting to know what malingering is, and measuring or attempting to measure it, will need to proceed in kind. Unfortunately, many efforts in this area seem to focus almost exclusively on one or the other side of the problem, with Rogers's work (e.g., Rogers et al., 1992) perhaps being the most notable exception.

At present, the key ontological question seems to be whether, at the one extreme, the phenotypic variations of malingering reflect a few basic and interknit underlying dimensions that have substantial consistency across situations, persons, and feigned conditions, or whether, at the other extreme, we are dealing with multiple independent dimensions and loose conglomerations of behaviors that often change markedly depending on the person, situation, and condition being feigned. These two extremes would likely call for vast differences in measurement approaches, even as stark a difference as sampling across persons versus situations. Moving from ontology to epistemology, key measurement issues seem to include the development of methods that, to the extent possible, retain discriminatory power across persons, situations, and variations of falsification, and under conditions in which examinees learn their underlying design. Finally, we believe that the key interface between these conceptual and measurement issues involves the matter discussed under the prior heading, that is, the clinical discriminations of greatest relevance, or those that the practitioner is required to make but cannot accomplish so easily.

As noted, we believe that at least two basic dimensions, falsification and intentionality, are inherent or intrinsic components of malingering. It follows from this that to identify malingering, both dimensions will need to be assessed. However, one should not assume an isomorphic relation between the number of dimensions or types of things that need to be assessed and the number or types of specific scales that are required. For example, when attempting to detect the intentionality of misrepresentations, one might use a disjunctive strategy, in which a score above a certain point on any of a variety of measures is sufficient for a positive identification. Alternatively, an elevated score on some measure of plausibility might inform us that the results on this or other measures are not credible, but there may be different mechanisms by which such elevations are obtained and the scale, by itself, may not be particularly useful in separating one cause from another. The F Scale from the MMPI is one such example. Although lacking the capacity to separate among different explanations, such scales can serve a number of purposes. For example, they may provide entry points in branching procedures, with positive results signaling the need for more detailed assessment. Additionally, quantitative measurement can help in identifying qualitative differences or types. For example, if we believe there is a difference in type between, say, a "borderline" patient and a normal individual, cutting points on a measure assessing the frequency with which primitive defenses are used might aid categorization.

There are, of course, many approaches to studying the underlying nature or structure of entities in psychology, such as factor analysis and cluster analysis. We would like to alert readers to one set of procedures with which they might be less familiar, and which we believe can be very helpful in clarifying the nature of malingering. These are the taxometric procedures that Meehl has been the central figure in developing (Meehl, 1995; Meehl & Yonce, 1994). These methods involve a series of mathematical analyses aimed at determining whether or not something is a taxon or type. Meehl's method also provides a means for estimating underlying base rates and determining optimal cutting scores, even absent a gold standard for identifying the potential entity. We consider Meehl's approach to be the most advanced by far for determining taxonicity, and very well suited to work on malingering when a researcher has a sufficiently large sample. To our knowledge, R. I. Frederick (personal communication, April 1996) has made the first attempt to apply Meehl's methods to malingering research, with promising results.

Finally, studies attempting to determine taxonicity and the latent structure of malingering should avoid artificial constraints on its manifestations. Many malingering studies present subjects with only a few measures or options. Although there is nothing wrong with this per se or when conducting certain types of studies, artificial constraints on response options can create fatal problems when one is trying to capture the nature or structure of malingering. In the clinical situation, the malingerer has a much larger number of options and is almost never forced to fake on a predetermined, narrow range of tests. Rather, the malingerer can fabricate history and symptoms and is likely to be selective in faking test performances. If the researcher severely restrains the range of options for malingering and forces the individual to fake on a specific measure or narrow set of measures, a very distorted picture of malingering can emerge. It would not be that much different from attempting to determine the underlying characteristics of great decathlon athletes by asking them to perform one or a few aspects of one event (e.g., show me how you grip a javelin). None of this should be confused with an argument for considering or integrating all of the evidence in assessing malingering (which is often terrible advice; see Faust, 1989). Rather, an attempt to determine underlying structure should provide the opportunity for the thing to be discovered to manifest itself as it is and should not artificially, and severely, constrain its expression.

FIDELITY/GENERALIZATION

Perhaps the greatest number of methodological criticisms, questions, and prescriptions relating to malingering research address the issues of fidelity and generalization. What do the studies to date tell us about the capacities of clinicians to detect malingering? How well do methods developed in artificial settings generalize to practice settings? What modifications might be needed in measures and strategies when one moves to applied settings or across areas of disorder? What should we report to the courts about our capacity to detect malingering?

The scientific status of malingering assessment devices would not be too important an issue if we had clear and convincing evidence that most clinicians, or at least a sizable (and identifiable) subgroup, could identify malingering with a high degree of accuracy. Presently, there is no credentialing or related process that provides a direct and representative assessment of a neuropsychologist's capacity to detect malingering. Absent such a procedure and a body of literature that provides a fair and representative test of clinicians, we simply do not know how well clinicians in general or particular subgroups (e.g., those with special qualifications) perform on this task. Further, our personal experience, for all of the reasons detailed previously (e.g., lack of feedback, lack of representative feedback, ambiguous feedback), provides a weak basis for appraising our own detection capacities. For example, how could the clinician appraise her error rate if she usually lacks a basis for determining when erroneous (or correct) identifications have been made?

In addition, as already described, a body of research indicates that laypersons and professionals have difficulties recognizing lies, and studies that have directly examined the capacity of clinicians to detect malingering have yielded mixed results, at best. Some of the criticisms directed at these latter types of studies, in particular their questionable generalization to everyday practice, deserve serious consideration. However, it should be realized that these studies could have, and sometimes have, turned out differently (even in the face of the same types of methodological features pointed to when negative outcomes occurred were no less present) and that, in the Popperian sense, failure to confirm a certain prior belief does not help the health of that belief. Also, the reasons sometimes given to discount the studies, such as the failure to test generalization to everyday clinical practice directly, often apply equally, if not more so, to the methods that are being applied in clinical settings to detect malingering. For example, if one argues that one or another investigation was limited because it did not study clinicians' everyday work, it is then hard to justify using a malingering detection device that has been studied almost exclusively in the laboratory and has undergone minimal field testing. It would seem reasonable to conclude that whatever their limitations, the studies to date generally do not support the notion that clinicians are highly accurate in detecting malingering and, rather, raise questions about such capacities.

In the absence of solid research evidence demonstrating satisfactory accuracy levels, given problems learning to detect malingering via experience and the difficulties appraising one's own accuracy on this same basis, considering the negative research on the detection of lies and, at best, the mixed results of studies that have directly examined clinicians' success in detecting malingering, confident pronouncements would seem unwarranted. There may be especially gifted clinicians who are proficient at identifying malingering and from whom we all could learn, and this is one clear reason for extending studies on clinicians' detection capacities. However, very few practitioners have, or are in a position to gather, the type of evidence needed to accurately appraise their malingering detection abilities. Even if there is an especially talented group of clinicians who do not need better malingering detection methods or instruments, they cannot be everywhere and others could benefit from improved methods.

Stated another way, researchers' intensive efforts to develop malingering measures and detection procedures and the many concerns that have been raised about fidelity and generalization to applied settings seem well directed. We will address three basic issues in the remainder of this section. These include generalization across: (1) clinically relevant distinctions, (2) individuals and situations, and (3) differing base rates.

Generalization across Types of Clinical Distinctions

Suppose a researcher has uncovered a variable or method that works in an applied setting and that separates some group of malingerers from some other clinic group. It is then natural to ask whether the discriminating variable or method will generalize to other groups of malingerers and clientele. For example, a variable that helps to discriminate between those feigning a traumatic brain injury and those with actual, severe sequelae from head injuries may or may not identify those feigning dementia, or more so those feigning posttraumatic stress disorder, or may not separate such groups from those with genuine but more subtle forms of dysfunction. When considering generalization of malingering indicators and methods across clinically relevant distinctions, it is helpful to separate at least two partly independent dimensions: (1) consistency across falsified conditions or states and genuine conditions and states (which we will refer to as cross-conditional consistency) and (2) the relative difficulty of the discriminations examined in background studies.

Generalization across Genuine and Malingered Conditions

Many malingering studies involve the discrimination between normals doing their best versus those faking bad. This type of task would seemingly give clinicians little trouble in everyday practice. Whether the discriminating variables in these studies generalize to other and often highly contrasting types of clinical or forensic conditions is another question and cannot be settled by reflection (see further discussion in the next section), but it would seem clear that strong presumptions about generalization are hazardous. These studies are probably best viewed within the context of discovery relative to the types of discriminations clinicians really need to make.

It is hard to anticipate level of cross-conditional consistency. For example, knowing that Method X separates those faking psychosis from those with genuine psychosis might seem a feeble basis to expect that this same method will separate those faking brain damage from the genuinely injured. However, studies with the MMPI seem to show exactly such cross-conditional consistency (e.g., Greene, 1991; Heaton et al., 1978). It is worth considering the factors that would likely promote, versus impede, cross-conditional consistency, although the armchair will only get us so far here.

Let us first imagine circumstances in which cross-conditional consistency is likely to be maximized. Although the particulars might vary, the essential nature of these situations is about the same. One has a circumstance in which the various forms of malingering still have one or a few common elements, and these elements show minimal overlap with the manifestations of the disorders or genuine conditions one has to differentiate. For example, there might be a set of signs or indicators that are common among malingerers but very rarely, if ever, seen among nonmalingerers, something akin to pathognomonic indicators. Alternatively, if one has quantitative indicators, the distributions that are obtained among these indicators, or some subset of indicators, across the various subtypes of malingerers might show minimal overlap with those seen among nonmalingerers. It is also a given that we must have adequate ways of measuring standing on these variables.

How much nature departs from these idealized conditions is difficult to say. Currently, lacking the type of evidence needed on the possible taxonicity and structure of malingering, we are basically reduced to guessing. The issue is important to keep in mind, however, for there might be much greater cross-conditional generalization than many suspect, especially if malingering has taxonicity and can be mostly reduced to a few common dimensions whose presence or distributions tend to differ markedly across malingering and nonmalingering groups. For example, exaggeration would seem to be common to most forms of malingering, and quantitative differences on this dimension might very well separate most malingerers and nonmalingerers. Greater levels of generalization are highly advantageous, sharply reducing the needed research effort and, ultimately, the clinician's undertaking. Imagine a situation in which we have tools that are sensitive to malingering of various general categories of conditions (e.g., emotional disorder, brain disorder), various subtypes within general categories (e.g., head injury and toxin exposure), and various symptom presentations (e.g., memory disorder and impaired executive functions), in contrast to a situation in which we need a different measure or approach for nearly every possible presentation the clinician encounters.

The extent to which our assessment techniques generalize across conditions and presentations is not solely determined by the state of nature but also by our capacity to recognize possibilities that present themselves to us and to develop the knowledge and assessment tools that facilitate breadth. For example, if the various manifestations of malingering have both general and specific elements, then all other things being equal, we might decide to focus on the former so as to work toward more generally applicable measures. As we increase our knowledge of malingering and its underlying nature, we might keep especially mindful of the conditions that promote generalization in measurement and of chances to increase cross-conditional consistency.

The Difficulty of Discriminations

The extent of generalization will also depend on the relative difficulty of the discriminations that need to be made. Strangely, this basic psychometric principle is sometimes ignored completely when considering the generalization of research in psychology and neuropsychology. For example, a demonstration that some method can identify severe brain damage does not mean it will work just as well (or at all) with mild brain injury. One of the authors, who performs legal consultations, has read many courtroom transcripts in which apparently sincere neuropsychologists cite studies involving coarse or gross distinctions to support the capacity of the same measures to make much subtler distinctions, as if generalization was a given and did not merit concern. The converse point should also not be overlooked: If subtle distinctions can be made, then, barring qualitative shifts, the method should do at least as well, and most likely better, with more gross distinctions. There is no question that generalization in the first direction, or from easier to harder, is usually much riskier than generalization in the other direction.

To illustrate the relevance of difficulty in evaluating research and methods, imagine the typical study in which one group of normal individuals is instructed to do its best and another group to fake a serious disorder. Some of these studies use within-subject designs, and the contrasts between the two conditions can be enormous. Further, the base rates for faking and genuine effort are known to the researcher (or well approximated). Compare the difficulty involved in making these kinds of distinctions versus those required in separating an individual who truly does have subtle persisting problems following mild head injury from an individual who is well-coached in malingering detection strategies and who fakes mild symptoms, or who had problems, recovered, and is falsifying symptom continuation, all in the absence of decent base rate information. When deciding whether to use methods in an applied setting or when reporting to the courts on their accuracy, we might want some assurance that procedures have been tested under comparably tough conditions; where such studies are absent, we would like to see them undertaken.

Various dimensions might be used to evaluate difficulty. These could include: (1) the subtlety of the condition one is trying to detect; (2) the availability of independent methods for appraising injury severity that are scientifically respectable and difficult or impossible to manipulate (e.g., MRI findings); (3) level of knowledge about the condition in question (e.g., we know a lot more about sensory distributions than about the manifestations of many toxic agents); and, partly related to some of the factors above, (4) the level of separation that can be expected between those with the condition and those faking disorder. Certain conditions (e.g., early stage dementias versus stroke) are likely to show much greater overlap than are other conditions with malingered symptoms, normal variations, and other pathological conditions.

Rating the difficulty of discrimination not only should help in predicting effectiveness in the population or patient of interest, but it is also essential in selecting among alternative methods. A proper comparison of methods requires not only knowledge of their accuracy rates but also testing under conditions of equivalent difficulty, or a consistent yardstick. A measure that achieves 70% success when attempting very difficult discriminations may have much more to offer the clinician in her applied setting than one that achieves 90% accuracy under much easier conditions. The difficulty of the tests to which malingering indicators and methods are subjected can vary markedly. Currently, it is often difficult to make informed choices among alternatives given the rapid proliferation of malingering assessment devices and procedures, the frequent unavailability of comparable or equal tests, and the problems that may be involved trying to evaluate the relative severity of tests even should one have the issue in mind.

The seemingly obvious answer is to conduct direct comparisons of measures across various types of discriminations (conditions) so that one is not reduced to bald speculation. Indeed, as more and more malingering detection methods and approaches are becoming available, showing that a single measure has discriminating power under one or another condition is really minimally informative. Often, we will already have other measures that have passed the same test, and one really needs to know how the new measure compares with other available devices and whether it makes a unique contribution to predictive accuracy.

We cannot, however, perform all possible comparisons among measures and across conditions and variations of malingering. Blind empiricism is inefficient and usually ineffective in the long run. Rather, scientific efforts typically should be guided by principles, informed advice, and generalizations that usually hold. For example, it is completely impractical to test every conceivable comparison, and scientific and clinical practice often occur under conditions of uncertainty, in which there is no sure road. In such situations, however, one operating from well-founded guesses and principles has a huge advantage over someone operating blindly. Take the methodological guide: "A method shown to make fine discriminations should do even better making more gross distinctions." There are times this generalization is flat-out wrong (as might occur, for example, when the situation changes qualitatively), but we usually do not know this in advance, and rather we are trying to resolve a question under ambiguous conditions. In attempting to do so, our odds of being correct are much greater if we follow this generalization than if we guess randomly, and correct guesses can greatly enhance the productivity of our scientific efforts.

In deciding which comparisons to make, it would seem sensible to direct most efforts toward the strongest competitors. We should also compare different combinations of methods and approaches, keeping in mind the advantages gained by pooling nonredundant measures (see more about this topic of redundancy and data combination later). When direct comparisons have not been made, it would help to at least be explicit about how we are evaluating the difficulty of the hurdles that measures and methods have faced. Journal editors and reviewers might keep the need for comparative studies in mind when they examine yet one more study showing that Method X achieves modest accuracy in detecting malingering. We also may consider starting with extreme tests so that methods might be sized up quickly. For example, if an approach seems especially promising, we might subject it to a stern test right away rather than progressively subjecting it to more difficult tests, for all but the last test in that sequence is unnecessary should this final hurdle be passed in the first place. Also, when a new method is developed for which strong competitors already exist, there is often little point in exposing it to flabby tests (unless they will help in directing refinements), because their passage will get us no closer to determining relative merits.

Person and Situational Variables

The issue of generalization across persons and situations has probably occupied more coverage within methodological critiques than any other issue. Some commentators tend to assume that studies will generalize and others that they will not, and some seem to portray agnosticism, indicating that we must await research outcomes. There are still occasional others who seem to act as if the issue does not exist, showing minimal apparent restraints in applying methods developed with one population and under one set of circumstances to other individuals and circumstances.

Person Variables

As noted, many malingering studies compare normal individuals instructed to fake bad with those instructed to do their best or portray themselves normally, a distinction that is unlikely to give the clinician trouble or to apply to the courtroom. The obvious appeal of these studies is that we know subjects' true status (although the failure of a certain percentage of subjects to comply with instructions can create some problems, especially absent a manipulation check). The obvious problem is that one does not know whether the results generalize to those seen in applied settings, and until the matter is clarified, the studies are of limited practical utility. It could further be argued that once it is possible to check on the accuracy of approaches with real populations or in applied settings, the original studies with normal populations are moot.

Given these considerations, studies contrasting normal individuals doing their best and faking bad, and even studies including comparisons with patient groups, might best be viewed within the context of discovery, as one means for identifying candidate variables meriting analysis in applied settings. The argument one sometimes hears that results in such studies almost surely will not generalize, which often rests on citing some feature that distinguishes normals faking bad from real malingerers, usually seems unjustified. We would not say that measures of temperature that work in establishing normality among children will almost surely not work with adults because children and adults show some obvious differences.

There is good reason to expect a generally positive relation between discriminating variables in these types of studies with experimental simulators and discriminating variables in the field, as shown for example by investigations on the generalization of MMPI indicators (see Berry, Baer, & Harris, 1991; Rogers, Sewell, & Salekin, 1994). If variables that simulation studies find to be effective discriminators have a greater probability of working in the field than, say, random guesses, and perhaps in many cases hypotheses based on clinical experience, that is about all that is needed to justify efforts within the context of discovery (although just how much these probabilities must exceed the best guesses that could be made otherwise is far too complex a matter to enter into here). The main potential exception are situations in which there are strong reasons to assume *negative* correlations between features of the study sample that lead to their inclusion in the investigation and the characteristics of those that need to be identified in the applied setting, as can occur in studies limited to malingerers (or presumed malingerers) who have been detected by commonly used or weak methods. For now, if we had to bet on candidate variables, we would lean more toward well-conducted studies with normals faking bad than studies involving a very select group of malingerers who were caught on the basis of results that, although relatively certain or definitive, were highly atypical (except under conditions we will describe below). As detection methods continue to improve, the sample of caught malingerers will of course increasingly resemble the total group of malingerers.

Problems determining the generalization of results from research subjects to genuine cases would be resolved with relative ease if we could recruit representative samples of malingerers. The seeming paradox is that one would need to know how to identify malingerers before conducting the studies needed to learn how to identify malingerers, at which point one would not need to do the studies. Those we can identify as malingerers with relative certainty, taken together, are probably nonrepresentative of the overall group we need to detect. This problem with representativeness, although rather bland, is extremely important. The absence of a representative sample, or rather the inability to determine whether a sample is representative, greatly hinders efforts to identify and evaluate potential malingering indicators. Under such conditions, it is very easy to inadvertently adopt signs that are ineffectual or, even worse, increase the number of misidentifications.

There are at least two major ways in which "real life" malingerers might differ from subjects in studies, such as college students instructed to fake bad. Real malingerers may be more skilled than research subjects (we will usually be less concerned if they are less skilled), and they may differ in kind, or along any of a number of qualitative features. Qualitative differences could distort or entirely alter malingering indicators or change co-relations among variables. As one example, performance patterns on intellectual measures that indicate genuine effort among research subjects may occur fairly often among true malingerers. As another example, research subjects may be more likely to exhibit delayed reaction times when instructed to lie because lying may not be habitual with them or they may be trying out a particular story for the first time. Or, if malingering really does show a strong association with sociopathy (and hence with various other features of sociopathy), studies of college students faking bad would probably never uncover such relations.

A researcher worried about differences of the first type, or in skill, could address the issue in various ways. There is little reason to believe that skill in malingering is limited to those who do malinger, and in any case, malingerers emerge from the general population. As such, it should not be that hard for an investigator to create conditions in which this variable can be altered. We do have a series of fallible, but valid, measures of malingering. It is reasonable to believe that the more of these measures someone can beat (assuming the measures have some independence from one another and that one procedure does not tip the person off about the others), the greater is his skill in malingering, or at least the greater our problem is likely to be in detecting him. Hence, if I am testing new Method X and its relative level of success as malingerers become more skilled (or more able to beat our available measures), I can administer other measures of demonstrated validity and assign subjects some kind of malingering skill rating. We will need to perform these types of studies anyway, because they provide the basis for determining effective or optimal composites of malingering measures. Similarly, one could have clinicians attempt to classify subjects. Presumably, the frequency with which subjects beat the clinicians should correlate with their malingering skills (or at least the level of difficulty clinicians are likely to encounter when trying to detect them).

If one is working with naturalistic populations of malingerers who are caught, and especially if it is possible to compile some reasonably large samples (as could occur with data pooling), it may often be possible to approximate how many times or for how long or under what conditions individuals successfully malingered before they were detected. Although this approach would not circumvent some of the problems with representativeness we have already described, it would provide a means to alter the variable of skill and to examine its potential impact on malingering indicators and detection methods. There are many other possible approaches (e.g., identifying those in occupations in which level of success often correlates with the ability to deceive; using peer nomination techniques), and we are confident that our suggestions can be greatly expanded.

Perfect, or even highly accurate, separations into groups is not necessary to make progress in our investigations of skill. Although classification of skill level using the types of approaches we have described will be inexact, the main condition one needs to meet is a strong likelihood that the high-skill group is substantially more skilled than the low-skill group. If the researcher has a means for estimating the frequency of misclassification, that is all the better. In many circumstances, all that is required are these contrasting, or impure but different groups, to get on with the needed forms of validation. Dawes and Meehl (1966) described methods and conditions under which validation work can proceed even when groups are far from pure.

The problem with distortion or alteration of qualitative features is a very difficult one. We can suggest some strategies that might be helpful, and we again feel confident that others can add to this list. One way to examine generalization across subjects in research and applied settings is to test promising new methods against the results of procedures that have already been shown to have at least a modicum of validity in applied settings, a type of concurrent validation strategy. It is not as if we are starting from a complete research vacuum, and various analyses conducted within applied settings demonstrate the relative effectiveness of such measures as the MMPI (Berry et al., 1991; Rogers et al., 1994).

High correlations between new and previously validated methods would provide fairly strong evidence for generalization, although as correlations grow, the increasing level of redundancy impacts negatively on the new method's potential contribution to predictive power. At the extreme, if two measures yield perfectly correlated results, one adds nothing to the other and one or the other can be eliminated. One clear limitation of such types of studies is the minimal interpretability of null results. A new measure may show little or no correlation with validated measures, but because the validated measures against which it is being compared are themselves likely to show only modest relations with true status, that new measure may be just as potent a predictor of the outcome as the validated measures. For example, a new measure may tap into a component of true variance that an old measure does not at all detect. This is a potentially serious problem given our ultimate aim and our knowledge about how we are most likely to get there. That aim of course is to maximize accuracy in malingering detection, and achieving it will likely require a combination of measures or methods. Adding redundant elements to composites usually does little for predictive punch, and we can get dramatically stronger effects by combining minimally redundant variables (Goldberg, 1991). If our procedures for identifying candidate variables for inclusion in the composite systematically tend to eliminate those that are less redundant, we may miss the variables that (in combination) would contribute the most to predictive accuracy.

A second approach starts by identifying conditions in which we have strong grounds to believe that the frequency of malingering differs among groups. For example, one might have circumstances in which it is in the self-interest of some individuals to do their best and of others to perform poorly. Some investigators have mistakenly viewed these types of groups as offering a direct means for assessing the effectiveness of methods across research and applied settings. The problem with this approach is that one does not know the true rate of malingering and nonmalingering in the contrasting groups, and there is often little reason to think that the bases for guessing about these matters are any more valid than the methods that are being tested. Consequently, it is problematic to argue, for example, that the accuracy of a certain MMPI malingering index decreases from 90% in the laboratory to 60% in the field, when that conclusion is based on application to contrasting groups and the researcher lacks effective means for formulating estimates of actual frequencies within those groups.

Suppose that one has invented a perfect malingering detection device. In the laboratory, in which one might obtain uniform compliance among subjects, the researcher achieves a 100% accuracy rate. However, in the field, the motivated-to-malinger group (e.g., disability applicants with minimal injuries who are disputing a rejected claim) might contain only 50% malingerers and the motivated-to-do-their-best group (those applying to vocational rehabilitation for educational funds) might still contain 20% malingerers. We now obtain a 50% "accuracy" rate in the first group and an 80% rate in the second group, when in fact the method has made the correct identification every time. One could even have a situation in which a method works better in the field than in the laboratory but results suggest the opposite.

With contrasting group methods, we often cannot do much better at first than identifying situations in which there are strong grounds to assume differing frequencies across groups, although we may not have any good idea about true frequencies. Nevertheless, that knowledge alone can be very helpful in studying the generalization of malingering detection measures. If a measure has decent discriminating power, the chances are good that application to contrasting groups will produce contrasting scores. When this result is obtained, one has a form of corroboration, and vice versa. At the same time, there is always a chance that the factors that lead to group membership, although correlated with malingering status, will not be correlated with the results of a measure that does have validity as a malingering indicator, or that a measure that is not effective in identifying malingering will nevertheless be correlated with factors that influenced group membership. In research on contrasting groups, it should also be possible to uncover circumstances in which we expect increasingly large differences in rates of malingering and can examine whether results on malingering measures change accordingly.

Generalization can also be studied by examining stability and patterns of correlations when measures are applied across diverse groups or, when possible, by conducting longitudinal analyses. We would like to propose an additional approach that we believe offers promise for obtaining a representative, or more representative, group of real-world malingerers. We will label this the Group Membership by Chance (GMC) strategy, and we believe it can be applied to a range of situations in the social sciences in which conventional methods of random selection are problematic either because of ethical constraints (e.g., head injury studies) or because means for identifying individuals with the condition in question are weak or lack adequate validation.

As is widely recognized, a fundamental problem with malingering research is that one cannot identify a representative sample of real-life malingerers to study. Ideally, one would want to sample randomly from the population of real malingerers and then compare that group with other groups the clinician needs to distinguish. The problem with current studies using real-life malingerers who have been caught is that, as noted, there are compelling reasons to believe that such individuals are not representative, and very possibly systematically misrepresentative, of malingerers as a whole. The more basic problem is the absence of a method for evaluating just how representative that subgroup might be. Without such a method, even if one happens to obtain a representative group, one cannot determine that this good piece of fortune has occurred, and hence it really does no good.

Some malingerers are caught primarily because they are lousy malingerers. Others are caught primarily because they are unlucky. Take the following case in which one of the authors consulted. One of the professional staff, who had left the treatment setting at an unscheduled hour as a result of an unexpected personal circumstance, just happened to observe a malingerer, who momentarily let down his guard once he was blocks away from the hospital, exactly at the moment he engaged in an activity he absolutely should not have been able to do. Or a plaintiff may have just happened to run into an unusually skilled and determined detective who caught him acting normally, whereas seven other malingering co-workers happen to have been assigned to more mediocre sleuths.

In the idealized instance, an individual who is caught entirely as a result of bad luck is directly parallel to a malingerer drawn randomly from the pool of malingerers, that is, he represents in essence an instance of random selection. If one can identify enough such individuals, one should be able to comprise a group that is likely to be representative of malingerers as a whole, or at least a good approximation. This allows not only for analysis of the group, but also for comparisons of groups formed in other ways to check their representativeness, such as malingerers caught by other means or cases compiled via contrasting group methods. In the latter case, it might also be possible to estimate the relative purity or base rates for malingering in contrasting groups, which offers major benefits, especially when studying generalization or the accuracy of measures in applied settings. For example, using methods designed by Dawes and Meehl (1966), if one can determine the relative impurity of validation groups, one can then correct for cases of false inclusion or the mixture of properly and improperly included individuals.

There are a number of questions and issues one might raise about such an approach, some of which can be touched on here (for further details see Faust, 1997). One question involves the methods used for determining the level of chance in identification. We believe that this is really not too difficult a methodological problem because: (1) the method does not require perfect indicators (one does not have to be particularly concerned about some impurity), (2) rational analysis should provide reasonable accuracy in estimating the contribution of chance, (3) failures of inclusion (false-negative errors) do not have distorting influences (one can be conservative if need be without worrying too much about consequential problems with representativeness), (4) the approach described here is an initial approximation to what has been a longstanding and very difficult problem and can be much further refined, and (5) a variety of checks can be built into the procedure. For example, a series of risky predictions can be made that should hold if the method works.

The second problem is not conceptual or methodological but practical. How could one possibly find enough caught-by-chance subjects? Data pooling would seem essential. On a national level, there are surely many such cases. The question is how to garner them. This is one of various domains of malingering research in which efforts would be helped greatly if more funding were available to researchers. Given the presumed cost of fraud, these might be dollars well invested.

A final approach would be to try to recruit malingerers who have immunity of some sort or who could be absolutely guaranteed anonymity. For example, one might attempt to study individuals who were granted lifetime benefits with no chance of reversal (as has sometimes been given to entire classes of workers, such as police officers in some areas of the country). With such approaches, one would still worry about who volunteers to participate. However, a circumstance in which all individuals were granted immunity might allow for a representative sample of malingerers and nonmalingerers, were it possible to definitely ensure anonymity and guarantee subjects that the results could not come back and harm others they cared about (such as co-workers who had not yet filed claims or whose benefits could be altered). For example, the researcher might have to find some way of keeping study sites secret. None of these are easy problems to resolve.

Situational Variables

Malingering studies have often been criticized because the circumstances under which research subjects falsify differ from those under which real malingerers operate. A frequently mentioned concern is the lack of incentives for subjects. In response, some researchers have provided monetary rewards, the impact of which has often been unimpressive (e.g., Bernard, 1990). It is really questionable how much the types of incentives that are offered bring investigators closer to real life. If the intent is to increase compliance and effort, manipulation checks may be as or more effective.

Beyond their role in fostering cooperation with the experimenter's instructions, we may need to think a little more broadly about incentives. First, the positive incentives for malingering in real-life situations can be enormously larger; researchers can hardly afford to offer each successful subject a million dollars. Second, not all malingerers have positive incentives to falsify, and instead the primary motive may be to avoid something bad, such as a jail term. Additionally, whether or not positive incentives are present, there are almost always negative consequences for malingerers who fail (e.g., public exposure, debt). In a case in which one of the authors consulted, a lawyer claimed that because of neurocognitive deficits, he could no longer continue in what had been a successful practice. If he was malingering and if he lost his case, he would have been faced with financial disaster, for he could not have resumed his practice. The potential of negative consequences, and sometimes severe ones, changes the dynamics of the situation. For example, it may well alter who tries to malinger, and may greatly magnify the intensity of the whole situation. As is well known, incentives may increase or decrease performance levels. In some circumstances, when motivation is extreme, effort is extreme but performance suffers. For example, as negative contingencies build, the resultant anxiety may impede performance.

Third, incentives may not be important so much for how they alter effort in the examination setting, but rather for what they lead individuals to do before they get there. An individual who stands to gain lifetime financial security may spend considerable time preparing to malinger. For example, she may read extensively about the disorder she will fake and about psychological assessment instruments. In fact, she may be the only one in the entire case who knows what the "F" in the

MMPI F Scale stands for. Additionally, positive and negative incentives may impact greatly on the level of inconvenience, and pain and suffering, an individual might be willing to tolerate in an effort to present a convincing picture. It is doubtful that the typical small reward that researchers offer would lead many individuals to load their bodies with anticonvulsants or submit to painful medical procedures. An individual who might avoid the electric chair by faking mental incompetence has a cost-benefit ledger from another universe.

Although subject to obvious limitations, it would be interesting to ask individuals about the conditions under which they would and would not malinger (or have and have not malingered). For example, have they, or would they, ever fake being sick so as to avoid school or work or a social outing? In contrast, would they fake injury in a medical malpractice case in which they would stand to benefit enormously, but only by hurting an innocent physician? How would the presence and extent of negative incentives, or the need to undergo painful or negative experiences, alter their judgments about the likelihood they would malinger? Under what conditions might they feel that faking disorder was justified?

If the modest incentives offered in studies do not invoke or re-create elements that are probably of greatest importance in increasing fidelity, or in coming closer to the malingerer's real situation, we will need to use other or supplemental approaches. Preparation would not seem too difficult a variable with which to deal because the researcher can mimic and telescope experience. Two of the dimensions to be addressed are knowledge about (1) the disorder to be faked and (2) the strategies for malingering detection. The safest approach, or at least a way to test the limits of methods, is to provide subjects with high-quality information about one or both dimensions (although a researcher might be interested in altering level or type on these variables). Fortunately, there is an increasing number of studies examining the influence of knowledge on malingerers' success (e.g., Cliffe, 1992; Frederick & Foster, 1991; Hayward, Hall, Hunt, & Zubrick, 1987; Rogers, Bagby, & Chakraborty, 1993; Wetter, Baer, Berry, & Reynolds, 1994). Studies with the MMPI, for example, suggest that knowledge of detection strategies is of considerably greater assistance than knowledge of symptom presentation (Rogers, Bagley, & Chakraborty, 1993; Wetter et al., 1994).

There seem very likely to be interactions between forms of knowledge and assessment methods. For example, although knowledge of disorder might provide little aid in beating the MMPI, it might well be very helpful on interview. Someone with intimate knowledge about head injury, including features that fall outside general knowledge (e.g., "I've been seasoning my food a lot more"), would seem more likely than a naive individual to fool an interviewer. This is one reason why studies examining general knowledge of disorder (what most people know even if they do not prepare themselves) are potentially so useful and can also inform the researcher about how much has to be done to mimic conditions of preparedness. Along these lines, researchers might make a systematic effort to assess baseline knowledge of subjects asked to malinger or who are about to be educated, and might also check on the understanding or mastery of the information that has been provided.

Related mainly to ethical reasons, the researcher faces a much more difficult task when trying to mimic negative incentives. The Institutional Review Board is not likely to feel very Rogerian should they review a research proposal that calls for incarcerating subjects who flunk the malingering test. Negative incentives do not really mean much unless there is real suffering or the threat of such, and it is hard to imagine any circumstance that would justify their inclusion in studies. It might be possible and ethical to offer subjects various financial options for their participation in a study, one being a guaranteed amount for participation versus an arrangement in which they receive an attractive amount of additional money if they succeed in faking but lose all funds if they fail (one might still give them the base amount whatever the outcome).

Strangely enough, given the extent to which the researcher's hands are tied manipulating negative incentives, manipulating imaginary negative incentives may have more impact, given the predilection of individuals to get highly involved in role-playing if the situation is set up properly. For example, one could have research subjects presume that the costs of being detected were great, or set up a situation in which they role-play a prisoner who is likely to face a long jail term unless he is found to be impaired. Such scenarios could also incorporate positive incentives to examine whether they lower or enhance proficiency. All this said, there seems little doubt that these types of approaches have serious shortcomings, and that they are merely preliminary attempts to understand how alterations in conditions may influence malingerers' efforts in real life.

A number of other situational variables may also separate typical research conditions from real life. Many malingerers, especially in brain damage cases, have experienced an injurious or potentially injurious event. Thus, for example, one might try to recruit subjects in the Emergency Room who were in car accidents but did not suffer head injuries. Also, some malingerers have been exposed to models or mentors (e.g., a relative who really has been injured or someone who has malingered successfully, such as a fellow prisoner). Many malingerers have met with attorneys prior to undergoing examinations. A sincere attorney may provide inadvertent cues through leading questions about head injury, or may warn the client about some of the tricks the independent examiner might try. Many malingerers have also been subjected to multiple medical examinations, including those in which feedback or "education" about injury is provided. For example, a neuropsychologist who discusses results with examinees may provide detailed information about head injury, about the examinee's typical and atypical features, or even about his reasons for questioning the examinee's cooperation. If the attorney is unhappy with the results, a new examination might be sought and the prior examination kept secret, with the plaintiff now far better forearmed. All of these types of variables are amenable to study and generally could be addressed through analogue designs.

Base Rates

Although estimates (guesses) have sometimes differed by many orders of magnitude, no one really knows the base rates for malingering, and they are almost sure to vary widely depending on setting and circumstance and where one draws the line. For example, if we equate almost any form of exaggeration with malingering, then we are likely to uncover extraordinarily high rates.

One reason why frequency information is so important is that the utility of diagnostic signs is not absolute but varies in relation to base rates (Meehl & Rosen, 1955; Wedding & Faust, 1989). Frequency data alone may be the best predictor of the relevant condition and may produce far superior results than classification based on one or another diagnostic sign. Assume, for example, that the rate of malingering is 1% in a certain setting and that a particular diagnostic sign provides correct identification in 75% of cases overall. Consequently, if I play the base rates (i.e., always assume that the more frequent circumstance holds) and diagnose everyone as not malingering, I will be right in 99% of cases. Thus, to do better, I would need a diagnostic sign that is correct more than 99% of the time, a level my diagnostic indicator does not even approach. In contrast, if the base rate is 50%, then my diagnostic indicator will do better than playing the base rates. As frequencies diverge in either direction from 50%, and hence one can achieve greater and greater accuracy by playing the base rates and always guessing that a condition is (or is not) present, then so too must diagnostic signs become more and more accurate if they are to assist us.

When some researchers suggest that the base rates for malingering are 50% and others that they are 1%, we do not know if we should believe that we are helped by diagnostic indicators that perform only a little better than chance or not helped by indicators that are right over 95% of the time! Of course, the fundamental problem is that we do not know which guesses are correct and hence are often in a dilemma when trying to determine whether our diagnostic indicators should be used. We almost never can make such determinations unless we have at least some idea about base rates, and in some situations more exacting knowledge of frequencies is required. Further, we cannot really determine the success or utility achieved by diagnostic indicators, because this is a product of a condition's base rate together with the frequency of false-negative and false-positive errors. For readers who may be less familiar with this terminology, false-negative errors represent instances in which the condition is missed when it is present, and false-positive errors instances in which the condition is identified when it is not present.

Suppose a diagnostic indicator for malingering has a 5% false-positive rate. If 50% of a population is malingering, then 5% of the 50% who are not malingering will be falsely identified, or 2–3 people in a series of 100. However, if only 1% of the population is malingering, about twice the number of individuals, or 5% of the remaining 99%, will be falsely called malingerers. Further, even if we assume that the measure never misses a true malingerer, the ratio of correct to incorrect positive identifications of malingering will shift in a very unfavorable fashion. In the first instance, we will misidentify about 2–3 nonmalingerers for every 50 malingerers we identify correctly, giving us a ratio of about 20 correct identifications for every error. In the second instance, we will misidentify about 5 nonmalingerers for every true malingerer we identify, or make far more errors than correct identifications. Thus, shifts in base rates alter ratios between true-positive and false-positive, and true-negative and false-negative identifications. The consequences can be disastrous when one type of error is far worse than the other, and it is just that type of error that increases in frequency, such as missing individuals with suicidal intent. In summary, then, base rate information is needed to determine whether we should use signs at all, the accuracy that signs achieve, and whether and how we should adjust cutting scores.

We return here to the same type of paradox we encounter when attempting to determine how to best measure malingering—we need to know more than we know if we are to find out what we need to know. We need base rate information to appraise the accuracy of our diagnostic methods, and yet to determine base rates we need accurate measures of malingering. Many of the points made earlier apply to this situation as well and to the strategies that might be applied in developing base rate information, such as recognition of the dialectical relation between measurement and conceptualization of the thing to be identified (see the prior section, "Relation between the Nature of the Beast and Measurement").

There is at least one way researchers should be able to determine the lower limits of base rates. If one applies a measure with a very high true-positive rate, or measures on which positive results offer something close to prima facie evidence of malingering (at least on that task), then the obtained rate of positive identifications should provide a good estimate of minimum frequencies. For example, suppose performances that are well below chance on a forced-choice procedure could be taken as strong evidence for malingering. If this method was applied, say, to a group of disability applicants, the frequency of positive results should provide a minimal estimate of malingering rates. Of course, the true base rate might be substantially higher, but we would at least have a good approximation of the lower limit, and anything that allows us to start narrowing ranges is helpful. In many circumstances, even obtaining a very rough estimate of upper and lower ranges can give us clear pragmatic guidance. For example, some signs would prove effective, and some ineffective, anywhere within the range. Application of the strategy suggested here would probably uncover some situations in which our minimal estimates are erroneous, permitting us to sharpen our knowledge of base rates.

We might be able to do a good deal better in estimating minimal frequencies if we use multiple assessment devices or approaches with high true-positive rates, taking positive results of any of these measures as evidence of malingering. For example, we might look for positive results on symptom validity testing, direct evidence that the individual can perform normally in areas in which disability is claimed (e.g., videotapes), and confessions. Some individuals might confess at the time of evaluation, and others might confess if granted absolute assurances about immunity or after a nonreversible determination is reached. When formulating estimates on this basis, the conjunctive false-positive error rate of the measures would need to be taken into account. The major advantage of such a combined approach is reduction in the false-negative rate because, at present, approaches that appear to have high true-positive rates also seem to have high false-negative rates. We do not suggest that these types of combined approaches are a cinch to pursue; but the effort would seem to be justified by the enormous benefits we gain if we are able to formulate reasonable estimates of the base rates. One would also think that the value of such knowledge should lead to favorable funding decisions.

In this context, we would reiterate the potential merit of Meehl's (1995) taxometric methods. It is precisely in this type of situation, in which we lack gold standards for identifying an entity or instances of a category and rather are limited to fallible indicators, that Meehl's method provides a viable means for estimating base rates.

DATA COMBINATION

Consider a situation in which you select stocks on your own and make excellent choices 30% of the time. You then seek out the advice of two stockbrokers, one who makes excellent selections 60% of the time and the other 75% of the time. Although going with the second person's advice more or less assures excellent selections in 75% of cases, you naturally would like to bolster this rate. This is the type of situation the psychologist often faces when attempting to integrate data. There may be one or more relatively strong indicators, but they do not attain a satisfactory level of accuracy when taken in isolation. There are additional indicators that, although not as strong, do show valid relations with the criterion. Finally, there are usually a variety of weaker or invalid so-called indicators.

Psychologists are typically advised to integrate or combine "all of the data." It is sometimes difficult to see how this can be done. If all indicators point in the same direction, there is no problem. However, in many cases, if for no reason other than measurement error, variables conflict. This does not necessarily reflect superficial inconsistency that deeper analysis would show to have an underlying order indicative of the patient's true characteristics. Rather, commonly, some variables provide accurate information about the case at hand and others do not.

Also, we are often faced with what are essentially, or plainly, dichotomous choices, e.g., pick or don't pick Stock A, brain damaged or not, capable or not capable of maintaining gainful employment. If one variable indicates that Stock A will beat Stock B over the next year and another variable produces the opposite prediction, it is hard to imagine that at a deeper level the contradiction evaporates.

To return to the stockbrokers, in some cases they will disagree. If you simply go with the broker who is right 75% of the time, you will have a 75% accuracy rate. Alternatively, you might look for exceptions, or instances in which you would defer to Broker 2 who, after all, is sometimes right when Broker 1 is wrong. The problem with this approach is that, at the outset at least, you have no trustworthy way of identifying exceptions, for that would usually require knowledge superior to that of the better consultant. And if you had such knowledge from the start, the consultants probably would not have been needed. If, instead, you defer to your own judgment to identify exceptions, you are using a weaker predictor to override stronger predictors, a strategy almost guaranteed to fail in the long run. Therefore, at least at first, the best strategy is almost surely to defer to the superior broker in all or almost all cases. You can carefully study cases of disagreement over time to see whether certain ways of combining information from the two brokers enhances accuracy. For example, you might find that for stocks in the electronics field Broker 2 usually beats Broker 1 and, in those instances, you should generally defer to Broker 2 in cases of disagreement. Augmenting decision procedures by identifying exceptions, however, seems to be much more difficult business than we think and frequently backfires (Faust, 1984; Meehl, 1986).

As we expand the number of valid malingering indicators, we will be faced with circumstances in which data combination can become more and more complicated. Fortunately, there is considerable research on this topic, which is of great practical utility and should lead to a rethinking of many common beliefs about data combination (see Dawes et al., 1989; Faust, 1984; Faust & Willis, in preparation).

Research on data integration suggests the following guidelines. First, it is often counterproductive to try to use all of the data. For example, when weak predictors are added to stronger predictors, they often decrease overall accuracy. Second, adding redundant predictors does little or nothing to increase accuracy. A second measure that is highly correlated with a first measure will give us little additional predictive punch. Third, for specific predictive tasks, we often approach or reach the ceiling in accuracy once we have properly combined our two or three or four best, nonredundant predictors. It follows from these three principles that if we have even a relatively small set of strong, minimally redundant predictors, we should be conservative about adding further predictors. We will tend to exclude relatively weak predictors or those whose quality is uncertain, because even if we happen to be lucky and the additional predictor is alright, it probably still will do little for us; but if we get unlucky and the variable is a weak or poor one, it can greatly compromise accuracy. Fourth, in many situations, a linear composite of variables, or even simply weighting all variables equally, approaches or matches the accuracy achieved through optimal weighting of variables or consideration of configural relations among variables, especially if the configural analysis is performed subjectively (Dawes & Corrigan, 1974; Dawes et al., 1989).

These principles of data integration suggest a certain agenda for researchers. Given the number of malingering indicators we now have that have been supported through research, it would be helpful to examine indicators that have not been studied adequately (or at all) but that still seem to be used frequently in clinical practice. Frequency of use could easily be identified through surveys. Examining these indicators might add to the pool of validated methods, but as importantly, if not more so, it will help us to identify variables that appear to be valid but are not. Again, when other valid methods are available, failing to include one more valid predictor is usually not nearly so bad a mistake as inadvertently adding an invalid variable.

There is limited utility in identifying or developing indicators that are redundant with previously available methods. Rather, we should be trying to uncover variables that are likely to contribute unique predictive variance. This might be achieved by seeking new classes of predictors (see the next section). It would also be very beneficial if far greater effort was made to assess incremental validity, that is, any improvement gained by adding a new predictor to the best predictors that are already available. Many studies involve single predictors or a few predictors. Although there is nothing wrong with this per se, we need to take the next step and examine incremental validity. Given the number of malingering indicators that are now available, one could argue that a study limited to showing that a new variable has discriminating power is of negligible help because we cannot evaluate whether that variable will have a negative, positive, or neutral effect on predictive accuracy when combined with other variables. Some investigators have examined multiple variables and their combined effects, which is a start; but too often these studies do not do all that much more than add to the innumerable demonstrations of a matter not at issue, that is, that the statistical combination of multiple valid predictors will usually outperform a single valid predictor. What these studies do not examine is the effect of combining new predictors with the best available predictors.

Given the inordinate demands that can be placed on subjective judgment, including the need to separate predictive and nonpredictive variables, gauge the strength of association between predictors and criterion, determine level of redundancy among predictors, and examine most or all possible ways of combining variables, it would be very helpful to have formal methods of data combination, and particularly actuarial or statistical procedures. There have been few *direct* comparisons of clinical versus actuarial approaches to malingering detection. However, given the overwhelming evidence for the superiority of actuarial methods in general (Dawes et al., 1989; Grove & Meehl, 1996; Meehl, 1954) and the contrasts in success that have been achieved thus far across separate studies examining actuarial methods (e.g., MMPI malingering indices) versus those examining subjective methods of malingering detection, one outcome seems much more likely than the other.

Finally, it is difficult to know how to best identify something you do not know that much about. The homogeneity of malingering or its structure, if it has one, will bear greatly on our methods of identification. For example, the types of decision procedures we need will likely differ greatly if malingering represents a number of orthogonal dimensions or a few unified dimensions. The development of actuarial methods will be partly bound by our overall knowledge of malingering. It is often easiest to develop highly accurate actuarial procedures where we least need them, such as methods that distinguish normal individuals doing their best versus faking bad. However, it is a major philosophical error to believe that one needs a gold standard or nearly infallible criteria to develop useful knowledge or decision rules, for were this the case, much of science could never have progressed. What if Galileo had concluded that peering through the telescope was useless because he had no final authority to test the accuracy of his observations?

It can be difficult, but not impossible, to develop useful actuarial methods for malingering detection absent a highly accurate method for identifying its presence. In fact, one theme of this chapter is that there are many ways to push the boundaries of knowledge, even if we seemingly need to know more than we know so as to do so. Views on philosophy of science that many psychologists have been taught, such as the need for operational definitions and rock solid criteria, and the desirability of minimizing theory (and other such components of methodological behaviorism), are often misrepresentations of positions that have been rejected anyway by mainstream philosophers decades ago (Meehl, 1991; Weimer, 1979).

CURRENT APPROACHES TO MALINGERING DETECTION: SOME THOUGHTS ON REFINING METHODS AND IDENTIFYING ADDITIONAL DISCRIMINATING VARIABLES OR STRATEGIES

Most methods of malingering detection fall into one of four groups: they either (1) look for instances in which individuals perform less well than they can, (2) less well than they should, or (3) differently than they ought to, or they (4) capitalize on stereotypic misconceptions about pathology. Methods that look for below-chance performance, such as symptom validity testing, provide an example of the first approach. The second approach might involve attempts to establish lower bounds on performance, even among severely injured individuals, or to uncover wide separations between plausibly and implausibly bad performance. For example, some researchers (e.g., Guilmette, Hart, & Giuliano, 1993) have examined the performance of seriously injured patients on forced-choice methods. Examples of the third approach include comparison of performance patterns among malingerers and nonmalingerers, such as relative proficiency across memory and attentional measures (e.g., Mittenberg, Azrin, Millsaps, & Heilbronner, 1993), or patterns of successes and failures in relation to item difficulty (e.g., Frederick & Foster, 1991). An example of the fourth approach is the F Scale of the MMPI. The F Scale items tend to work because the way one would think that individuals with severe pathology will respond and the way they do respond often differ.

These various approaches usually require examinees to hold some type of faulty belief, or attempt to induce some false assumption: They depend on tricking the individual. The depth and difficulty of the tricks vary. In some cases, an examinee is told that a test that is practically shouting out, "Try me, I'm easy," is really difficult, and then must bomb the measure in order to be identified as a possible malingerer. In contrast, the F Scale depends on false stereotypes about disorder, which may be shared by laypersons and mental health professionals alike (e.g., see Gough, 1954). As such, attempts to educate oneself about disorder might not help. Rather, one needs to find out how the F Scale works and how to identify F Scale items, and one then needs to endorse enough of them to portray disorder but not so many that one is caught. (However, given the extremely conservative approach to malingering identification that some clinicians bring from the clinic to the courtroom, this might not be too difficult to pull off.) Of course, in a brain damage case, the malingerer may justifiably feel no need to exaggerate emotional disorder and might play the MMPI straight or even dissimulate. Overall, for many methods of malingering detection, should the instructions fail to create misbelief, should examinees not try to overplay disorder grossly, or should they grasp one concept, they stand a good chance of beating the procedure. And if the clinician interprets anything short of clearly malingered performance on one or a few such measures as presumptive evidence of good effort, the examinee is likely to beat the clinician as well. Many of our methods are much too transparent and are likely to lose much of the effectiveness they might have as word circulates.

Decreasing the transparency of malingering detection methods or making them much more resistant to knowledge about their design would seem to be among the utmost research priorities. There has been considerable debate concerning the circulation of information about malingering detection and testing methods. Whatever one's view on this matter, the problem would be largely resolved if knowledge of the methods provided malingerers with no advantage. Also, given such realities as the exceptional motivation of some malingerers, the public nature of legal proceedings, and the wide latitude given cross-examiners in challenging the underlying bases of conclusions, it is naive to believe that trade secrets will not leak out.

We can think of various means to counter transparency, and we are confident that others can expand and improve on the ideas provided here. First, problems with the transparency of forced-choice methods would be immediately improved by increasing the number of foils. Further gains would be realized by varying the number of foils across items and randomizing the order in which items with varying numbers of foils appear. For example, suppose one had items with two to four foils. Suppose that each of these items required the individual to identify a previously presented word on a memory test. Further suppose that the order of the two-, three-, and four-foil items was randomized, such that one did not complete the items with any particular number of foils in a group. The task of producing plausible rates of successes and failures when trying to portray a serious memory disorder would seem to be immensely more difficult under such conditions than those in which, for example, the individual just needs to aim for about a 50% failure rate. This and other approaches can capitalize on limits in human cognition, such as restrictions in the ability to track multiple dimensions of a problem simultaneously.

In a related vein, we might also take advantage of limits in human memory. For example, if inconsistency in presentation does help to differentiate between malingerers and the genuinely disordered, we can create circumstances in which fakers likely must resort to making it up as they go along and will probably have extreme difficulty reproducing their performances at a later time. Suppose we compile a large number of items with low face validity that call for fairly rapid responses and have reasonable stability among honest reporters. A malingerer who does not know how she should answer but is trying to alter her presentation will most likely fall into an arbitrary pattern of responding that is very difficult to repeat on a subsequent occasion given normal limits in recall. There are many other ways one could attempt to design procedures that require extraordinary or impossible memory feats if one is to produce plausible performances over time.

There are some cognitive and physiological functions that are difficult to monitor or control consciously and that offer other possible approaches to the transparency problem. For example, it would seem difficult to consciously control certain priming effects. Suppose, for example, someone was complaining of severe perceptual deficits. Prior to exposing subjects to perceptual ambiguities (e.g., a drawing that could be seen as a face or a goblet), one would present visual information that substantially altered the perception of these subsequent materials. Suppose further that perceptually impaired patients did not show priming effects on some of the materials as a result of their disorders, it was difficult for examinees to judge which materials would and would not produce such effects by looking at them, different sets of test materials were available, and items were ordered randomly. One could also introduce other dimensions, such as changing the number of foils used in follow-up if individuals produced certain responses. Developments in physiological measurement and wide adaptation of the computer also create many new possibilities, as illustrated by efforts to study such variables as reaction time and other functions that computers easily measure and record (D. Schretlen, personal communication, February 3, 1997).

Current attempts to create mental sets about item difficulty might be checked directly against subjects' perceptions. For example, how hard does an item seem at first blush and to what extent do suggestions about item difficulty alter perceptions (especially among those warned that the examiner may sometimes mislead them)? If we are going to pursue such approaches, we might try to expand and refine our methods for creating misperceptions. Indirect verbal suggestion might sometimes be as or more effective than direct suggestion (e.g., telling someone that they will get five chances at materials versus telling them something is hard). Also, there would seem to be ways to alter perceptual impressions of difficulty without really changing objective difficulty, or in fact changing it in the opposing direction. For example, various perceptual illusions might be exploited to create misimpressions.

We are not suggesting that researchers abandon attempts to create measures that tap into false stereotypes. This type of approach has a long history of success, at least with the MMPI, and we certainly should not demand from malingering detection devices that they catch everyone. Many malingerers will not invest the time and effort needed to learn what they should do to effectively portray disorder, others will have difficulty mastering the needed knowledge and strategies, and initial evaluations may be performed before someone really has a chance to become educated. Additionally, methods that tap commonly held but false stereotypes may show limited redundancy with other approaches, which, as noted, increases their potential utility when combined with other predictors. Further, if methods and approaches are consistently updated as knowledge advances, it may be possible to stay a step ahead of many malingerers. For these reasons, efforts to extend this type of approach to structured and semistructured interview techniques and questionnaires that are specifically targeted at neuropsychological and related disorders seem very much worthwhile, as well as continuing efforts to study lay perception of head injury and other neurological disorders (e.g., Wong, Regennitter, & Barrios, 1994). Such research can help in identifying candidate items for these types of malingering detection approaches.

We would like to briefly describe some variables or approaches that would seem to have promise for malingering detection. Many of these represent an attempt to take commonsense considerations that many practitioners might already apply impressionistically and place them on a more explicit, systematic, and formal basis so as to facilitate scientific testing and comparison.

Some disorders would seem to have relatively predictable outcomes, or outcomes that are far more probable than others. For example, with mild head injury, we would not expect catastrophic symptoms or a 6-month delay in symptom onset, and we would be much more likely to see problems in new learning rather than difficulties remembering major life events that occurred preinjury. If we could develop better measures of prototypic outcome and range of expected variation from that prototypicality among those with genuine disorder, and if the level of variation was not too great, we would be in much better shape to say that some outcome does not fall within expectations or is not plausible. Such measurements should be reducible to one or a few dimensions, with studies then conducted to look at distributions among those with and without the disorder (including those feigning). One might call these types of measures indices of prototypicality. If outcome was so varied that most anything was about equally possible, it would serve as a more general warning about formulating causal judgments. A few words of caution are necessary here. We should be very careful about measures of severity, because one does not want to systematically identify those with genuine but atypically bad outcomes as malingerers. Also, failure to fit expectations for a particular type of injury only suggests that the person does not have that type of injury, not necessarily that they are malingering. For example, it may just be something else that ails them.

Inconsistency within and across assessments is frequently mentioned as an indicator of malingering. However, there are presently few formal measures of consistency, subjective judgments often seem to substantially underestimate normal levels of variation (e.g., see Chapter 2 of Faust, Ziskin, & Hiers, 1991), and inconsistency is often viewed as a symptom of brain damage. Putting aside some of the complexities involved here, one is simply looking for instances in which inconsistencies are implausible. For example, there should be some systematic quality to the difficulty of the items someone passes and fails (absent, for example, serious attentional problems or a rapidly fluctuating condition), some cognitive functions are not expected to get dramatically worse across assessments even if the individual has the problems he says he has, and someone's personal history should not change in an increasingly self-interested manner. In one case in which one of the authors consulted, an individual told eight different stories about her head injury over the course of about 3 years, and, without exception, every new story conveyed a more serious event than the last one. The literature documenting the marked difficulties involved in appraising scatter subjectively (in large part reflecting clinicians' skewed exposure to the human population) makes a strong case for developing formal measures and conducting systematic study examining their discriminatory potential.

Some intentional symptom production requires constant attention. A patient who portrays a severe tremor may have difficulty doing so when fencing with the attorney on cross-examination. Using analogue approaches, we can examine what happens to intentionally produced symptoms under distracting conditions.

It may be possible to get at the intentionality of misrepresentations if we could create some type of index that compares the expected odds of misrepresentations working for or against the individual's self-interests and the examinee's obtained distribution. Some examinees misrepresent matters in a way that could cost them large settlement dollars. For example, some seriously impaired individuals deny problems, even when they have much to gain from accurate reporting. Other individuals show a very different pattern. For example, when it comes to remembering preinjury events, they seem to systematically forget all of their shortcomings but remember all of their strengths; the pattern is reversed when it comes to postinjury events, in which case they show remarkable recall of their shortcomings but profound loss of memory for their accomplishments. Misrepresentations that are unintentional are not likely to work systematically in the direction of serving the person's legal case or self-interests. It would not seem that difficult a matter to come up with methods for grading level of self-interest and classifying responses. Approaches that indicate deviation from expected patterns of error might be similarly useful in identifying when individuals have underrepresented their problems in a manner that could greatly impede fair resolution of their case.

A related type of index would provide some measure of negative consequences or events that have occurred in proportion to the negative consequences claimed. Take an individual, for example, who reports intolerable pain but will not take a medication with mild side effects. One would expect some correlation between the level of suffering someone has and is experiencing and the level of suffering someone has and will tolerate in an effort to try to improve her lot. The examinee who claims to be deeply distressed by being off the job but will not participate in a work hardening program or even send out applications, has experienced no loss of income as a result of a generous benefit package, and has maintained an active recreational life, would seem much more likely to be a malingerer than the individual who has voluntarily undergone multiple painful operations, has had his house repossessed, and almost never goes out with friends. This type of index bears some resemblance to comparisons between subjective complaints and hard examination findings, although it is obviously problematic that some serious physical disorders or conditions often cannot be detected objectively. Therefore, it might be more helpful to examine the relation between claimed distress and the level of negative consequences that have occurred or to which the individual has willingly submitted, such as reduction in income, pleasurable activities, and personal freedoms; and exposure to painful and/or dangerous medical procedures. Such indices might also consider what individuals have to gain if their legal cases are concluded in their favor.

In some situations it is to an individual's advantage to be (or appear) impaired, and in other (most) instances it is advantageous to be unimpaired. For example, if an individual is feigning paralysis of a limb to obtain a large settlement, a burning building can suddenly alter the contingencies. In the course of assessment, treatment, and day-to-day living, the relative balance of incentive and disincentive for competence and impairment can shift dramatically, and in some circumstances individuals who have something to gain by being competent may not realize that their behavior could be detected or that they are falling out of role. The anecdotes about such matters are legion. Thus, the patient feigning neurological deficit suddenly becomes extremely competent when appearing in a separate custody dispute. The individual with severe spatial deficits suddenly regains abilities when taking a driving exam. Other times matters are less obvious. The patient with supposed problems in word finding becomes highly articulate when needing to defend herself during cross-examination, or the individual who appears to struggle with the motoric aspects of writing signs the release form for the office secretary with stellar penmanship. It seems worthwhile to try to identify instances in which the contingencies for proficiency shift and to examine the extent to which level of performance shifts accordingly.

Thus far, much of the work on malingering detection in neuropsychology has gone into identifying *inadequate* effort. *Sufficient* effort is often identified by default, an approach with serious limitations. Measures of inadequate effort often have high false-negative error rates; level of effort is not all or none and is better represented along a continuum; and organic and affective conditions can impede effort, especially over time. In fact, in many instances, level, consistency, and maintenance of effort are among the most important factors in determining what a patient can do.

If someone passes, say, symptom validity testing, about all we usually can say is that she was not grossly underrepresenting her abilities on that procedure. It is not sound to conclude that because effort was not bad, it was fine or good. Particularly when such leanings move beyond the clinic and into the courtroom, it can seem like clinicians are operating from inconsistent standards of evidence: They are very quick to assume sufficient effort and very slow to identify suboptimal effort. It is almost as if, having freed themselves from the worry of obvious or gross deficiencies on this matter, they turn away from the issue entirely. Such a mind-set may explain why so little work has been directed toward constructing indices of positive effort (as opposed to those indicating lack of effort or the lack of lack of effort).

We should try to develop formal, validated procedures for assessing level of effort, rather than having to depend largely on subjective judgments. One approach would be to obtain the best possible indicators of prior functioning, ideally in areas unlikely to be affected by the condition of interest and, even better, in areas that malingerers are likely to believe ought to be affected. One also would prefer measures of prior ability that were obtained in situations in which individuals would likely be motivated to do their best (e.g., pre-employment ability testing). Based on these indicators, such as scores on past aptitude testing, one can predict level of performance. When these predictions are met or exceeded, one would have potentially strong evidence of adequate effort. As a simplified example, if an individual who had received a Full Scale IQ of 100 on a preinjury administration of one of the Wechsler Intelligence Scales obtained a score of 105 on postinjury testing, we would have good reason to assume that adequate effort was made on the test. Decreased scores are ambiguous, but the point of this method is not necessarily to identify inadequate effort, because we already have methods to do that, but rather to identify good effort.

Past indicators of ability, even those unlikely to be altered by the condition at issue, are fallible indicators of postinjury abilities. The trick is to combine multiple fallible indicators properly (empirically and statistically) so as to construct a much stronger composite and to make predictions across a range of functions. In turn, one should be able to formulate error terms or distributions of expected results. We could then examine the match between expected and obtained results. For example, we might make predictions in five domains that should be unaltered by, say, mild to moderate head injury, and then look at the correspondence between the distribution of expected performance levels and that of obtained performances. In some cases at least, we might be able to obtain powerful evidence of good effort. These methods might well turn out to have excellent true-positive rates, giving us something roughly equivalent to symptom validity testing in the domain of good effort, that is, a procedure that more often than not yields evidence of limited use (related to low sensitivity), but one in which the value of the exceptions makes it well worthwhile.

We realize that a number of issues would need to be addressed (e.g., identifying the best predictors of later performance, difficulties interpreting performance that is lower than expected, identifying areas that are unlikely to be affected by injury), but we do not see these problems as insurmountable. The potential utility that measures of effort would have for legal and nonlegal assessment and the relative neglect of this area by researchers would seem to warrant the attempt.

Finally, certain forms of misrepresentation are most likely to occur outside of formal testing. For example, individuals might simply misrepresent the cause of their problems or their past history. Historical, collateral, and interview information can provide valuable, nonredundant evidence for assessing malingering, although extensive research shows that subjective means for combining such data are very error prone and that formal methods do better (see Dawes et al., 1989; Sawyer, 1966). Further, recent research, especially by Rogers and colleagues, suggests that structured interview methods that are interpreted using empirically derived decision rules, in contrast to unstructured interviews that are analyzed subjectively, offer considerable promise for malingering detection (Rogers, 1995). Rogers, Bagby, and Dickens's *Structured Interview of Reported Symptoms* is one such example, and has, in a few short years, generated a number of positive studies (Rogers et al., 1992). The instrument seeks to measure endorsement of various types of symptoms and symptom patterns that may be indicative of malingering, such as improbable symptoms and combinations of legitimate symptoms that, however, rarely co-occur. This type of approach and format could easily be adapted to interviews that neuropsychologists conduct.

We strongly suggest efforts to measure and *formally* combine information from multiple sources, such as tests, interview, and history. The task here is not to "analyze all of the information," but rather to garner from these various informational sources the variables that are most predictive and to derive formal, scientifically validated means of data combination. Some individuals think that debates about clinical and actuarial judgment pertain to type of information, such as interview versus test data; but this is not true, they pertain only to how information, from whatever source, is best combined. Among the three or four predictors that work best in combination, it would not be surprising if one came from interview data, one from historical data, and one from test data. Alternatively, the single most powerful predictor might be some measure of consistency across different forms of information. In any case, some of the predictors that seem most promising and likely to generalize to real life, such as the direction of misrepresentations and indices of suffering/inconvenience, all seem to require information that goes beyond test data.

SOME FURTHER RESEARCH SUGGESTIONS

This final section highlights and synthesizes a few of the research ideas we have provided throughout this chapter. Most importantly, we believe that the most central task in malingering detection research, at least for now, is one of construct validation (Cronbach & Meehl, 1955). Thus, we should be preoccupied with questions such as, "Just what is it we are trying to measure?" "Is malingering a taxon?" "What are the intercorrelations between different possible indicators of malingering?" "Is there enough continuity among forms of malingering that indices are likely to generalize broadly, or do we need many different assessment devices?"

Appraising construct validation is much like evaluating a theory, and, ultimately, we know if we are getting somewhere by the orderliness of the data revealed, as shown by a variety of methods, such as the accuracy of prediction. When the task is construct validation, we do not fool ourselves into thinking that operational definitions will solve our conceptual problems or that we can work on one or another facet of the problem, such as measurement or conceptualization, in isolation from one another. Nor do we demand or expect the attainment of near-perfect solutions in one area so as to solve problems in other areas. For example, we do not yet really know how to conceptualize malingering, but this problem need not be fully worked out, by any means, for us to increase our knowledge of base rates or improve our measurement techniques. In all of these domains, firmer footing would greatly accelerate progress and save us from guessing so much. It might sometimes seem as if we have to know more than we know in order to learn what we need to learn or advance knowledge, but these seeming paradoxes are commonplace in the development of a scientific field and there is usually some way to plod through. Indeed, we are making excellent progress in the area of malingering detection.

It seems essential to recognize the tremendous obstacles involved in learning to identify malingering through experience alone, and the very complex cognitive task that faces the clinician, who must try to sort out the predictive and nonpredictive variables, and also determine relative levels of validity, redundancy among predictors, and the best possible combination of predictors. This is an undertaking almost surely best accomplished through formal scientific knowledge and method. Most likely, the essential task is not to try to uncover every possible predictive variable and discern some master underlying pattern that integrates them all. Rather, it is to identify a limited—perhaps very limited—number of predictors that, when acting in concert and combined properly, maximize predictive accuracy.

It is still unclear what sources of information, in combination, might be most helpful in detecting malingering. The identification of these variables requires us to consider not only their individual predictive strengths but also their relative redundancy. Our ultimate list will probably not consist of the three or four or five strongest predictors, when taken one at a time, but the three to five predictors that make up the strongest combination. As such, we should continue, and perhaps broaden, our inquiries into different types of information and their potential utility in malingering detection, such as test performance, history, and interview. We have made a number of suggestions that could help to formalize some of the dimensions that are currently appraised via impressionistic judgment and that seem promising in malingering detection. Researchers might also want to perform more extensive studies of clinicians' abilities to detect malingering to aid their search for those with special talents from whom we might learn. For example, as has been done successfully in other clinical areas, we might be able to construct mathematical models that reproduce their judgments and make their methods more accessible to others (see Goldberg, 1968). It would probably be a significant error to ignore powerful and rapidly advancing technologies that help determine the presence or probability of brain injury, such as volumetric analysis (Blatter et al., 1995). It is hard to believe that information from such sources will not enter into formulaes for appraising malingering.

When planning, interpreting, and critiquing research, we should remain cognizant of the distinction between the context of discovery and the context of justification, or between uncovering promising methods and predictors and verifying them. There is still good reason to search for new discriminating variables. However, our efforts need to go well beyond identifying still one more possible discriminator, given the number that are already available and the ultimate need to develop composites of the most predictive variables in an effort to maximize accuracy in applied settings. Thus, studies that examine the effectiveness of combined variables, and particularly incremental validity, would seem essential.

The evaluation of malingering detection devices require an equal yardstick. It can be problematic to compare methods that have been subjected to separate tests of widely varying or uncertain difficulty. If we conducted equal horse races with different techniques, more informed selections would be possible. When such direct comparisons are not available, we should at least try to be as clear and explicit as possible about the difficulty of the tests to which various methods have been subjected. For example, we would not want to conclude that two methods that have produced similar hit rates have equal merits if one has been subjected to much sterner tests.

It appears that many or most malingering detection techniques can be beaten with relative ease by individuals who gain a little knowledge about their underlying design. We strongly encourage efforts to decrease the transparency of methods and to make them more knowledge proof, or tougher to beat even should someone possess awareness of their underlying rationale. Efforts to do so might capitalize on the limits of the human mind, such as restrictions in the capacity to track multiple dimensions of a problem simultaneously or to maintain exact memories of highly detailed information, or might emphasize areas of human performance for which we have limited awareness or control.

Concerns that have been raised about fidelity and particularly about generalization often seem to be well founded; these issues create difficult, but seemingly not insurmountable, problems. All other things being equal, methods that cut across conditions and forms of malingering provide tremendous advantages, and as our understanding increases we should be vigilant for opportunities to maximize the breadth of methods. Testing the representativeness of samples and gathering representative samples also create methodological stomachaches and will require considerable effort. We believe the method we have proposed that considers the element of chance in detection and Meehl's taxometric methods may provide some inroads toward solving these problems. Pooling of data and sufficient funding would also make a big difference. Given the assumed cost of malingered disorder to taxpayers and insurance companies, we would think that the right types of proposals presented to the right groups might eventually gain substantial financial support.

When examining generalization, it is important to maintain a consistent standard. If reviewers exercise rigorous methodological standards with studies that examine the capacity of clinicians to detect malingering, and we can see how someone might justify such an approach, the same standards should be applied to analysis of methods used in practice to detect malingering. We would also argue for explicit and open methodological standards, not only in scientific publications but also in courtroom testimony. For example, if a clinician demands much stronger evidence to conclude that malingering is present than not present (or vice versa), then just stating the conclusion and failing to openly acknowledge the underlying approach, at least on cross-examination, can be very misleading.

Finally, there may be nothing more helpful to malingering detection than increasing our knowledge about neuropsychological disorders and techniques for measuring them. Surely it is much easier to know what is unexpected when one knows just what to expect.

Acknowledgments

The authors extend their most sincere appreciation to P. E. Meehl and L. J. Yonce for their many helpful suggestions and ideas.

REFERENCES

Albert, S., Fox, H. M., & Kahn, M. W. (1980). Faking psychosis on the Rorschach: Can expert judges detect malingering? *Journal of Personality Assessment*, *44*, 115–119.

Bernard, L. C. (1990). Prospects for faking believable memory deficits on neuropsychological tests and the use of incentives in simulation research. *Journal of Clinical and Experimental Neuropsychology*, *12*, 715–728.

Berry, D. T. R., Baer, R. A., & Harris, M. J. (1991). Detection of malingering on the MMPI: A meta-analysis. *Clinical Psychology Review*, *11* 585–598.

Bigler, E. D. (1990). Neuropsychology and malingering: Comment on Faust, Hart, and Guilmette (1988). *Journal of Consulting and Clinical Psychology*, *58*, 244–247.

Blatter, D. D., Bigler, E. D., Gale, S. D., Johnson, S. C., Anderson, C. V., Burnett, B. M., Parker, N., Kurth, S., & Horn, S. D. (1995). Quantitative volumetric analysis of brain MR: Normative database spanning 5 decades of life. *American Journal of Neuroradiology*, *16*, 241–251.

Butcher, J. N., Dahlstrom, W. G., Graham, J. R., Tellegen, A., & Kaemmer, B. (1989). *Minnesota Multiphasic Personality Inventory-2 (MMPI-2): Manual for administration and scoring*. Minneapolis: University of Minnesota Press.

Chapman, L. J., & Chapman, J. P. (1967). Genesis of popular but erroneous psychodiagnostic observations. *Journal of Abnormal Psychology*, *72*, 193–204.

Chapman, L. J., & Chapman, J. P. (1969). Illusory correlation as an obstacle to the use of valid psychodiagnostic signs. *Journal of Abnormal Psychology*, *74*, 271–280.

Cliffe, M. J. (1992). Symptom-validity testing of feigned sensory or memory deficits: A further elaboration for subjects who understand the rationale. *British Journal of Clinical Psychology*, *31*, 207–209.

Cronback, L. J., & Meehl, P. E. (1955). Construct validity in psychological tests. *Psychological Bulletin*, *52*, 281–302.

Dawes, R. M. (1989). Experience and validity of clinical judgment: The illusory correlation. *Behavioral Sciences & the Law*, *7*, 457–467.

Dawes, R. M., & Corrigan, B. (1974). Linear models in decision making. *Psychological Bulletin*, *81*, 95–106.

Dawes, R. M., Faust, D., & Meehl, P. E. (1989). Clinical versus actuarial judgment. *Science*, *243*, 1668–1674.

Dawes, R. M., & Meehl, P. E. (1966). Mixed group validation: A method for determining the validity of diagnostic signs without using criterion groups. *Psychological Bulletin*, *66*, 63–67.

DePaulo, B. M. (1994). Spotting lies: Can humans learn to do better? *Current Directions in Psychological Science*, *3*, 83–86.

Ekman, P., & O'Sullivan, M. (1991). Who can catch a liar? *American Psychologist*, *46*, 913–920.

Faust, D. (1984). *The limits of scientific reasoning*. Minneapolis: University of Minnesota Press.

Faust, D. (1989). Data integration in legal evaluations. Can clinicians deliver on their premises? *Behavioral Sciences & the Law*, *7*, 469–483.

Faust, D. (1997). Of science, meta-science, and clinical practice: The generalization of a generalization to a particular. *Journal of Personality Assessment*, *68*, 331–354.

Faust, D., & Guilmette, T. J. (1990). To say it's not so doesn't prove that it isn't: Research on the detection of malingering. Reply to Bigler. *Journal of Consulting and Clinical Psychology*, *58*, 248–250.

Faust, D., Hart, K., & Guilmette, T. J. (1988). Pediatric malingering: The capacity of children to fake believable deficits on neuropsychological testing. *Journal of Consulting and Clinical Psychology*, *56*, 578–582.

Faust, D., Hart, K., Guilmette, T. J., & Arkes, H. R. (1988). Neuropsychologists' capacity to detect adolescent malingerers. *Professional Psychology: Research and Practice*, *19*, 508–515.

Faust, D., & Meehl, P. E. (1992). Using scientific methods to resolve questions in the history and philosophy of science: Some illustrations. *Behavior Therapy*, *23*, 195–211.

Faust, D., & Willis, W. G. (In preparation). *Counterintuitive imperatives: A guide to improving clinical assessment and care by predicting more accurately*. Boston: Allyn & Bacon.

Faust, D., Ziskin, J., & Hiers, J. B. (1991). *Brain damage claims: Coping with neuropsychological evidence* (Vol. 1). Los Angeles: Law and Psychology Press.

Frederick, R. I., & Foster, H. G., Jr. (1991). Multiple measures of malingering on a forced-choice test of cognitive ability. *Psychological Assessment*, *3*, 596–602.

Frederick, R. I., Sarfaty, S. D., Johnston, J. D., & Powell, J. (1994). Validation of a detector of response bias on a forced-choice test of nonverbal ability. *Neuropsychology*, *8*, 118–125.

Goldberg, L. R. (1968). Simple models or simple processes? Some research on clinical judgments. *American Psychologist*, *23*, 483–496.

Goldberg, L. R. (1991). Human mind versus regression equation: Five contrasts. In D. Cicchetti & W. M. Grove (Eds.), *Thinking clearly about psychology: Essays in honor of Paul E. Meehl: Vol. 1. Matters of public interest* (pp. 173–184). Minneapolis: University of Minnesota Press.

Gough, H. G. (1954). Some common misconceptions about neuroticism. *Journal of Consulting Psychology*, *18*, 287–292.

Greene, R. L. (1991). *MMPI-2/MMPI: An interpretive manual*. Boston: Allyn & Bacon.

Grove, W. M., & Meehl, P. E. (1996). Comparative efficiency of informal (subjective, impressionistic) and formal (mechanical, algorithmic) prediction procedures: The clinical–statistical controversy. *Psychology, Public Policy, and Law*, *2*, 293–323.

Guilmette, T. J., Hart, K. J., & Giuliano, A. J. (1993). Malingering detection: The use of a forced-choice method in identifying organic versus simulated memory impairment. *The Clinical Neuropsychologist*, *7*, 59–69.

Hathaway, S. R., & McKinley, J. C. (1983). *Minnesota Multiphasic Personality Inventory manual*. New York: Psychological Corporation.

Hayward, L., Hall, W., Hunt, M., & Zubrick, S. R. (1987). Can localized brain impairment be simulated on neuropsychological test profiles? *Australian and New Zealand Journal of Psychiatry*, *21*, 87–93.

Heaton, R. K., Smith, H. H., Jr., Lehman, R. A. W., & Vogt, A. T. (1978). Prospects for faking believable deficits on neuropsychological testing. *Journal of Consulting and Clinical Psychology*, *46*, 892–900.

Meehl, P. E. (1954). *Clinical versus statistical prediction: A theoretical analysis and a review of the evidence*. Minneapolis: University of Minnesota Press.

Meehl, P. E. (1986). Causes and effects of my disturbing little book. *Journal of Personality Assessment*, *50*, 370–375.

Meehl, P. E. (1991). *Selected philosophical and methodological papers* (C. A. Anderson & K. Gunderson, Eds.). Minneapolis: University of Minnesota Press.

Meehl, P. E. (1992). Needs (Murry, 1938) and state-variables (Skinner, 1938). *Psychological Reports*, *70*, 407–451.

Meehl, P. E. (1995). Bootstraps taxometrics: Solving the classification problem in psychopathology. *American Psychologist*, *50*, 266–275.

Meehl, P. E., & Rosen, A. (1955). Antecedent probability and the efficiency of psychometric signs, patterns, or cutting scores. *Psychological Bulletin*, *52*, 194–216.

Meehl, P. E., & Yonce, L. J. (1994). Taxometric analysis: I. Detecting taxonicity with two quantitative indicators using means above and below a sliding cut (MAMBAC procedure) [Special issue]. *Psychological Reports*, *74*(Pt. 2), 1059–1274.

Mittenberg, W., Azrin, R., Millsaps, C., & Heilbronner, R. (1993). Identification of malingered head injury on the Wechsler Memory Scale–Revised. *Psychological Assessment*, *5*, 34–40.

Mittenberg, W., DiGiulio, D. V., Perrin, S., & Bass, A. E. (1992) Symptoms following mild head injury: Expectation as etiology. *Journal of Neurology, Neurosurgery, and Psychiatry*, *55*, 200–204.

Reichenbach, H. (1938). *Experience and prediction*. Chicago: University of Chicago Press.

Reitan, R. M. (1992, August). *Clinical neuropsychology: We've arrived, but do we want to stay?* Paper presented at the annual meeting of the American Psychological Association, Washington, DC.

Reitan, R. M., & Wolfson, D. (193). *The Halstead–Reitan Neuropsychological Test Battery: Theory and clinical interpretation* (2nd ed.). Tucson, AZ: Neuropsychology Press.

Rogers, R. (Ed.). (1988). *Clinical assessment of malingering and deception*. New York: Guilford Press.

Rogers, R. (1995). *Diagnostic and structured interviewing: A handbook for psychologists*. Odessa, FL: Psychological Assessment Resources.

Rogers, R., Bagby, R. M., & Chakraborty, D. (1993). Feigning schizophrenic disorders on the MMPI-2: Detection of coached simulators. *Journal of Personality Assessment*, *60*, 215–226.

Rogers, R., Bagby, R. M., & Dickens, S. E. (1992). *SIRS: Structured Interview of Reported Symptoms: Professional manual*. Odessa, FL: Psychological Assessment Resources.

Rogers, R., Harrell, E. H., & Liff, C. D. (1993). Feigning neuropsychological impairment: A critical review of methodological and clinical considerations. *Clinical Psychology Review*, *13*, 255–274.

Rogers, R., Sewell, K. W., & Salekin, R. T. (1994). A meta-analysis of malingering on the MMPI-2. *Assessment*, *1*, 227–237.

Rogers, R., Sewell, K. W., & Ustad, L. L. (1995). Feigning among chronic outpatients on the MMPI-2: A systematic examination of fake-bad indicators. *Assessment*, *2*, 81–89.

Sawyer, J. (1966). Measurement *and* prediction, clinical *and* statistical. *Psychological Bulletin*, *66*, 178–200.

Wedding, D., & Faust, D. (1989). Clinical judgment and decision making in neuropsychology. *Archives of Clinical Neuropsychology*, *4*, 233–265.

Weimer, W. B. (1979). *Notes on the methodology of scientific research*. Hillsdale, NJ: Erlbaum.

Wetter, M. W., Baer, R. A., Berry, D. T. R., & Reynolds, S. K. (1994). The effect of symptom information on faking on the MMI-2. *Assessment*, *1*, 199–207

Wiggins, E. C., & Brandt, J. (1988). The detection of simulated amnesia. *Law and Human Behavior*, *12*, 57–78.

Wong, J. L., Regennitter, R. P., & Barrio, F. (1994). Base rates and simulated symptoms of mild head injury among normals. *Archives of Clinical Neuropsychology*, *9*, 411–425.

2

The Significance of Base Rates, Test Sensitivity, Test Specificity, and Subjects' Knowledge of Symptoms in Assessing TBI Sequelae and Malingering

WM. DREW GOUVIER, JILL S. HAYES, AND BRANDI B. SMIROLDO

Three factors are often overlooked in the interpretation of neuropsychological test data collected from patients with head injury. These factors are base rate information regarding symptom sequelae commonly associated with head injury, base rate information regarding test performance passes and failures, and subject knowledge of traumatic brain injury. This chapter is intended to provide information regarding these issues in an attempt to aid the neuropsychologist in conducting and interpreting the neuropsychological assessment. Although base rate data are typically overlooked or ignored in making clinical judgments, specific suggestions for overcoming this base rate fallacy are offered. These include history taking and records review, selection of tests varying along a continuum of sensitivity, and the use of retrospective self-report and collateral interviews. Additionally, misconceptions regarding symptoms following traumatic brain injury will be discussed along with the actual sequelae of mild head injury. The ability of neuropsychologists to

---

WM. DREW GOUVIER, JILL S. HAYES, AND BRANDI B. SMIROLDO • Department of Psychology, Louisiana State University, Baton Rouge, Lousiana 70803.

Detection of Malingering during Head Injury Litigation, edited by Reynolds. Plenum Press, New York, 1998.

identify accurately malingering on neuropsychological tests/batteries will be examined, and the present-day usage of malingering detection tests will be considered in light of the base rate fallacy.

NORMATIVE DATA/BASE RATES

In a discussion of base rates, several commonly used terms must be explained. Base rates are different from the epidemiologists' incidence and lifetime prevalence statistics (Bar-Hillel, 1980; Gordon, 1977). They are best regarded as a *current* population prevalence. Base rate data are a priori. The subject comes in with them already in the background; his or her behavior has nothing to do with them beyond perhaps allowing more and more precise specification of the subclass within the population to which that subject belongs. Base rate information is prior probability information (Bar-Hillel, 1980).

Base rates can be used to help the clinician in data interpretation (e.g., what is the clinical/diagnostic meaning of a particular sign/symptom?). Base rate information could be collected and used to give a better understanding about the meaning of symptom complaints, test scores, or classification situations (Arkes, 1981; Carroll & Siegler, 1977; Davidson & Hirtle, 1990; Duncan & Snow, 1987).

Research examining base rate information has been conducted almost exclusively in the context of interpreting the significance of diagnostic test findings (Bar-Hillel, 1980; Duncan & Snow, 1987; Faust & Nurcombe, 1989; Meehl & Rosen, 1955; Willis, 1984). Such data are essential in establishing the validity of clinical assessment procedures.

Validity Testing Using Base Rates

Establishing the validity of any assessment procedure involves examining sensitivity, specificity, and the false-positive and false-negative error rates for that procedure (Bar-Hillel, 1980; Duncan & Snow, 1987; Willis, 1984). Sensitivity refers to the correct detection of the problem/disease by the test or other measure, and specificity relates to accurately identifying those individuals without the problem or disease.

Clinicians should always be cognizant that no test is perfect; there is always the possibility of error (Bar-Hillel, 1980; Duncan & Snow, 1987; Hinkle, Wiersma & Jurs, 1994; Willis, 1984). Error can be one of two types. The first is often termed Type I error or a false positive. This occurs when a test indicates that the individual has the disease/problem, when in actuality he or she does not. Conversely, a Type II or false negative error occurs when the disease is present and the test does not identify the problem.

Although clinicians often overlook base rates, they are directly applicable to validity testing and psychological evaluations (Bar-Hillel, 1980; Duncan & Snow, 1987; Willis, 1984). Imagine for example that Dr. Brown has developed a measure to aid in identifying individuals with leprosy, and he wishes to investigate the validity of his new instrument. The base rate for leprosy is near zero. The validation of the instrument will be nearly impossible because there will be no subjects with the disease (cells 1 and 2 in Figure 1). In the absence of individuals with this disorder, the sensitivity and false-negative error rate cannot be investigated. The most that could possibly be investigated is its specificity and false-positive error rate. The specifics of what one is interested in can vary widely, but the manner in which this should be examined applies across all situations. Although this example is extremely simplistic, it gives us a foundation on which our later examples can be built, and provides a preview of the sorts of diagnostic problems that occur when studying conditions that present with extremely low base rates.

Base rates for any condition are based on a ratio computed as follows:

$$\frac{\text{No. of cases with the condition}}{\text{No. of cases in the population}}$$

So, for a condition that exists in 5 people for every 1000, the base rate for that condition is 5/1000 = .5%. Before continuing, a philosophical crisis must be resolved. Is it acceptable in psychology to make inferences from class membership? For example, if little Johnny, a delinquent, is from a broken home, and it is known that 80% of all delinquents from broken homes become recidivists, is it fair to say that Johnny has an 80% chance of committing another crime? How does one go from the nomothetic to the ideographic? Any particular delinquent has a 100%

		STATE INDICATOR +	STATE INDICATOR -
TRUE STATE	+	HIT SENSITIVITY VALID POSITIVE TRUE POSITIVE 1	MISS FALSE NEGATIVE TYPE II ERROR 2
	-	3 FALSE ALARM FALSE POSITIVE TYPE I ERROR	4 CORRECT REJECT VALID NEGATIVE TRUE NEGATIVE SPECIFICITY

FIGURE 1. Two-by-two contingency table for evaluating test performance characteristics.

chance of either going straight or being a recidivist. That is, for each individual, only one of the situations can occur; therefore, even though statistical data allow one to compute a percentage, the percentage is actuarial, not personal. The key to solving this problem lies in what Meehl (1954) called the person–situation interaction. As class membership is more precisely specified, behavioral likelihoods can be predicted more accurately.

No predictions/classifications about any single case are certain, but all have some probability of being true. This probabilistic relationship is inherently tied to frequency—the frequency of occurrence of events within a class. Even predictions/ classifications involving individuals make implicit references to the personal characteristics among people in the category to which the individual belongs. This category might be other individuals from the same background, with similar circumstances or with the same complaints, or it might be the past behavior of the same person in similar, previous circumstances. The more precisely we can define this reference population for comparison, the better we can use base rate information to enhance our diagnostic accuracy.

To understand better how to compute and use base rates, examples will be offered beginning with the *cab problem*, (Kahneman & Tversky, 1982; Lyon & Slovic, 1976) and some variants that will let us look at effects of base rates and test sensitivity on diagnostic judgments.

Cab Problem

Two cab companies, the Blue and the Green, operate in Narnia. Eighty-five of the cabs are Blue and 15 are Green. A cab was involved in a hit-and-run accident last night, and an eyewitness identified it as a Green cab. The court tested the witness's ability to distinguish Blue and Green cabs at night. Viewing films of five Blue cabs and five Green cabs, she identified 4 of 5 for each. What is the probability that the hit and run cab was Green? To determine this probability, the following formula should be used (refer to Figure 2). The formula is based on the number of correct Green calls over the total number of Green calls:

$$\frac{\text{Cell 4}}{\text{Cell 2 + Cell 4}} \quad \text{thus} \quad \frac{17}{17 + 12} = 0.414$$

Therefore, the probability that the cab was Green is 41%. Had the witness said it was Blue, the probability that she was correct would be 96%, using the formula shown below.

$$\frac{\text{Cell 1}}{\text{Cell 1 + Cell 3}} \quad \text{thus} \quad \frac{68}{68 + 3} = 0.958$$

		WITNESS SAYS (Test Data, Symptoms, or Signs)		
		Blue	**Green**	
TRUE COLOR	**Blue**	68	17	85
(Disease State)	**Green**	3	12	15

FIGURE 2. Cab problem contingency table; base rate for Green = 15%.

This disproportionate skewing of predictive accuracy does not remain when $p = q$ and the base rate of Green cabs goes up from 15% to 50%.

Under the conditions where the base rates for $p = q$, if the witness said the cab was Green, the probability she is correct = 40/(40 + 10) = 80%. The same is true had the witness said the cab was Blue. It is clear that when the probability of both states is equal (Green cabs = Blue cabs), test accuracy determines diagnostic accuracy. However, when the base rates for the two conditions are not equal, diagnostic accuracy consistently changes with a boost in the prediction of the more common condition and a reduction in the accuracy of prediction of the rarer condition, and test accuracy alone no longer determines diagnostic accuracy.

This phenomenon can be illustrated once again using the same problem but looking at the situation just before the Green cab company goes out of business, and only five Green cabs are on the street. Seeing the market opportunity, the Blue cab company increases their fleet accordingly so that they now have 95 cabs. If the witness said the cab was Green, the probability this is true is 4/(19 + 4) = 17%. Had the witness said the cab was Blue, the probability she is correct is 76/(76 + 1) = 99%.

What should one do with the witness's data? Eighty percent is relatively accurate at detecting color, but the usefulness of the accuracy data varies as a function of what the witness says and the base rates for what is actually out there. Clearly, in this case it is difficult to place much faith in the report that the cab was Green. As Table 1 displays, the tendency of base rate skew to improve classifica

		WITNESS SAYS		
		Blue	**Green**	
TRUE	**Blue**	40	10	50
COLOR	**Green**	10	40	50
		50	50	

FIGURE 3. Cab problem contingency table; base rate for Green = 50%.

		WITNESS SAYS		
		Blue	Green	
TRUE	Blue	76	19	95
COLOR	Green	1	4	5
		77	23	

FIGURE 4. Cab problem contingency table; base rate for Green = 5%.

tion into the more common category and detract from classification accuracy into the rarer group can be seen across a range of test sensitivity. Even with extremely good tests (90% accuracy), at 15% base rates, classification is only a little better than chance and nowhere close to the overall diagnostic accuracy that could be achieved using base rate information alone.

What does this mean in the diagnosis of rare or unusual cases in the clinic? In light of the data presented in Table 1, using test indicators for the diagnosis of rare conditions provides a relevant context in which to discuss the importance of base rates.

TABLE 1. Cab Problem Overall Diagnostic Accuracy across Different Base Rates and Observer Accuracies

		Base rate for Green cabs		
Observer accuracy 80%		.5	.15	.05
Likelihood of correct identification	Green	80%	41%	17%
	Blue	80%	96%	99%
		Base rate for Green cabs		
Observer accuracy 60%		.5	.15	.05
Likelihood of correct identification	Green	60%	21%	7%
	Blue	60%	89%	97%
		Base rate for Green cabs		
Observer accuracy 90%		.5	.15	.05
Likelihood of correct identification	Green	90%	61%	32%
	Blue	90%	98%	99%

Base Rates in Clinical Practice

Clinicians are overconfident about what they are doing in their clinical practice, and probably do not even know it (Arkes, 1981; Faust & Nurcombe, 1989), except for some gnawing sense of uncertainty and exposure. How many clinicians get excited on hearing or seeing rare or unusual signs in testing and history? It is exciting to diagnose the first case of something never personally recognized. Beware of the odd and novel. The excitement of the strange may distract from the important but mundane information that would clinch the diagnosis more accurately (Chapman & Chapman, 1967, 1969; Kurtz & Garfield, 1978).

If many data are available, how does one make sure he or she does not get swayed by the dramatic and then ignore the essential information? Faust and Nurcombe (1989) suggested using "information that increases accuracy and discarding whatever does not" (p. 198). To do this, they assert that the data must pass two tests. These are validity and effectiveness. Validity asks, is this indicator something that is significantly related to my predictive/classification concern? For an indicator to possess validity:

$$\frac{\text{Cell 1}}{\text{Cell 3}} > \frac{\text{Cell 2}}{\text{Cell 4}}$$

Looking back at Figures 3 and 4 from the prior examples of the cab problem, it is clear that in every instance, the witness's report is a valid sign.

The results of this simple validity test indicate that anything that increases hits, decreases misses, decreases false alarms, or increases true negatives will increase the validity of the instrument.

Even in less clear-cut cases, where for example 90% of subjects with a diagnostic sign have the disorder while 75% of those without the disorder also have the sign, the sign is still valid.

Valid signs do not necessarily increase accuracy; this is where the question of

TRUE STATE	DIAGNOSTIC SIGN +	DIAGNOSTIC SIGN -
+	TS+ DS+ 1	2 TS+ DS-
-	3 TS- DS+	4 TS- DS-

FIGURE 5. Two-by-two contingency table cell composition.

		DIAGNOSTIC SIGN +	DIAGNOSTIC SIGN -	
TRUE STATE	+	90	75	165
	-	10	25	35
		100	100	

$\frac{90}{10} > \frac{75}{25}$ **Valid Sign**

FIGURE 6. Computation of test validity from contingency table information.

effectiveness is raised (Faust & Nurcombe, 1989). Thus, effectiveness asks, are predictions made more accurate when relying on the presence of the valid sign? The importance of effectiveness can be illustrated in Faust and Nurcombe's (1989) example of Drs. Smith and Jones attempting to diagnose Dissociative Identity Disorder (DID). Suppose the prevalence of DID is one per 1000. Dr. Smith always says no, whereas Dr. Jones makes the diagnosis with perfect sensitivity but imperfect specificity. Dr. Jones makes a single false-positive error for every 100 diagnostic judgments. In the final analysis, Dr. Jones makes 10 times more errors than Dr. Smith, even though he does identify the one case of DID in the reference population.

To determine the effectiveness of a valid sign, remember that a sign can increase accuracy *only when* the frequency of the condition exceeds the sign's combined error rate (false positives and false negatives) (Faust & Nurcombe, 1989). Conversely, if the combined false-positive and false-negative error rate exceeds the frequency of the condition to be diagnosed, the clinician will be more accurate using base rates alone. In quantitative terms, this relationship is expressed as follows: For base rates below 50%, relying on the sign will increase diagnostic accuracy when:

$$\text{Base rate} > \text{false positive} + \text{false negatives}$$

Taking Dr. Jones's approach to DID diagnosis,

$$.001 \text{ is not} > .01 + 0$$

Therefore, he ought not count on the diagnostic utility of his sign in circumstances where maximizing overall diagnostic is the tantamount issue. For base rates above 50%, the sign will increase diagnostic accuracy when

$$1 - \text{base rate} > \text{false positives} + \text{false negatives}$$

Once the validity and effectiveness of a diagnostic sign have been established, how does base rate information apply in clinical practice? Obviously, Dr. Jones's talent for identifying DID is of some merit, and the clinician must weigh the relative costs and benefits associated with Type I and Type II error rates. "Base rates should guide practice, not rule it" (Faust & Nurcombe, 1989, p. 201).

Here's where things get murky. Accuracy must be weighed against utility and the implications of different error types should be considered (Faust & Nurcombe, 1989; Gordon, 1977; MacLennan, 1988). If the question were diagnosis of brain tumor or prediction of suicide/homicide, Dr. Jones and his test would be preferable to Dr. Smith (who just plays base rates) every time, because he has the diagnostic sensitivity needed, even though he makes 10 times more errors than Dr. Smith. But even here, there's a weighing that has to take place. Dr. Jones's brain tumor error rate of 1:100 is acceptably low, but what would the neuroradiologist say if his error rate were 10:100 or 20:100? At what point does this become an exercise in "hollering wolf"? Sometimes the cost to the individual or the insurance company of following up the false positives outweighs the benefits of an occasional hit.

A similar example was given by MacLennan (1988) and looks at a population whose base rate for suicide is 10%, using a test that is 60% accurate in identifying potential suicides. Even though the correlation is only weak, there is a correct prediction of 82%; however, these results are not as good as those Dr. Smith would get with base rates alone. But Dr. Smith be damned; despite the decreased overall accuracy, 60% of the possible suicides would be identified, and hopefully prevented when Dr. Jones's test is used, while Dr. Smith would have identified none. Put in human terms, Dr. Jones may not win in the diagnostic box score, but his approach saves 6 otherwise wasted lives at the cost of inconveniencing 14 nonsuicidal patients.

Observations on the Disuse of Base Rate Information

Base rate data are not readily available. Despite the importance and usefulness of base rate information, clinicians and researchers rarely report them in the

		TEST		
		DEPRESSED	NONDEP	
BEHAVIOR	SUICIDE	6%	4%	10
	NO SUICIDE	14%	76%	90
		20	80	

Base rate = 10%
82% correct predictions
phi correlation = .33

FIGURE 7. Dr. Smith's 90% accuracy beats Dr. Jones's 82%, but Dr. Jones saves six lives.

literature or use them in their practice (Ajzen, 1977; Arkes, 1981; Bar-Hillel, 1980; Carroll & Siegler, 1977; Christensen-Szalawski & Beach, 1982; Davidson & Hirtle, 1990; Duncan & Snow, 1987; Einhorn & Hogarth, 1981; Faust & Nurcombe, 1989; Kahneman & Tversky, 1982; Lyon & Slovic, 1976; MacLennan, 1988; Manis, Dovalina, Avis, & Cardoze, 1980; Willis, 1984). Duncan and Snow (1987) observed that "thirty years after Meehl and Rosen (1955, p. 194) demonstrated the importance of base rates, we can reaffirm their statement that 'base rates are virtually never reported' " (p. 369). This statement is just as true today as it was then. Duncan and Snow (1987) noted in their review of 12 major validation studies of the Halstead–Reitan and Luria–Nebraska neuropsychological batteries that only one study (Malloy & Webster, 1981) even reported the base rate for organic brain syndrome among their referral population. So the first reason base rate information is not used is that even though it is readily available to the researchers, it is not widely reported in their research papers. Said Meehl and Rosen (1955), "Our ignorance of base rates is nothing more subtle than our failure to compute them" (p. 213).

A second reason for this disuse of base rate information is that such data are not particularly salient. In contrast to concrete and tangible descriptive data, base rate data are abstract and remote.

A third reason draws from this abstract and remote characteristic of base rate data. People do not know what to do with base rate information when they are given them. Christensen-Szalawski and Beach (1982) showed that if subjects received base rate information, they could estimate base rates relatively accurately, but still did not incorporate such data into their diagnostic decision making unless the base rate information was paired with the diagnostic test data. Only when the subjects "experienced" the association of base rate *and* test data did they begin to use base rate information to enhance their diagnostic accuracy.

A fourth reason for the disuse of base rate information is that we are overimpressed with our own clinical skills and often put far too much confidence in our tests. We see correlations even when there are none really there (Chapman & Chapman, 1967, 1969).

A fifth reason is another indictment against diagnostic practitioners. That is, we are lazy. It is easier to use cultural stereotypes (e.g., "representation heuristic" [Davidson & Hirtle, 1990]) than to have to take statistical data into account. Tversky and Kahneman (1982) invited us to take Steve: "Steve is a very shy and withdrawn, invariably helpful, but with little interest in people or in the world of reality. A meek and tidy soul, he has a need for order and a passion for detail" (p. 33). They ask us, is Steve a salesperson or a librarian? No matter what the representational heuristic says, odds are that Steve is a salesperson. On hearing this, one colleague grudgingly replied, "Yes, but he's probably a book salesman." Old beliefs die hard. Davidson and Hirtle (1990) showed that this habit could be broken only by presenting subjects with descriptive data that contradicted the stereotype, and only when this was done would the subjects use base rate information to enhance their classification accuracy.

The final reason to be considered is more personal, but it is felt by all of us at some times, namely, fear. Usually this is just some gnawing sense of uncertainty or exposure of vulnerability, and we usually can't put our finger on just why that feeling comes over us, but consider the implications of not considering a set of vital and important (albeit abstract and remote) diagnostic information that we don't know what to do with, have little experience with, and do not worry about because we are cocky, overconfident and lazy. It is the sort of thing that makes you want to hide your head in the sand. As Watterson (1992) observed, if ignorance is bliss and one is "willfully stupid," in pursuit of "short-term, stupid self-interest," one must be cautious about learning from experience. The basis for our fear can be found in the rhetorical question, for how many of us did the phrase "willfully stupid" ring a resonant chord?

Ways of Overcoming the Base Rate Fallacy

As it is apparent that base rate information is rarely used, how can clinicians conduct a thorough assessment that includes normative data? Three methods will be discussed including history and record reviews, using tests of differing sensitivity levels, and collecting retrospective self-report data on symptoms subsequent to the injury/disease.

Initially, a thorough developmental history should be gathered to determine any complications during the birthing process or any medical difficulties during childhood and adolescence (Allport, 1942; Spreen & Strauss, 1991). School records should also be obtained (Allport, 1942; Sattler, 1988; Spreen & Strauss, 1991). These records should include such useful information as transcripts, behavioral data sheets, and standardized testing. The latter is likely the most important information, given that this is likely to provide a relatively accurate indication of the individual's premorbid level of functioning. Finally, information regarding work history should be accumulated (Allport; 1942, Spreen & Strauss, 1991). If the individual was in the military, detailed records are often kept of work behaviors, attitude, and injuries. For hospital records, nurse's notes often contain the most detailed behavioral observations.

Once a thorough history and record review has been conducted, testing should begin. One method for improving diagnostic accuracy beyond base rate information alone is using multiple measures with differing sensitivity levels (Sattler, 1988; Spreen & Strauss, 1991). A funnel-type approach could be designed wherein a test that initially identifies a large number of individuals possibly exhibiting the disease/problem is used. A second more sensitive measure could then be administered to rule out those individuals with some presenting symptoms but without the disease/problem.

Finally, collecting information regarding the presence of symptoms prior to the head injury/disease allows the clinician to detect better those symptoms possibly resulting from the head injury/disease (Hartlage, 1995; Lees-Haley & Brown, 1993). Psychological and neuropsychological symptoms are commonly observed among undiagnosed individuals (Dunn, Brown, Lees-Haley, & Euglisi, 1993; Fox, Lees-Haley, Earnest, & Dolezal-Wood, 1993; Gouvier, Uddo-Crane, & Brown, 1988; Lees-Haley, 1992; Roberts et al., 1990). Because this is the case, the presence of the symptoms is not necessarily indicative of the disease/injury. Collecting retrospective information from the individual and significant others may help alleviate some confusion.

Using base rates in clinical practice for the diagnosis of neuropsychological disorders and also in malingering detection following traumatic brain injury is imperative for a thorough evaluation and diagnosis. To illustrate the importance of this factor, a discussion of the sequelae of traumatic brain injury, base rates in the general population, misconceptions of head injury, and knowledge of the general public will follow.

SEQUELAE OF TRAUMATIC BRAIN INJURY

Over 9 million new cases of traumatic brain injury per year are reported, making this a prominent health care concern with males age 16–25 (the most at-risk group) (Caveness, 1977; Kraus & Nourjah, 1989; Sorenson & Kraus, 1991). It is estimated that over 2 million of these cases will suffer some degree of permanent measurable cerebral damage from their head injury (Goldstein, 1990). Because so many cases of head injury are available for study, researchers have clearly identified physical signs and symptoms associated with traumatic brain injury, as well as neuropsychological progression of recovery (Levin, Benton, & Grossman, 1982).

As mild head injury constitutes the majority of individuals presenting with traumatic brain injury and is very well represented among personal injury claims, the sequelae associated with mild injuries are of greatest interest here. Mild head injury patients appear to have the most difficulties with tests tapping attention, verbal and visual memory, problem-solving skills, planning and judgment, and information processing speed (Barth et al., 1983; Rimel, Giordani, Barth, Boll & Jane, 1981). For example, Leininger, Gramling, Farrell, Kreutzer, and Peck (1990) found that individuals who sustained mild head injury performed significantly worse on a sensitive neuropsychological test battery than matched controls even at 6 months after injury. However, methodological difficulties abound, and longitudi-

TABLE 2. Neuropsychological Complaint Base Rates among Personal Injury Claimants and Controls

Controls	Claimants	Symptom
54%	93%	Anxiety or nervousness
52%	92%	Sleeping problems
32%	89%	Depression
62%	88%	Headaches
48%	80%	Back pain
58%	79%	Fatigue (mental or physical)
26%	78%	Concentration problems
36%	77%	Worried about health
38%	77%	Irritability
30%	74%	Neck pain
36%	65%	Impatience
18%	62%	Restlessness
24%	61%	Feeling disorganized
30%	60%	Loss of interest
16%	59%	Confusion
16%	56%	Loss of efficiency in carrying out everyday tasks
14%	55%	Shoulder pain
20%	53%	Memory problems
26%	44%	Dizziness
6%	41%	Sexual problems
12%	39%	Numbness
34%	38%	Nausea
20%	34%	Word finding difficulty
28%	32%	Diarrhea
22%	32%	"Visual problems, blurring or seeing double"
8%	30%	Trembling or tremors
18%	29%	Hearing problems
16%	29%	Constipation
22%	24%	Foot pain
12%	24%	Trouble reading
20%	21%	Bumping into things
12%	21%	Elbow pain
16%	18%	Speech problems
4%	15%	Impotence
12%	11%	Bleeding
2%	4%	Seizures
8%	2%	Broken bone or bones

From Lees-Haley & Brown, 1993, Neuropsychological complaint base rates of 170 personal injury claimants. *Archives of Clinical Neuropsychology*, *8*, 203–209. Adapted with permission.

nal research provides mixed results on the persistence of these symptoms over years (Dikmen, McLean, & Temkin, 1986; Ewing, McCarthy, Gronwall, & Wrightson, 1980).

Symptom Base Rates in Individuals without Traumatic Brain Injury

Although the symptoms noted in individuals after a head injury may be the result of the brain injury, these same symptoms are also often present in the general population (Gouvier, Uddo-Crane, & Brown, 1988). Such symptoms are even more common among personal injury claimants who have not sustained neuropsychological insults (Lees-Haley & Brown, 1993). Table 2 summarizes these results, showing rates of symptom endorsement among nonneuropsychological personal injury or other civil litigation plaintiffs and among a nonneuropsychological nonlitigant comparison group.

The presence of such symptoms in individuals without traumatic brain injury forces us to reconsider the diagnostic significance of the sign or symptom. For example, the most commonly reported difficulty among personal injury claimants is anxiety and nervousness (93%), but over half of control subjects complain of this problem as well. Two other symptom complaints commonly voiced following head injury, memory difficulties and headaches, are similarly confounded, with very little difference in symptom reports between personal injury claimants and controls, respectively.

Given these data (Lees-Haley & Brown, 1993), let us examine the validity and effectiveness of headache and memory complaints as diagnostic signs of being victimized. Base rate estimates for these complaints among victimized and nonvictimized populations were first generated by collapsing across the base rate estimates and victim complaints of Gouvier, Uddo-Crane, and Brown (1988), Lees-Haley, and Brown (1993) and Wong, Regennitter, and Barrios (1994). Using the validity test, both headache and memory complaints are valid indicators that a person has been victimized. With regard to the effectiveness, note that whereas headache is effective in the circumstance in which half of the subjects have been victimized and half have not ($p = q$; base rate = 50%), we can also see that it would not be an effective sign under circumstances where the base rates for victimization were outside the range between .335 and .665 in either direction. The effectiveness of headache as a diagnostic sign is limited by base rates for victimization status, and also by the rather high rate of headache endorsement among the nonvictimized subjects.

Turning our attention to the effectiveness of memory as a diagnostic sign for victimization (Figure 9), we see that it was less effective a sign than was headache. Note that its effectiveness is also affected by the arbitrary $p = q$ base rates set in this example, but the slightly lesser robustness of this sign can be seen by looking at the base rate limit at which it would no longer be effective. In this case, effectiveness

SYMPTOM COMPLAINT OF HEADACHE

TRUE STATE VICTIMIZED	+	-
+	85 (1)	15 (2)
-	52 (3)	48 (4)

Is it valid? $\frac{85}{52} > \frac{15}{48}$ Yes, it is valid!

But is it effective?

BR > FP + FN

.5 > .26 + .075

.5 > .033

Yes, headache is an effective sign, but only weakly so. Its effectiveness is due to the arbitrary assignment of p = q, and it would remain effective when base rates range between .335 and .665.

FIGURE 8. Computation of validity and effectiveness for the symptom complaint of headache.

SYMPTOM COMPLAINT OF MEMORY

TRUE STATE VICTIMIZED	+	-
+	55 (1)	45 (2)
-	29 (3)	71 (4)

Is it valid? $\frac{55}{29} > \frac{45}{71}$ Yes, it is valid!

But is it effective?

BR > FP + FN

Is .5 > .225 + .145

.5 > .38 Yes, memory complaints are effective, and would remain so anytime the base rates for memory complaints range between .38 and .62.

FIGURE 9. Computation of validity and effectiveness for the symptom complaint of memory dysfunction.

would be lost whenever the base rate for victimization fell outside the range between .38 and .62. Thus, for either sign to be effective, at least approximately one-third, but not more than two-thirds of the population of subjects under study must have victimization status.

Just as base rates allow clinicians to determine valid and effective symptom complaints as predictors for a disorder, base rates can be used to examine the validity and effectiveness of test scores in the same way (Bar-Hillel, 1980; Duncan & Snow, 1987; Willis, 1984). Suppose 30% of controls and 60% of individuals with traumatic brain injury do not pass a particular test. Is failure a valid indicator of traumatic brain injury? With the base rate for head injury set at 50%, and using the formula for validity testing described above, failure is a valid indicator of traumatic brain injury (60/30 > 40/70). However, it is not an effective predictor except in those situations where the base rate for traumatic brain injury falls within the range of .35 to .65. When the base rate for traumatic brain injury is set at 20%, test failure remains a valid sign (12/21 > 8/49), but it is not even close to being effective (.20 is not greater than .21 + .8).

Because there is a fairly high base rate for symptom complaints and test failures among the general population, and a fairly low base rate for many of the conditions we are asked to test for, accurate diagnosis is problematic. This is particularly true when one is confronted with the prospect of individuals who may not have the test sign or symptom complaint, but may act as if they do.

Misconceptions of Head Injury

Researchers have documented a surprising amount of ignorance in the general population about what happens in traumatic brain injury, particularly in areas related to cognitive and emotional changes (Aubrey, Dobbs, & Rule, 1989; Gouvier, Prestholdt, & Warner, 1988; Willer, Johnson, Rempel, & Linn, 1993). Aubrey et al. (1989) examined perceptions of college students regarding symptoms following head injury and whiplash. They presented evidence that the students typically thought physical symptoms were more common than cognitive symptoms following mild head injury. In light of these findings, the authors suggested that individuals attempting to simulate mild head injury would be unlikely to portray accurately the cognitive impairments associated with such an injury.

Common misconceptions about head injury (Gouvier, Prestholdt, & Warner, 1988; Willer et al., 1993) may serve as pathognomonic signs of malingering when they are given by the patient or collateral in an interview. Subjects who report prolonged retrograde amnesia, but little or no posttraumatic amnesia, or who report on the specific things they can remember and the specific things they cannot are examples of such deviant report patterns.

But individuals can be coached or trained to simulate more accurately the disorder they are faking, and these coaching interventions can be somewhat effective. Coached malingerers can fake symptom complaints accurately (Wong et al., 1994), and their neuropsychological test performance tends to be more like the test performance of real patients than is that of naive, uncoached malingerers (Martin, Bolter, Todd, Gouvier, & Niccolls, 1993; Martin, Gouvier, Todd, Bolter, & Niccolls, 1992) but even the coached malingerers tended to exaggerate their neuropsychological performance deficits. Furthermore, although pointed coaching can affect symptom complaints and test performance, subjects' native level of knowledge about head injury and its effects has been shown to be unrelated to their ability to simulate deficits (Hayes, Martin, & Gouvier, 1995).

Base Rates and the Detection of Malingering

If clinicians could better understand some of the possible reasons why patients complain more and perform worse on our tests, then a better understanding of what it means when a patient complains or does poorly could be achieved. In an attempt to explain why individuals may malinger, Rogers (1988, 1990) proposed that there are some instances in which the individual may perceive malingering as an adaptive response, causing the patient to file a personal injury suit.

Litigation influences complaints (Rogers, 1988, 1990). Even in patients with nonneuropsychological injuries, but also in patients with neuropsychological injuries, litigation status will lead to higher levels of symptom complaints. This is also seen in severe traumatic brain injury (McKinley, Brooks, & Bond, 1983) and in nonneuropsychological personal injury, sex discrimination, or wrongful termination cases (Lees-Haley & Brown, 1993).

In addition to the influence of litigation alone, repeated suggestions can aid the litigants in more closely and accurately presenting themselves as displaying the disorder they claim. As clinicians, it would be flagrantly unethical to help a patient obtain or learn information about head injury, psychological and neuropsychological testing so as to simulate deficits more effectively and appear more hurt than is truly the case. However, such simulation (faking bad when no disorder is present) and dissimulation (faking good when disorders are present) do occur. Youngjohn (personal communication, 1993) reported witnessing an attorney plead before the judge that "I'd consider it malpractice if I *did not* coach my client on how to take the MMPI."

The whole field of malingering research is moving toward refining our ability to tell normalcy against a background of pseudo-neuropsychopathology. Current procedures have not been examined with sufficient scrutiny to allow clinicians to make this distinction. The following examines some important issues regarding malingering testing and the use of base rates.

Estimates for the prevalence of malingering vary from low (2–7%) (Schretlen, 1988) to very high (64%) (Heaton, Smith, Lehman, & Vogt, 1978). Which is right? It depends on the population reference sample. Schretlen's figures are general clinic referrals, whereas Heaton and colleagues' are personal injury claimants. The Heaton et al. estimates may also be flawed by methodological problems of deriving a regression equation on simulators and then applying this to real patients. These authors incorrectly identified nearly one-fourth of the control sample as malingerers in their cross validation of this regression equation.

However, by choosing the appropriate reference population, a more accurate clinical picture can be derived. It is the present authors' opinion that Trueblood (1994) offered the best current estimate of base rates for malingering among a mild head injury sample, with clear malingering ($n = 12$) and questionable validity ($n = 10$) subjects identified out of a sample of 150 consecutive referrals. Based on Trueblood's (1994) data, using an estimate of the population base rate among mild traumatic brain injury for possible malingering, 22/150 or about 15%, the usefulness of two measures to detect malingering can be examined. It is purely a coincidence that this 15% estimate parallels the base rates used previously in examining the cab problem.

Suppose there are two malingering tests, one with high specificity but low sensitivity and one with high sensitivity and low specificity. For the sake of

MEMORY FOR FIFTEEN ITEMS FAILURE

MALINGERING STATUS		+	-
	+	5 (1)	10 (2)
	-	5 (3)	80 (4)

Is it valid? Yes ... $\frac{5}{5} > \frac{10}{80}$

Is it effective? (Better than base rate) BR > FP + FN

.15 > .10 + .05

No better than base rate only. 85% accuracy for MFIT, and 85% accuracy for base rates alone.

Overall accuracy of MFIT + calls is 56%.

FIGURE 10. Hypothetical computation of validity and effectiveness of malingering detection using the Memory for Fifteen Items Test.

DOT COUNTING TEST FAILURE

		+	-
MALINGERING STATUS	+	10 (1)	5 (2)
	-	17 (3)	68 (4)

Is it valid? Yes ... $\frac{10}{17} > \frac{5}{68}$

Is it effective? BR > FP + FN

.15 > .17 + .05

.15 > .22

Overall accuracy for the DCT = 78%.
Base rate accuracy = .85%.
Accuracy of DCT + calls = 37%.

FIGURE 11. Hypothetical computation of validity and effectiveness of malingering detection using the Dot Counting Test.

example, and recognizing that these sensitivity and specificity figures are purely hypothetical, let's call the former test the Memory for Fifteen Items Test (MFIT) and the latter test the Dot Counting Test (DCT). As indicated in Figure 10, the test with high specificity is a valid sign, but is only effective when the malingering base rate is between 15% and 85%. Likewise, the measure with high sensitivity shown in Figure 11 is valid, but only effective when malingerers have a base rate of incidence between .22 and .78. In either case, base rate prediction would be on par with or superior in overall accuracy, but no malingerers would be identified.

Although it is desirable to identify malingerers whenever we can, one must consider the consequences of misdiagnosis. In the context of the "do no harm" principle, one can clearly see that the consequences of a false-positive error in malingering detection will likely do more harm than a false-negative error, particularly on a forensic unit where the false-positive error might lead to a lethal injection or similar nonreversible consequence. This same argument applies in civil proceedings in which a deserving plaintiff may be "zeroed out" because he or she was incorrectly labeled as a malingerer. Considering this, there is a way we can improve our chances of being correct when we call somebody a malingerer.

Diagnoses of malingering based on MFIT findings alone are no better than chance. Diagnoses made on DCT failure are worse than chance; that is, they are more probably than not *wrong*. Now obviously, neither the DCT nor the MFIT is

DOT COUNTING TEST SIGN

MALINGERING STATUS		+	-
	+	10 (1)	5 (2)
	-	17 (3)	68 (4)

MEMORY FOR FIFTEEN ITEMS SIGN

MALINGERING STATUS		+	-
	+	3 (1)	7 (2)
	-	1 (3)	16 (4)

FIGURE 12. Two-tiered malingering strategy reduces false-positive errors, but lets more malingerers escape detection.

going to hang the moon, and base rate prediction would match or exceed either one, but then no malingerers would ever be identified until we get to the point where malingerers outnumber the real patients, and then Dr. Smith would say that *all* are malingerers. However, if we take these two tests together, we can use them in tandem to pick up some malingerers and still reduce the likelihood of misclassifying the nonmalingerers as well.

Among the DCT respondents, 27 out of 100 failed the test; of these, 10 were malingerers and 17 were not. If these 27 subjects were run through a second pass using the MFIT, 3 of the 10 true malingerers would be identified and only 1 nonmalingerer would be misclassified. Our probability of being correct when we classify someone as a malingerer exceeds the more probably than not standard, and stands at 75%. The same outcome results when the MFIT is used for the first pass and the nine MFIT failures are given the DCT in the second pass. In this example, three of the 15 malingerers (20%) are correctly identified, and 80% of the malingerers get away with deception. But this approach, and the alarming 80% false-negative rate that goes along with it, is the only way we can really honor our oath to tell the truth and more probably than not be accurate when we call someone a malingerer. Such is the impact of base rates, test sensitivity, and test specificity on our diagnostic judgments. And even here, with lethal injection or financial ruin as a possible wrongful consequence of making a false-positive error, 75% accuracy is woefully poor protection for the accused or afflicted.

CONCLUSION

In light of the importance of the detection of malingering and the necessity of incorporating base rate information into the process, the following guidelines are recommended for clinicians.

Tests of different sensitivities to tap a range of possible deficits should be administered. Spreen and Strauss (1991) is an excellent review of the reliability and validity of numerous measures. Second, pre- and postinjury data should be collected at every opportunity from multiple sources. Next, the risks of misses and false positives should be weighed. Sometimes using base rate information alone may be best, but at other times, clinicians may be better served to leave base rates behind and trust their assessment measures and their clinical judgment. Accordingly, when rendering diagnosis, clinicians should be cautious. Multiple indices should be used to ensure the presence of any symptom/disease, and the possibility of misses should be acknowledged. Research efforts in the field need to be realigned to guarantee better collection and reporting of base rates and test sensitivity/specificity data. Finally, clinicians and researchers should look in new directions. In the same way, drug companies need constantly to devise new drugs to combat increasingly drug resistant strains that mutate so as to survive the last generation of antibiotics. This pathogen/antibiotic analogy will require new generations of detection strategies to be developed on an ongoing basis. Such new approaches may include implicit measures, hidden manipulations (e.g., varying the meaningfulness or imagery), studies of situations, and development of situational taxonomy and situational criteria value of the test stimuli. These new tests

		WITNESS SAYS		
		Blue	**Green**	
TRUE	**Blue**	85	0	85
COLOR	**Green**	3	12	15
		88	12	

$\frac{12}{12} = 1.0$ Probability that "Green" call is correct

$\frac{85}{88} = .966$ Probability that "Blue" call is correct

97% overall accuracy

Base rate for "Green" is 15%

FIGURE 13. Cab problem contingency table with perfect accuracy in identifying blue cabs.

should include norms and specifications for sensitivity and specificity, and need to be evaluated on appropriate reference groups, including blue collar and other workers who are employed in occupations that are likely to be related to increased risk of traumatic brain injury.

TOWARD AN IMPROVED TECHNOLOGY

Returning to the cab problem, in real life our tests are not always equally accurate in the detection of Blue and Green cabs. In circumstances where we have perfect detection of one class and imperfect detection of the other, we may see a way to solve the problem of the wrongly labeled malingerer. Figure 13 outlines a situation in which Blue cabs are identified with perfect accuracy and the identification of Green cabs remains imperfect at 80%. Paradoxically, this situation ensures 100% likelihood that Green calls are correct. As Reitan and Wolfson (1994) observed, neuropsychologists struggle with understanding what "normal" is. If as a profession, we could become more accurate in identifying normalcy, then we could worry less about ruining lives with diagnostic misclassification.

Acknowledgments

The authors gratefully acknowledge David Faust and John Courtney, whose writing and comments have greatly influenced this work.

REFERENCES

Ajzen, I. (1977). Intuitive theories of events and the effects of base-rate information on prediction. *Journal of Personality and Social Psychology*, *35*(5), 303–314.

Allport, G. W. (1942). *The use of personal documents in psychological science*. SSRC Bulletin #49. (Cited in Meehl, 1954)

Arkes, H. (1981). Impediments to accurate clinical judgment and possible ways to minimize their impact. *Journal of Consulting and Clinical Psychology*, *49*(3), 323–330.

Aubrey, J., Dobbs, A., & Rule, B. (1989). Layperson's knowledge about the sequelae of minor head injury and whiplash. *Journal of Neurology, Neurosurgery and Psychiatry*, *52*, 842–846.

Bar-Hillel, M. (1980). The base-rate fallacy in probability judgments. *Acta Psychologica*, *44*, 211–233.

Barth, J., Macciocchi, S., Giordani, B., Rimel, R., Jane, J., & Boll, T. (1983). Neuropsychological sequelae of minor head injury. *Neurosurgery*, *13*, 529–533.

Carroll, J., & Siegler, R. (1977). Strategies for use of base-rate information. *Organizational Behavior and Human Performance*, *19*, 392–402.

Caveness, W. (1977). Incidence of craniocerebral trauma in the United States, 1970 - 1975. *Annals of Neurology*, *1*, 507.

Chapman, L., & Chapman J. (1967). Genesis of popular but erroneous psychodiagnostic observations. *Journal of Abnormal Psychology*, *72*, 193–204.

Chapman, L., & Chapman, J. (1969), Illusory correlation as an obstacle to the use of valid psychodiagnostic signs. *Journal of Abnormal Psychology*, *74*, 271–280.Christensen-Szalawski, J., & Beach, L. (1982). Experience and the base rate fallacy. *Organizational Behavior and Human Performance*, *29*, 270–278.

Davidson, D., & Hirtle, S. (1990). Effects of nondiscrepant and discrepant information on the use of base rates. *American Journal of Psychology*, *103*(3), 343–357.

Dikmen, S., McLean, A., & Temkin, N. (1986). Neuropsychological and psychosocial consequences of minor head injury. *Journal of Neurology, Neurosurgery and Psychiatry*, *49*, 1227–1232.

Duncan, D., & Snow, W. (1987). Base rates in neuropsychology. *Professional Psychology: Research and Practice*, *18* (4), 368–370.

Dunn, J., Brown, R., Lees-Haley, P., & Euglisi, L. (1993, November). *Neurotoxic and neuropsychological symptoms base rates: A comparison of three groups*. Presented at the 13th meeting of the National Academy of Neuropsychology, Phoenix, AZ.

Einhorn, H. & Hogarth, R. (1981). Behavioral decision theory: Process of judgment and choice. *Annual Review of Psychology*, *32*, 53–88.

Ewing, R., McCarthy, D., Gronwall, D., & Wrightson, P. (1980). Persisting effects of minor head injury observable during hypoxic stress. *Journal of Clinical Neuropsychology*, *2*, 147–155.

Faust, D., & Nurcombe, B. (1989). Improving the accuracy of clinical judgment. *Psychiatry*, *52*, 197–208.

Fox, D., Lees-Haley, P., Earnest, K., & Dolezal-Wood, S. (1993, November). *Post concussive symptoms: Base rates and etiology in psychiatric patients*. Presented at the 13th meeting of the National Academy of Neuropsychology, Phoenix, AZ.

Goldstein, M. (1990). Traumatic brain injury: A silent epidemic. Editorial. *Annals of Neurology*, *27*, 327.

Gordon, N. (1977). Base rates and the decision making model in clinical neuropsychology. *Cortex*, *13*, 3–10.

Gouvier, W., Prestholdt, P., & Warner, M. (1988). A survey of common misconceptions about head injury and recovery. *Archives of Clinical Neuropsychology*, *3*, 331–343.

Gouvier, W., Uddo-Crane, M., & Brown, L. (1988). Base rates of postconcussional symptoms. *Archives of Clinical Neuropsychology*, *3*, 273–278.

Hartlage, L. (1995). Neuropsychological complaint base rates in personal injury, revisited. *Archives of Clinical Neuropsychology*, *10* (3), 279–280.

Hayes, J., Martin, R., & Gouvier, W. (1995). Influence of prior knowledge and experience on the ability to feign mild head injury symptoms in head injured and non head injured college students. *Applied Neuropsychology*, *2*, 63–66.

Heaton, R., Smith, H., Lehman, R., & Vogt, A. (1978). Prospects for faking believable deficits on neuropsychological testing. *Journal of Consulting and Clinical Psychology*, *46*, 892–900.

Hinkle, D., Wiersma, W., & Jurs, S. (1994). *Applied statistics for the behavioral sciences*. Boston: Houghton Mifflin.

Kahneman, D., & Tversky, A. (1982). On the psychology of prediction. In D. Kahneman, P. Slovic, & A. Tversky (Eds.), *Judgment under uncertainty: Heuristics and biases* (pp. 48–68). London: Cambridge University Press.

Kraus, J., & Nourjah, P. (1989). The epidemiology of mild head injury. In H. S. Levin, H. M. Eisenberg, & A. L. Benton (Eds.), *Mild head injury* (pp. 8–22). New York: Oxford University Press.

Kurtz, R., & Garfield, S. (1978). Illusory correlation: A further exploration of Chapman's Paradigm. *Journal of Consulting and Clinical Psychology*, *46*, 1009–1015.

Lees-Haley, P. (1992). Neuropsychological complaint base rates of personal injury claimants. *Forensic Reports*, *5*, 385–391.

Lees-Haley, P., & Brown R. (1993). Neuropsychological complaint base rates of 170 personal injury claimants. *Archives of Clinical Neuropsychology*, *8*, 203–209.

Leininger, B., Gramling, S., Farrell, A., Kreutzer, J., & Peck, E. (1990). Neuropsychological deficits in symptomatic minor head injury patients after concussion and mild concussion. *Journal of Neurology, Neurosurgery and Psychiatry*, *53*, 293–296.

Levin, H., Benton, A. & Grossman, R. (1982). *Neurobehavioral consequences of closed head injury*. London: Oxford University Press.

Lyon, D., & Slovic P. (1976). Dominance of accuracy information and neglect of base rates in probability estimation. *Acta Psychologica*, *40*, 287–298.

MacLennan, R. (1988). Correlation, base-rates, and the predictability of behaviour. *Personality and Individual Differences*, *9*(3), 675–684.

Malloy, P., & Webster, J. (1981). Detecting mild brain impairment using the Luria–Nebraska Neuropsychological Battery. *Journal of Consulting and Clinical Psychology*, *49*, 768–770.

Manis, M., Dovalina, I., Avis, N., & Cardoze, S. (1980). Base rates can affect individual predictions. *Journal of Personality and Social Psychology*, *38*, 231–248.

Martin, R., Bolter, J., Todd, M. Gouvier, W., & Niccolls, R. (1993). Effects of sophistication and motivation on the detection of malingered memory performance using a computerized forced choice task. *Journal of Clinical and Experimental Neuropsychology*, *15*, 867–888.

Martin, R., Gouvier, W., Todd, M., Bolter, J., & Niccolls, R. (1992). Effects of task instruction on malingered memory performance. *Forensic Reports*, *5*, 393–397.

McKinley, W., Brooks, D., & Bond, M. (1983). Post-concussional symptoms, financial compensation and outcome of severe blunt head injury. *Journal of Neurology, Neurosurgery and Psychiatry*, *46*, 1084–1091.

Meehl, P. (1954). *Clinical vs. statistical prediction*. Minneapolis: University of Minnesota Press.

Meehl, P., & Rosen, A. (1955). Antecedent probability and the efficiency of psychometric signs, patterns, or cutting scores. *Psychological Bulletin*, *52*, 194–216.

Reitan, R., & Wolfson, D. (1994, November). *Practical approaches to puzzling problems in neuropsychology using the Halstead–Reitan Battery*. Workshop presented at the 14th meeting of the national Academy of Neuropsychology, Orlando, FL.

Rimel, R., Giordani, B., Barth, J., Boll, T., & Jane, J. (1981). Disability caused by minor head injury. *Neurosurgery*, *9*, 221–228.

Roberts, R., Varney, N., Hulbert, J., Paulsen, J., Richardson, E., Springer, J., Shepherd, J., Swan, C., Legrand, J., Harvey, J., & Struchen, M. (1990). The neuropathology of everyday life: The frequency of partial seizure symptoms among normals. *Neuropsychology*, *4*, 65–85.

Rogers, R. (1988). *Clinical assessment of malingering and deception*. New York: Guilford Press.

Rogers, R. (1990). Models of feigned mental illness. *Professional Psychology: Research and Practice*, *21*(3), 182–188.

Sattler, J. (1988). *Assessment of children* (3rd ed.) San Diego: Author.

Schretlen, D. (1988). The use of psychological tests to identify malingered symptoms of mental disorders. *Clinical Psychology Review*, *8*, 451–476.

Sorenson, S., & Kraus, J. (1991). Occurrence, severity and outcomes of brain injury. *The Journal of Head Trauma Rehabilitation*, *6*, 1–10

Spreen, O., & Strauss, E. (1991). *A compendium of neuropsychological tests: Administration, norms, and commentary*. London: Oxford University Press.

Trueblood, W. (1994). Qualitative and quantitative characteristics of malingered and other invalid WAIS-R and clinical memory data. *Journal of Clinical and Experimental Neuropsychology*, *16*, 597–607.

Tversky, A., & Kahneman, D. (1971). Belief in the law of small numbers. *Psychological Bulletin*, *76*, 105–110.

Tversky, A., & Kahneman, D. (1982). Judgment under uncertainty. Heuristics and biases. In D. Kahneman, P. Slovic, & A. Tversky (Eds.), *Judgment under uncertainty: Heuristics and biases* (pp. 3–20). New York: Cambridge University Press.

Watterson, W. (1992, May 17). *Calvin and Hobbes*. Universal Press Syndicate.

Willer, B., Johnson, W., Rempel, R., & Linn, R. (1993). A note concerning misconceptions of the general public about brain injury. *Archives of Clinical Neuropsychology*, *8*, 461–465.

Willis, W. (1984) Reanalysis of an actuarial approach to neuropsychological diagnosis in consideration of base rates. *Journal of Consulting and Clinical Psychology*, *52*(4), 567–569.

Wong, J., Regennitter, R., & Barrios, F. (1994). Base rate and simulated symptoms of mild head injury among normals. *Archives of Clinical Neuropsychology*, *9*, 411–425.

3

Detection of Malingering Using Forced-Choice Techniques

JUAN MANUEL GUTIÉRREZ AND RUBEN C. GUR

Neuropsychology has become a significant contributor in legal proceedings. For example, a legal manual for examining psychological testimony recommends that neuropsychological assessment accompany neurological evaluation in cases where brain damage is claimed (Ziskin & Faust, 1988). Further, in the case of *Horne v. Marvin L. Goodson Logging Company* (1986), the Supreme Court of the State of North Carolina ultimately ruled positively in a case in which a neuropsychologist's opinion was deemed admissible in court, despite the medical community's protest that the neuropsychologist was not a physician. Finally, the Supreme Court case of *Daubert v. Merrell Dow Pharmaceuticals, Inc.* (1993) solidified support for neuropsychological evaluations and testimony.

Many (perhaps most) cases involving cerebral dysfunction are not considered res ipsa loquitur, where it is clear even to laypeople that some act has caused damage to a patient (e.g., a sponge left in after surgery; Kraus, 1985). Therefore, clinical neuropsychologists are needed to assess the presence and extent of neuropsychological damage. Many applications can be readily imagined: a variety of personal injury cases (e.g., motor vehicle accidents, work-related accidents, industrial electrical injuries), trauma resulting in the lack of oxygen to the brain caused by complications from surgery, impairment from long-term exposure to toxic substances, and criminal cases involving defendants with documented cerebral insult or disease. Even exotic cases may fall within the realm of neuropsychology:

JUAN MANUEL GUTIÉRREZ AND RUBEN C. GUR • Brain Behavior Laboratory and the Neuropsychiatry Section, Department of Psychiatry, University of Pennsylvania, Philadelphia, Pennsylvania 19104.

Detection of Malingering during Head Injury Litigation, edited by Reynolds. Plenum Press, New York, 1998.

for example, the determination of the testamentary capacity of a deceased woman by reviewing records and relating them to cognitive dysfunction secondary to alcohol abuse (Kurylchek, 1984).

However, recent review of trial cases within the United States indicates that the amount of litigation within our court system hinders its performance. Depending on the source cited, it is estimated that there will be somewhere between 3 million head injuries per year (Beers, 1992) and 10 million mild head injuries per year (Colohan, Dacey, Alves, Rimel, & Jane, 1986). Regardless of the exact number of injuries, it has become obvious that many of these cases will lead to litigation, and as such, will add to the work load of an already overburdened court system.

Therefore, neuropsychologists are being called on more and more to become part of the medical-legal team (Barth, Gideon, Sciara, Hulsey, & Anchor, 1986; Satz, 1988), and the onus falls on those practicing neuropsychological assessment to assure the court systems and the public that their assessments are valid. Guilmette, Hart, and Giuliano (1993) went even further. These authors noted that neuropsychologists are required to demonstrate, empirically, the validity of techniques that reveal inadequate effort and symptom exaggeration. Thus, clinicians in neuropsychology need to feel confident regarding their patients' claims and they need to be able to show support for those claims (Faust, Ziskin, & Hiers, 1991).

The question remains, how is this task to be best completed? Can neuropsychologists claim, with any degree of certainty, that those people who seek their services are truly injured and not malingering? Moreover, do neuropsychologists feel confident in making this estimation in a courtroom? In the end, these rather lofty questions are not for neuropsychologists to answer alone. Although we may attempt to create tests and instruments to the best of our ability, to validate them, and to continue to refine them, we will never make the final judgments in isolation. We will work in conjunction with other medical professions, and most importantly, with the legal system and the public. But, as stated by Nies and Sweet (1994), although malingering is not easily detected, it is *possible* to detect, as long as adequate effort is made to do so.

GUIDELINES FOR THE DEVELOPMENT OF MALINGERING SCREENS

As Wedding (1991) noted, practitioners in neuropsychology are not immune to poor clinical decision making, and therefore we must search for ground rules that will assist the clinician in making sound decisions, especially in the forensic area and in regard to malingering. Pankratz (1988) described a paradigm that the neuropsychologist may use to distinguish the legitimate patient from someone presenting in an exaggerated manner. For example, observing that a patient exhibits near misses to simple questions should serve as a warning, and a more thorough evaluation should be considered. This guideline is based on the notion that it would seem atypical for the patient to exhibit near misses to simple probes, yet be able to respond easily to overlearned questions (e.g., name, date of birth). Similarly, if a patient exhibits gross discrepancies from the expected norms, the clinician is cautioned to evaluate for exaggeration. Although we are mindful that not all of the literature agrees on this point, we are also careful to consider that at least some authors indicate that extreme impairments were reported by subjects who were asked to simulate malingering, as well as by patients who were eventually diagnosed as malingerers (Larrabee, 1990).

Inconsistency between diagnosis and neuropsychological findings can also be considered an indication of exaggeration. In cases where results are mixed or puzzling, intensive assessment of malingering frequently proves useful. Inconsistencies between reported and observed symptoms are also a sign that the patient may be exaggerating. For example, a patient who complains of severe short-term memory loss, yet can recall events quite well when information is needed to better evaluate his case, or such things as medications, procedures, names, location of the examiner's office, and even things such as where he had left his hat.

Resistance, avoidance, and bizarre responses to standard tests are further clues that the patient may be exaggerating her symptoms. Additionally, any marked discrepancies between measures that evaluate similar cognitive abilities must be scrutinized. Lastly, the most significant indicator of deception is, of course, the failure of a patient on a specific measure of neuropsychological malingering.

BASE RATES OF NEUROPSYCHOLOGICAL COMPLAINTS

As a result of the above-noted prompts, a neuropsychologist must be careful to examine and rule out poor motivation and effort as hindering performance. However, we must also be familiar with what could be the profile of legitimate symptoms, or base rates. By determining the rates at which symptoms are presented, we can develop a better picture of the individuals who seek our services and an awareness of the needs these people have. The first task in beginning to assess a possible malingerer would be to obtain an understanding of the extent of the public's knowledge of neurology and neuropsychology (Lees-Haley & Brown, 1993; McCaffrey, Williams, Fisher, & Laing, 1993). Using these base rates, we can educate juries through our courtroom testimony, as has been advocated by leading professionals in this area (Blau, 1994). With such information we can dispel myths, replacing them with the best knowledge available.

Aubrey, Dobbs, and Rule (1989) demonstrated the general public's unfamiliarity with neurological and neuropsychological sequelae to minor head injury. They noted that only 50% of their subjects felt that cognitive symptoms were common in head injury. Additionally, Gouvier, Prestholdt, and Warner (1988) and Willer, Johnson, Rempel, and Linn (1993) noted that subjects indicated implausible symptoms, extreme severity of symptoms, and rather improbable reactions to head injury. For example, the majority of subjects answering these surveys endorsed the following statement: "If a person is struck on the head, and loses memory as a result, another strike to the head will most likely help that person regain memory." Several of the authors cited slapstick comedy as the reason for these beliefs. Incredibly, the belief behind the above statement has continued to be exhibited on popular television (*Full House*, ABC, 1995).

Further complicating the neuropsychologist's task is the fact that many commonly presented symptoms occur with significant frequency among the general public, and many common instruments for assessing these symptoms are vulnerable to dissimulation on the part of a variety of patients. For example, Wong, Regennitter, and Barrios (1994) noted that even though non-head-injured simulators in their study did underestimate the severity, range, and permanence of head injury patients, they were nevertheless misclassified as head-injured by several of the symptom checklists used in the study. Adding to this complex picture is the finding by Gouvier, Uddo-Crane, and Brown (1988), as well as Lees-Haley and Brown (1993), that malingering-simulation subjects do not present with a unique constellation of symptoms. Indeed, Gouvier, Cubic, Jones, and Brantley (1992) reported that the non-head-injured subjects in their study did not present a significantly different number of symptoms compared with head-injured subjects, and that symptoms considered indicative of head injury are also common among healthy, normal subjects experiencing significant stress. In summary, it is evident that neuropsychologists need to assess whether a malingering evaluation is necessary in light of the patient's situation and symptoms, and gauge whether those symptoms are plausible and not exaggerated.

THE DEVELOPMENT OF FORCED-CHOICE TECHNIQUES

It can readily be seen that individuals are quite varied in their knowledge and beliefs regarding head injury, and as neuropsychologists, we are obligated to enter the legal arena with the intent of demystifying the effects of head injury for the courtroom and the public. With many people reporting such a varied range of severity and types of symptoms, the clinician must make every effort to ascertain the veracity of the reported deficits. However, commonly held misconceptions and beliefs among laypeople can actually be quite helpful to the neuropsychologist. These misconceptions are the very basis for procedures collectively referred to as *symptom validity testing* (Pankratz, 1988). This method of detecting malingering has shown promise and is considered simple yet effective (Faust et al., 1991).

The forced-choice technique is based on the binomial distribution theory. The clearest example is that of the old-fashioned coin toss. Over a large set of trials, it is expected that as long as the coin and all other conditions are fair, 50% of the coin tosses will result in the coin coming up heads (there are two alternatives and there must be an answer, a forced choice). A deviation from that distribution is considered significant if it is beyond chance expectations, and should caution the person conducting the coin tosses that something is wrong. The idea for a forced-choice malingering test is to establish a clinical procedure producing below-chance level of performance that can be considered indicative of malingering.

Pankratz (1979, 1988) stated that a review of work conducted in psychiatric populations generated what ultimately became this clinical procedure. The work of Brady and Lind (1961) has been a key to the advancement of the forced-choice techniques. They described a patient who presented with hysterical blindness. The patient was treated with operant techniques to develop rather dramatic improvements in vision. Three years later, Grosz and Zimmerman (1965) described following the same patient, who had once again developed the blindness, claiming disability status. At that time, he denied that the previous treatment had been beneficial. However, in the hospital, he could avoid objects in his path, was childish, disruptive, and manipulative. Ironically, he had stated to the nursing staff that he could see somewhat, but he never intended to work hard again, and intended to live on social security disability and a disability pension. Therefore, a visual discrimination task was developed and the patient was asked to respond each time a buzzer sounded. The identification of one stimulus (triangle) as being different would allow him to turn off the buzzer, and the task was presented over many trials. The patient performed at significantly less than chance levels, suggesting he had to see the stimulus so as to avoid responding to it. He was then told the expectation of a truly blind person was at least 50% correct, or chance. Once he was informed of the expected response rates, he suddenly improved to within a chance level. Additionally, Theodore and Mandelcorn (1973) helped Pankratz realize that the forced-choice procedure could be altered and adapted to assess a variety of sensory or memory deficits.

The technique was successfully utilized to assess a large variety of complaints. Pankratz, Fausti, and Peed (1975) described the assessment of symptom exaggeration in a psychiatric patient who presented with deafness. The patient was a 27-year-old male with a long history of psychiatric admissions. Medical records indicated a manipulative personality and that he was generally a disruptive patient. The hospital staff also related their concerns that the patient had exaggerated his symptoms to his advantage. This patient presented with bilateral auditory loss among numerous other complaints. Previous examinations proved to be inconsistent but the patient suddenly recovered from all symptoms, with the exception of the deafness. Ironically, traditional auditory testing discovered that he could hear, at least to some degree, in his left ear. An elaborate paradigm was consequently established in which the patient was tested using a tone in conjunction with a set of lights. His task was simply to indicate with which light stimulus the tone had been paired (two alternatives, forced choice). This established the necessary conditions in which he could respond at chance levels. That is, if the patient could not hear at all, and thus responded randomly, he would still perform at roughly the 50% level. However, his performance was limited to a 36% accuracy rate. The probability of obtaining such a score, calculated by the normal approximation to the binomial distribution, was reported as being less than one in 4000 ($p < .004$). Therefore, it appeared probable that this patient had indeed heard the tone, but selectively chose the wrong answer, so as to give the appearance of impairment.

Given the initial success, work on symptom validity testing continued. In 1983, Pankratz adapted the technique for use with three psychiatric patients, suspected of feigning a memory deficit. The first patient was seated at a table, with both a red light and a white light in view (again, the two alternatives). The lights were attached to the ceiling, approximately 10 feet from the patient. The task was to recall which light was flashed (forced choice). To make the test appear more difficult, the examiner added an interference task. The patient was to respond after being distracted while he completed portions of the Symbol Digit Modalities Test (Smith, 1968). This symptom validity testing did not support the patient's claims. The second case was similar to the first. The third patient was tested utilizing the forced-choice procedure, but in this case, the patient had sought to minimize his deficits. Thus, the procedure helped examiners support the veracity of complaints, discovering the opposite of what it was designed to do.

Binder and Pankratz (1987) cited the forced-choice procedure as assisting in the evaluation of a patient feigning a memory complaint. The case involved a patient complaining of severe memory loss, yet the examiners discovered that to arrive at the testing location the patient had traveled hundreds of miles by public transport. This discrepancy aroused suspicion, and when forced-choice procedures were utilized, the results created doubt regarding the patient's effort. After presentation of the target, the patient was simply asked to recall which object had been displayed, a black pen or a yellow pencil. Over several trials, this patient performed at only a 37% rate, significantly below chance at the $p < .01$ level (less than 1 in 100).

Pankratz, Binder, and Wilcox (1987) reported a patient who described numbness over his entire body. The medical record indicated a history of viral encephalitis and abnormal EMG readings in the upper extremities. Poor conceptualization, cognitive inflexibility, and impaired visuoconstructive skills were noted against a background of otherwise normal neuropsychological abilities. However, hospital staff related suspicions regarding deception and because the case was so complicated, there was a need to evaluate the veracity of the patient's claims. The investigators utilized symptom validity testing, and found little support for his claims. They suspected deception because the patient identified lateralized touch to the hand at significantly below chance levels.

The key feature of these evaluations was that the tests were constructed precisely for the complaint of the individual and to anticipate the responses of the reluctant patient. The test necessitates the use of a reproducible stimulus for which the patient claims a deficit. The patient is then presented with the stimulus over a large set of trials using the two-alternative, forced-choice design. As Pankratz (1988) stated, "symptom validity testing provides an opportunity to show more than a low score. It has the potential to demonstrate that the patient performed below the probabilities of chance" (p. 185).

A patient attempting to malinger on a forced-choice test can find himself in a rather perplexing quandary. If the patient wishes to continue the deception he may realize that the structure of the test puts him at risk of exposure as a fraud. However, if the patient suddenly performs properly, the performance becomes an admission that the deficit was not as serious as had been previously claimed, which would be undesirable for someone seeking financial compensation or some other reward. Procedures such as the forced-choice paradigm permit neuropsychologists to exploit the lack of knowledge within the general public so as to assess patients who may be attempting to exaggerate.

VARIATIONS OF THE FORCED-CHOICE PROCEDURE

The forced-choice procedure was described as being adaptable to a plethora of situations, limited only by the imagination of the examiner. Memory deficits have been the focus of the literature, but these are not the only area of research using such procedures (e.g., Miller, 1986; Pankratz, 1979; Pankratz et al., 1987)

Binder (1990, 1993a,b; Binder & Willis, 1991) described the Portland Digit Recognition Test (PDRT), a forced-choice procedure consisting of 72 items of digit recognition modeled after the Hiscock and Hiscock (1989) task. The subject hears five-digit numbers at the rate of one digit per second. Following presentation, the patient counts backward aloud until interrupted with a visual recognition card. Each recognition card has only one distractor (two alternatives), and the subject must provide an answer for each trial (a forced choice). The task is seemingly made even more difficult by having 5 seconds of interpolated activity of counting backward for the first 18 trials, then counting backward for 15 seconds for the next 18 trials. The third and fourth trials involve counting backward for 30 seconds. Although there are 72 trials in total, there are actually only 18 different correct target items, and 36 recognition cards (the 18 items are administered four times). It is noteworthy that because of the complexity of such a task, results can be variable, and some differences can be driven by either actual brain dysfunction or educational differences. Further, average time needed to complete this test is approximately 45 minutes.

In response to concerns that the PDRT was time consuming, Binder (1993a) developed an abbreviated version by specifying criteria for discontinuation of the PDRT when the patient is performing in a well-motivated fashion. However, the test would be continued if the patient was at risk for performing significantly below chance or below the cutoff scores previously established for the PDRT. It appeared that a conservative criterion for discontinuation was six correct out of the nine longer-delay items. It was noted that using this procedure would cut administration time significantly, at least for the difficult item trials.

Prigatano and Amin (1993) used the Digit Memory Test, a forced-choice procedure to distinguish malingerers from brain-injured patients. Performance of 27 unequivocally brain-injured patients with enduring and severe memory loss resulted in an 85 to 100% correct rate. The test was also administered to 5 patients with postconcussional syndrome and 6 patients suspected of malingering. The patients suspected of malingering performed at a level significantly lower than that of the other groups (74% accuracy rate). Even patients with severe but static dysfunction and unequivocal memory disorder outperformed the suspected malingerers. This performance was not below chance, but given the performance of the suspected malingerers relative to the cerebrally challenged patients, this test may still be helpful in evaluating patients suspected of malingering.

Frederick and Foster (1991) described a three-part study of a forced-choice procedure. The first part utilized a two-alternative format with 199 incomplete picture puzzle items based on the Test of Nonverbal Intelligence. The test items were arranged in a hierarchy of difficulty and were then presented in a random order (these items are normally presented with four choices, but in this study choices were limited to only two). In a simulation study, decision rules regarding performance, consistency, and the product of the slope and consistency ratings resulted in high discriminability among the results of normal controls, cognitively impaired controls, and simulators. The latter subjects were told to act as if they were brain damaged, but not to do so in any obvious manner. Phase two of the study replicated the first phase. In phase three, malingering simulators were either naive, or coached on how to malinger successfully. The coached simulators were told to obtain at least a 50% correct score, to answer the easy items correctly, and to miss on only the more difficult items. Support was found for the decision rules derived during the first phase, and 73.2% of the informed malingerers were correctly classified.

Brandt, Rubinsky, and Lassen (1985) adapted the forced-choice paradigm to a verbal memory task. A 20-item word list was administered to normal controls, memory-disordered subjects, and simulators. On free recall of the word list, the controls scored higher than the simulators and the memory-impaired subjects. Then a recognition task was given, in which the subjects were administered each word from the original list and a distractor, and were asked to select the word they felt had been on the original list. In this case, chance performance fell within a range of 6–14 correct, at a 95% confidence level. The controls and memory-disordered subjects consistently scored better than would be expected from random responding. In contrast, only the simulators performed at or below chance.

Iverson, Franzen, and McCracken (1991) modified the procedure slightly, using 21 items with similar results. They continued with their simulation studies (Iverson, Franzen, & McCracken, 1994) using community volunteers, psychiatric patients, and neuropsychological patients. One-half of the psychiatric and community volunteer groups were given instructions to malinger. A discriminant function analysis indicated that the forced-choice measure was the strongest predictor of group membership.

Hiscock and Hiscock (1989) revised the forced-choice strategy by adding time delays. They noted that without an additional factor the test might appear too simple to the malingering patient, allowing her to respond correctly and thereby defeating the purpose of the test. The addition of time delays creates an appearance of difficulty, which could easily be manipulated without changing the actual difficulty level. The basic format of the procedure was to present the patient with a five-digit number for 5 seconds. The examiner then waits 5 seconds, and next shows the patient another card with two five-digit numbers, one a distractor, the other the originally presented number. The patient is then given feedback as to whether she is correct. This procedure is followed for 24 trials. Once the patient reaches the 24th trial, she is told that because she has done so well, she will have to take the test in a manner that is more difficult. Therefore, the patient is asked to conduct another 24 trials, but instead of a 5-second delay, the patient will need to retain the stimulus for 10 seconds. After 24 trials at the 10-second delay, patients are again told that their performance was better than expected, and that the delay will be increased to 15 seconds. As can be seen, the true difficulty of the task is not changed significantly, but the *perception* of the degree of difficulty may be manipulated. There is a paucity of reliability and normative data for this (and we would say, most) forced-choice procedures. Nevertheless, these authors did relate a case study utilizing this procedure, which resulted in a suspected malingerer performing not at the 50% level, but 21 out of 72, or the 29% level, which is highly significant ($p = .002$). By comparison, a severely demented 53-year-old woman obtained a 51% accuracy rate and a 5-year-old performed at an 82% correct rate. An important aspect of the task is the trial-by-trial feedback, which the authors felt would make the malingering patients prone to feel as if they were doing too well, or too poorly. By dividing the test into blocks, the deceptive patient may feel as if the test is indeed becoming harder. Thus, the malingering patient may adjust performance to allow the outcome to be what that patient perceives as a poor performance (this, again, is where the public's lack of knowledge regarding base rates and sequelae to head injury comes even more into play).

Guilmette et al. (1993) used the above procedures to assess malingering in brain-impaired patients, psychiatric patients, and two groups of nonpatients. One group was asked to simulate brain damage and the other to perform to the best of their ability. The results suggested that the level of accuracy for the simulators was less than that of the other groups, but not necessarily below chance. Further, the variability of the scores for the simulators was much greater. These results led the investigators to note that the deceptive patient may understand the need to score at or above the 50% correct rate, thus defeating the test. They suggested that less than 75% correct would be a better cutoff. Lastly, they also suggested that a shorter version of the Hiscock and Hiscock (1989) forced-choice procedure could be equally effective.

Niccolls and Bolter (1991) described a test based on the Hiscock and Hiscock (1991) procedure. The Multi-Digit Memory Test was developed in much the same manner as any forced-choice test and is considered a recognition test for the purpose of assessing deception. This test is readily adaptable to computerization, and we now move on to this format.

FORCED-CHOICE TESTING: THE NEXT PHASE IS COMPUTERIZED

We are at the threshold of a new century, yet most test procedures utilized by the majority of clinicians and researchers in our profession were developed early in the present century. Newly developed computerized neuropsychological tests and batteries have been described in detail by Kane and Kay (1992). Over the last 15 years, the lower costs of computers, their greater efficiency, and precise test scoring and administration options have made computerized neuropsychological testing more of a reality than ever before. They raise the following considerations.

Standardized Administration

The most basic step in test administration for any examination is that the test be administered in the same manner to each patient, as it was intended by the test constructors (Anastasi, 1980; Sattler, 1988). This provides the ability to compare the results from each test administration with results from previous administrations. Otherwise, the test and its results will be biased. For example, the nonstandardized examination is known to be susceptible to "halo effects" and a variety of other sources of contamination. Hence, each examiner must assess her ability to be objective in the administration of tests, and if not objective, she is ethically obligated to exclude herself from testing the individual patient. This problem obviously can be avoided, to a large degree, by the use of a computer. The program can run with very little examiner involvement (in some cases, none at all).

Ease of Scoring

Our experience has shown that although a paper test can be easily administered, the examiner is often required to take several steps in the scoring procedure. Limited data are often derived and there is occasionally a need to transform the scores from simple raw data into rather complicated formulas. It is quite common to translate a raw score into a scaled score and then an age-adjusted score, and then further at times into a *T* score or percentile. These transformations can be associated with errors (e.g., number transposing, simple addition or subtraction errors). The use of a computerized program enables the examiner to bypass the steps where the mistakes are most likely. If a program is arranged in a manner that not only will accept the raw scores, but also will facilitate the transformation of raw data, it can easily assist in greater efficiency and precision in scoring.

Data Collection

Data derived from traditional testing is usually transposed onto a summary sheet, and then examined for test interpretation or data entry. Data collected in such a way have always been bulky and required a substantial amount of space in archives. Once again, the use of computerized data can eliminate this need, allowing easy storage of substantial amounts of data. Data stored in this manner can be copied with very little effort, and more importantly, can be loaded up onto larger mainframe computers for comparison with other databases using sophisticated data analysis procedures.

Generation of Alternate Forms

For an investigator wishing to establish reliability, alternate forms of the same test can much more easily be developed through the use of a computer (e.g., split half tests). Thus, speed and efficiency are key advantages to alternate form generation on computers.

Use of Technicians

According to Adams and Rourke (1992), there is a longstanding history of utilizing technical assistants in many fields (such as use of radiology technicians to administer x-rays). The same can be said for the administration of neuropsychological testing, leaving the neuropsychologist free to conduct the activities that require more training (i.e., interpreting the test data). With computerized testing, the neuropsychologist can be further freed from the mechanical aspect of the traditional examination by allowing a technician to operate a computerized battery. The advantages of a computerized battery can therefore be translated into lower costs and greater efficiency.

Superior Testing Environment

It is believed that a less adversarial testing situation for the patient exists if a computer rather than a human examiner is utilized. The social psychology literature indicates that when a human runs a race against a machine (a clock), he will not exert as much effort as when running a race against another human. Thus, there seems to be an inherent need to compete against other humans. There does not seem to be as much pressure on an examinee when that examinee is taking a test from a computer. There is lessened perception that judgment is being cast on the examinee, and there is less competitiveness between the examinee and the computer.

Stimulus Presentation and the Tracking of Various Responses

We have noted throughout this chapter that the forced-choice procedure typically requires the presentation of a stimulus that can be replicated and displayed for a set time. For example, the Hiscock and Hiscock (1989) procedure requires that an examiner display the five-digit number for exactly 5 seconds. Further, there is a time delay of 5, 10, and 15 seconds on the first, second, and third trials, respectively. Hence, on this test (and many others), it is incumbent on the examiner not only to observe the patient, but also to monitor the time of exposure for the stimulus and the time of the delays. In contrast, the computer can time the reaction latencies down to a millisecond, with great accuracy. Further, the computer can report averages within a few moments, and again, the examiner can be assured of accuracy.

Faust et al. (1991) cited the possibility that lawyers, preparing clients for court in the case of possible neuropsychological disorders, might inadvertently cue litigants as to the kinds of symptoms that it would be to their advantage to present. On a forced-choice procedure, the patient may understand that a 50% correct rate is necessary to avoid suspicion. However, even if a patient knew to perform within a certain reaction time, it is hard to image how the deceptive patient would calculate that time.

THE DEVELOPMENT OF A COMPUTERIZED FORCED-CHOICE TEST

We are aware of the development of a computerized version of the Binder (1990) Portland Digit Recognition Test, but we will leave the discussion of this test to our esteemed colleague. Martin, Bolter, Todd, Gouvier, and Niccolls (1993) examined the use of the Multi-Digit Memory Test in a computerized format. The basic idea of a two-alternative, forced response format with built-in time delays was modeled after the Hiscock and Hiscock (1989) procedure. They studied 119 undergraduates and 33 head-injured rehabilitation patients. To simulate more closely real-world situations, there were two levels of monetary rewards (high, low) and three levels of malingering instructions (eventually collapsed into "coached" and "uncoached"). All subjects were administered the test on a similar computer, using similar screens, with distance, brightness, and contrast settings for the screen adjusted to the desire of each subject. Subjects responded by reading the screen and following the written directions. Responses were generated by use of the right and left arrow keys to highlight the choice. Once the response was highlighted, the subject was to hit the enter key. The subject would hear a high-pitched beep if the answer was correct, and a low-pitched beep if the answer was incorrect. On-screen instructions were provided during the actual test, and another beep would sound when the instructions changed. At the completion of the tasks more directions and prompts would appear on the screen.

Significant differences were noted between the head-injured and non-head-injured groups. Sophisticated malingering subjects showed a relative performance decline over time, most pronounced at the third interval. Many non-head-injured simulators consistently performed above chance levels, but below the levels of head-injured patients. Lastly, 45% of the naive simulators did perform below chance levels. The authors suggested that it was best to compare simulators with head-injured patients so as to more fully understand the pattern of performance of these two groups. This allows for a better evaluation of the deceptive patient.

This is arguably the best computerized test available for the assessment of malingering, but it raises several concerns. No reliability data were reported by the authors, and they state at the end of their report that they would like to see such data generated. Therefore, we cannot be certain how the computerized test relates to the paper-and-pencil version. It is unclear whether there was a history of computer use among the subjects. The test required several key strokes, and may not have afforded subjects who were unfamiliar with computers the same opportunity to respond as those who were computer literate. As Kane and Kay (1992) noted, when there are numerous instructions and key strokes to be made, familiarization with the computer allows a subject to handle the test more easily. Lastly, it would seem that a computerized version of a paper-and-pencil test should parallel, wherever possible, the original test. However, the subjects were required to go through several steps in order to respond. In contrast, the standard forced-choice procedure allows for the patient to respond even by a simple pointing of a finger.

COMPUTERIZED FORCED-CHOICE DESCRIPTION

We have taken the recommendations made by Kane and Kay (1992) and attempted to incorporate them into the design of our computerized forced-choice (CFC) test. This is a preliminary design, and we need to continue to improve the test.

We used a software program (MACLAB 2.0®) for Macintosh based computer platforms (Chute, 1990), and attempted to create a computerized version that was as similar to the original as possible. The basic format was that a patient viewed the opening screen (title) and then the instructions page. The instructions read as follows:

> You will be shown a FIVE DIGIT number for only a FEW SECONDS. Then you will be shown a pair of numbers. If the number you had previously seen is on the right, as quickly as you can, press the "/" key; if the number you have previously seen is on the left, press the letter "z" as quickly as you can.
>
> PLACE A FINGER ON THE "/" KEY AND ANOTHER ON THE "z" KEY AND PRESS THE LETTER "z" WHEN READY TO BEGIN.

The patient is exposed to the target stimuli (Figure 1) for 3 seconds. After exposure to the target, the patient immediately chooses from two stimuli, one a distractor.

After 60 such trials, the patient is confronted with another instruction screen:

> Because you have done so well, we will continue, but this time there will be a delay of 10 seconds between the first number you see and the pair of numbers from which you will make your choice.
>
> All other instructions remain the same. As quickly as you can, press "/" if the number is on the right, and the "z" key if the number is on the left.
>
> PRESS "z" WHEN YOU ARE READY TO BEGIN.

After 20 trials, the patient was once again confronted by an instruction screen:

> WELL DONE!
>
> Because you continue to do so well, we will continue, but now there will be a delay of 30 seconds between the first number and the pair of numbers from which you will make your choice.
>
> All other instructions remain the same; if the number is on the right, then quickly press the "/" key; if the number is on the left, then quickly press the "z" key.
>
> PLACE ONE FINGER ON THE "/" KEY AND ANOTHER ON THE "z" KEY AND PRESS "z" WHEN READY TO BEGIN.

Screen 1:

1 0 5 6 2

Screen 2:

1 0 5 6 2 **9 6 4 1 8**

FIGURE 1. Stimuli set-up.

After 20 more trials, the test ended, and a screen instructing the patient to stop was shown. The examiner can then save the data.

The standard forced-choice test presents the stimuli for 5 seconds, with an immediate 5-second delay, followed by the 10- and 15-second delays. Note that the program on the CFC presented the stimuli for only 3 seconds, whereas this is 5 seconds for the paper-and-pencil version. Lest the reader finds this to contradict our recommendation that computerized tests parallel the standard tests, we note that our experience with computers has made us realize that the presentation of stimuli can be quite different from that of paper-and-pencil tasks and a 3-second presentation for simple stimuli is considered optimal (Chute, 1990). Thus, using the presentation times of a paper-and-pencil test would seem unjustifiably long on a computer screen. It does seem that subjects lose interest rather quickly when a screen is presented for a longer time with few stimuli on it.

In addition, the subject was given 60 trials with no delay. We felt that this would help the subject unfamiliar with computers by allowing an adjustment period. This helps alleviate the fears that some people present regarding computers (especially geriatric patients). However, the basic format of the three levels of delay, built into a forced-choice procedure, is preserved.

The presentation of the stimuli is especially important for a computerized test. Our computer screens incorporate black digits on a white background. They have adjustable brightness and contrast and the viewing angle can be altered to reduce glare as the subject wishes, for optimum visibility. We used the Macintosh Geneva font, because it does not decay as readily as many other fonts and the stimuli are preserved despite changes in size (Chute, 1990). For example, the size of the spaces within the numbers can sometimes seem to collapse on themselves whenever a stimulus is made smaller than the font in which it was originally constructed. The size chosen for our stimuli is that of the Macintosh 24 point. This ensured that older patients could see the stimuli as easily as our younger patients.

When constructing the actual stimulus, we used the MACLAB system menus to establish the stimulus height and position. After defining the four end points of the field, we placed our field in the middle of the screen. The field was located at the following settings: top, 220; bottom, 254; right side, 217; left side, 431. The stimuli themselves were placed in the center of those four points. When constructing the two-stimulus screen for response, the top and bottom settings were the same, but the left stimuli were flush against the left side of the screen (right setting: 20; left setting: 229). The right stimuli were flush against the right side of the screen (right setting: 428; left setting: 633).

The above format enable presenting the stimuli on the response screens as far apart as possible, with the hope of avoiding any confusion on the part of the respondent. The response format uses several computer and keyboard combinations, allowing the greatest adaptability for the test. Another goal was to circumvent fears of interacting with the computer by making the response as easy as possible. Patients were able to respond without looking down at the keys. Furthermore, selecting eligible response keys (not all keys are eligible in MACLAB) that were as far apart as possible enabled the subjects to respond more easily and seemed to better mimic the original test format. It also allowed the subjects to rest their hands on the bases of the several keyboards we tested.

The five-digit numbers are arranged in a manner so that each number (0–9) is equally represented as the first digit (roughly). The remaining numbers were then generated by random selection. Distractors were generated in much the same manner, although care was taken not to start the two numbers (the target and the distractor) with the same numeral. We also wish to point out that on the two-stimulus screens (when the patient was to respond) the target five-digit numbers were presented in a balanced order, such that the correct answer was equally represented on the right and on the left, in a random order (to avoid response sets).

These lead to another advantage: portability. The stimulus is generally presented to the patient on a 14-inch screen. However, the CFC program can employ an Apple Powerbook as well as larger screens. This allows the examiner to move the test to the patient (e.g., the patient's bedside).

Timing is milliseconds, and is achieved through a pulse method, built into the MACLAB software. The program is extremely easy to run, and saving data requires only a few strokes, or simple maneuvering of the pointing device (mouse or trackball). Of course, the examiner stores the data; the patient is not required to do any of this. We observed that even an examiner with minimal exposure to computers can easily learn to do this procedure.

CFC: A PILOT STUDY

The goal of the pilot study was to compare a paper-and-pencil malingering test with the computerized version we have developed. This required normal healthy individuals to take the Hiscock and Hiscock (1989) procedure along with the CFC.

The subjects consisted of 20 healthy, normal volunteers (11 males and 9 females, all native English speakers). Age ranged between 18 and 59, with a mean of 33.73. Education ranged from 5 to 22 years, with a mean of 14.27, and it was noted that only the higher-educated subjects had moderate exposure to the use of computers. Cronbach's alpha for this 100-item version was quite high at .94.

Subjects were recruited by the first author using the technique of establishing a relationship with a key member within charitable organizations (churches and social service advocacy programs). Our goal was to recruit subjects from a wide range of age and education levels. The subjects were screened and found to have no neurological or psychiatric history. They were paid a small fee ($10) for answering a few questions and taking both tests. Each subject was administered both the standard procedure and the CFC, in a counterbalanced order.

The first goal was to assess the comparability of performance on the paper test with that of the CFC. As both procedures are designed to yield nearly perfect performance, successful implementation would result in extremely truncated variability. This would attenuate a correlation coefficient and accentuate the significance of any mean difference. The results showed very close means (mean $\pm$ SD 99.73 $\pm$ 0.58 for the paper-and-pencil version; 99.40 $\pm$ 0.89 for the computer version), which were nonetheless significantly different by the paired t-test ($t = 2.408$, $df = 29$, $p = .02$). However, despite the truncated range, performance in the two tests was significantly correlated, $r(28) = .54$. This yields an attenuation-corrected estimate of reliability of .70, which is psychometrically acceptable.

To examine the internal consistency of the tests, Cronbach's coefficient alpha statistics were calculated. These were .97 and .94 for the paper test and the CFC, respectively, and can be considered satisfactory.

A second pilot study was performed to gain some understanding of the potential influence of language and culture in this test. Instructions were translated into Spanish by a native English speaker with Spanish expertise, and then back-translated by a native Spanish speaker with English expertise. A group of 10 Spanish-speaking subjects (4 females, 6 males) was then examined. For these subjects, age ranged from 18 to 59 (mean 31.7). Five had 12 to 20 years of education and five had 5 to 9 years of education (mean 12.0). There was no statistically significant difference between the standard and the CFC procedures of the Spanish speakers ($t = 0.788$, $df = 09$, $p = .44$). Standard test percentage correct mean for the Spanish-speaking subjects was 99.80 (SD = 0.42), nearly identical to the CFC (percentage correct mean = 99.60, SD = 0.69). Neither score differed significantly from that of the English speakers ($t = -0.86$, $df = 28$, $p = .39$). Thus, we can tentatively conclude that the test is valid for the Latino population.

The pilot study raised several concerns. The CFC was a long test, taking approximately 22 minutes for total administration. Our pilot study subjects were frustrated at the time it took to complete the test; the subjects uniformly stated that the delays felt too long and that the test should be shortened. Many felt it was close to a vigilance task and found it to be fatiguing. However, technically, the test ran well and no major flaws were observed.

Fortunately, the CFC can be easily manipulated, and alternate forms could be generated. Thus, it was decided that because the computer version resulted in such similar power and patterns (all groups scored nearly 100% correct), we could afford to shorten the test. Therefore, the test was shortened to half its original length, with only 50 responses total. The resulting test had the same instructions for the subjects but now had only 30 trials in the first phase, and 10 trials in both the second and third phases. By reducing the test in half, it now required only 11 minutes in total test time. We considered this to be a feasible experimental procedure.

CFC: AN EXPERIMENTAL TASK

The purpose of the third experiment was to evaluate the performance of the shortened version of the CFC when administered in the context of a battery of other computerized neuropsychological measures. We also wanted to examine reaction times on the CFC, and begin to establish a response time profile, which could augment the traditional number correct score and perhaps prove useful in better describing normal performance. The sample consisted of Drexel University undergraduate students ($N = 37$; 17 women and 20 men) who were freshmen in a psychology class (mean age = 19.3). They were asked to take the tests for class credit. Subjects in this group were not given any special instruction other than to try their best on each test.

We also wished to establish a profile of malingering on this version of the CFC, and therefore an additional sample of 10 subjects (6 men, 4 women, mean age = 19.1, mean education = 12.2) was asked to simulate that they had endured a head injury. These subjects were given instructions to respond as if they had endured a severe brain injury.

TABLE 1. Number Correct (out of 50 Items) and Reaction Times for Controls and Simulators

	Controls		Simulators	
	Mean	SD	Mean	SD
Number correct	49.19	1.20	32.70	12.23
Reaction time	988.55	313.81	1398.99	495.65

The results of this experiment are summarized in Table 1. Instructions to simulate resulted in decrement of performance seen both in reduced number of correct responses and in increased reaction time. Because of the nature of the data (negatively skewed and substantially different variances between the controls and simulators), Mann–Whitney *U* tests were used. The difference between the control and simulator group means is significant for number correct ($z = 3.96, p < .01$) as well as for reaction time ($z = 2.50$, $p = .01$).

Consider the differences in demographics between the pilot study subjects and the experimental subjects. The pilot study mean age was 33.7 and the experimental study group 19.3. Despite such differences and the fact that the test was shortened, the results were essentially the same (98/100 for the pilot study and 49/50 for the experimental study, or 98% for both). This suggests that the CFC is consistent, and not susceptible to varying subject characteristics.

A Cronbach alpha coefficient was calculated to be .96. This indicated that subjects did not reply significantly differently to any items. This would imply that there were no items that were significantly more difficult than any other and therefore that the items were very similar in difficulty.

We also examined performance decay over the three delay periods on the CFC, as noted by other investigators employing forced-choice tasks with time delays (Prigatano & Amin, 1993). Analysis of both number correct and reaction times over the three time delays (no delay, 10-second delay, and 30-second delay) was conducted. A two-way repeated-measures ANOVA compared normal controls and simulators (grouping factor) for number correct over the three time delays (repeated-measures factors, three levels). The ANOVA showed a main effect of grouping, simulators performing more poorly, and a main effect of time delay, performance deteriorating with delay. Most importantly, however, the group × time delay interaction was significant ($F(2,90) = 5.50$, $p < .001$). For controls, percent correct remained stable for all time delays, whereas simulators showed a decline in performance for the long-delay condition.

The same ANOVA was applied to the reaction time data. Here too there was a main effect for group, simulators had longer reaction times, an effect of time delay, reaction time slowed with increased delay, and a group × time delay interaction ($F(2,90) - 3.74, p < .03$). This interaction indicated that reaction time slowing over time delays was more pronounced in simulators than in controls.

In summary, the CFC did differentiate between normal controls and subjects asked to simulate head injury, and we were able to begin to develop a profile of normal versus malingering performance on this test. It can be deduced that many naive simulators felt a need to demonstrate impairments in their accuracy rate and slowed reaction times. These same subjects were compelled to make more errors as time delays were implemented and this further delayed their responses. Simulators were slower also because they may have needed to assess which digit was the target, and then decide to strike the key corresponding to the distractor stimulus, in keeping with conjecture by previous investigators (Hiscock & Hiscock, 1989; Pankratz, 1988). It should also be noted that only some subjects, all from the simulator group, performed below chance levels.

Further, we indicated that resistance, avoidance, and bizarre responding should caution the evaluator to attempt to assess any possible patient deception. Therefore, still another level of analysis is required in assessing malingering on the CFC. Lezak (1983) indicated that although malingerers have a tendency simply to omit items, it was also recommended that type of error rather than absolute level of performance be considered to avoid false-positive errors. Binder (1990) and Pankratz (1988) noted that there are numerous indications of malingering, including distortions, evasiveness, and explaining away the successes obtained by the deceptive patient. This received empirical support in a study by Bernard (1990). Additionally, Malloy (1994) noted that numerous "Other" responses on the Wisconsin Card Sorting Test may serve as an indicator of exaggeration because these types of responses are very rare. On the CFC, unusual responses (e.g., selecting a series of keys that were not discussed in the instructions or alternating rapidly between the two acceptable keys as a response) were found *only* within the simulator group. These bizarre responses were coupled with a performance decay over the last two phases, with the majority of the bizarre responses occurring within these two intervals.

CONCLUSION

Because of an increase in litigation, the courts need to be assured that work done in neuropsychology and other biomedical disciplines is of the best quality (Faust, Zisking, & Hiers, 1991). As clinicians and researchers we must be willing to stand behind our work, and we therefore need to be able to discern the veracity of our patients claims. Our hope is that instruments such as the CFC will be of assistance in this endeavor. Although some believe that patient performance below the expected norm on a forced-choice test is highly suspicious, others believe performing below chance levels is irrefutable evidence of poor motivation and exaggeration (Binder, 1990). Hiscock and Hiscock (1989) noted that it is always preferable to view poor performance on forced-choice testing as creating the *inference* of poor motivation on other neuropsychological tests, not as objective proof. Further, Cliffe (1992) noted that response styles are also to be examined carefully. For example, his work studied not only whether the simulators gave lower-than-chance responses, but also if the responses were random. He indicated that anyone who gave systematic responses was most likely malingering. Pankratz (1988) as well as Beetar and Williams (1994) noted similar response styles as being quite important in assessing malingering.

Lastly, we turn to the issue of ethics. The ethical dilemma of deception in assessment is raised by some (Ben-Porath, 1994; Berry, Lamb, Wetter, Baer, & Widiger, 1994) and we feel it quite important to discuss this issue. Some may criticize the work that contributed to creating this chapter because of the belief that it is unethical for a clinician to mislead the patient in an attempt to assess effort (i.e., telling the subject the he or she is doing better than expected and therefore the test will be made more difficult). On the other hand, this deception is used as a countermeasure for possibly motivated responding by subjects, which can result in the miscarriage of justice. The justice system has a long tradition of justifying such maneuvers, dating perhaps back to King Solomon's handling of a dispute over the parenthood of a child.

In consultation with our university's Biomedical Ethics Center, we have been told that it may very well be ethical to deceive a patient who is suspected of malingering, but it must be done in a manner that affords the patient the opportunity to deny any deficit and perform well on any given test (Caplan, 1995). This conforms to Pankratz's (1979) study, in which he related that a patient should be given every opportunity to save face, and deny previously claimed deficits. We agree with this recommendation and hope that colleagues in our field can make use of tests such as the CFC not only to help expose malingering, but also to treat the malingerer.

Nonetheless, it is worth noting that the success of deception is contingent on the subject's gullibility and ultimately it is impossible with such maneuvers to eliminate the potential for successful countermeasures by the more savvy subject. This, of course, could be addressed with increasingly complex deceptive schemes, but perhaps computerized testing can offer an alternative that needs careful exploration. Conceivably, multiple measures can be derived from a computerized neuropsychological battery, administered without any deceptive instructions, which could show subtle and complex differences between malingerers and truly impaired individuals. For example, differences between recognition and recall, reaction times for correct and incorrect responses, and the several indicators such as we have identified on the CFC, can be systematically evaluated. Conceivably, with such measures even a scale designed specifically for detection of malingering can be administered without deception. Patients can be truthfully told that the CFC is designed to detect malingering, yet they would be unable to reproduce the response pattern characteristic of the truly impaired. We suggest that this would be a fruitful avenue to advance future work in this area.

Our study underscores the fact that if patients do not attempt to deceive, they will all maximize their performance on instruments such as the CFC. Our future effort will focus on developing additional response parameters as well as more extensive normal control and simulator data. Thus far, we have observed performances on the CFC by patients of minimal intellectual abilities (Mildly Mentally Retarded, Borderline intellectual ability), and can report preliminarily that these patients have performed well (above 90% correct for all cases). We are currently augmenting this by examining the performance of patients with mild to moderate cerebral dysfunctions, such as closed head injuries and cerebrovascular disease, so as to compare their performance with that of healthy subjects and simulators.

ACKNOWLEDGMENTS

Supported by NIH Grants 5-T32-MH19112 and 5-P50-MH43880. We thank Drs. Paul Moberg, J. Daniel Ragland, James Holdnack, Richard Mahr, and Adam Sherman for comments and help and Helen Mitchell-Sears for manuscript preparation.

REFERENCES

Adams, K. M., & Rourke, B. P. (1992). *The TCN guide to professional practice in clinical neuropsychology*. Berwyn, PA: Swets & Zeitlinger.

Anastasi, A. (1980). Abilities and the measurement of achievement. *New Directions for Testing and Measurements*, *5*, 1–10.

Audrey, J. B., Dobbs, A. R., & Rule, B. G. (1989). Laypersons' knowledge about the sequelae of minor head injury and whiplash. *Journal of Neurology, Neurosurgery and Psychiatry*, *52*, 842–846.

Barth, J. T., Gideon, D. A., Sciara, A. D., Hulsey, P. H., & Anchor, K. N. (1986). Forensic aspects of mild head trauma. *Journal of Head Trauma Rehabilitation*, *1*(2), 63–70.

Beers, S. R. (1992). Effects of mild head injury in children and adolescents. *Neuropsychology Review*, *3*, 281–320.

Beetar, J. T., & Williams, J. M. (1994). Malingering response styles on the Memory Assessment Scales and Symptom Validity Tests. *Archives of Clinical Neuropsychology* *10*(1), 57–72.

Ben-Porath, Y. S. (1994). The ethical dilemma of coached malingering research. *Psychological Assessment*, *6*(1), 14–15.

Bernard, L. C. (1990). The detection of faked deficits on the Rey Auditory Verbal Learning Test: The effect of a serial position. *Archives of Clinical Neuropsychology*, *6*, 81–88.

Berry, D. T. R., Lamb, D. G., Wetter, M. W., Baer, R. A., & Widiger, T. A. (1994). Ethical considerations in research on coached malingering. *Psychological Assessment*, *6*(1), 16–17.

Binder, L. M. (1990). Malingering following minor head trauma. *The Clinical Neuropsychologist*, *4*, 25–36.

Binder, L. M. (1993a). An abbreviated form of the Portland Digit Recognition Test. *The Clinical Neuropsychologist*, *7*(1), 104–107.

Binder, L. M. (1993b). Assessment of malingering after mild head trauma with the Portland Digit Recognition Test. *Journal of Clinical and Experimental Neuropsychology*, *15*, 170–182.

Binder, L. M., & Pankratz, L. (1987). Neuropsychological evidence of a factitious memory complaint. *Journal of Clinical and Experimental Neuropsychology*, *9*, 167–171.

Binder, L. M., & Willis, S. C. (1991). Assessment of motivation after financially compensable minor head trauma. *Journal of Consulting and Clinical Psychology*, *3*(2). 175–181.

Blau, T. (1994). *The expert witness—current perspectives*. Presentation at the 14th Annual Conference of the National Academy of Neuropsychology, Orlando, FL.

Brady, J. P., & Lind, D. L. (1961). Experimental analysis of hysterical blindness. *Archives of General Psychiatry*, *4*, 331–339.

Brandt, J., Rubinsky, E., & Lassen, G. (1985). Uncovering malingered amnesia. *Annals of the New York Academy of Science*, *44*, 502–503.

Caplan, A. (1995). *Ethics in biomedical research* Presentation at the University of Pennsylvania, Philadelphia.

Chute, D. L. (1990). *MacLaboratory for psychology: Software documentation.* Devon, PA: Maclaboratory Inc.

Cliffe, M. J. (1992). Symptom-validity testing of feigned sensory or memory deficits: A further elaboration for the subjects who understand the rationale. *British Journal of Clinical Psychology 31*, 207–209.

Colohan, A. R. T., Dacey, R. G., Jr., Alves, W. M., Rimel, R. W., & Jane, J. A. (1986). Neurologic and neurosurgical implications of mild head injury. *Journal of Head Trauma Rehabilitation, 1*(2), 13–21.

Daubert v. Merrell Dow Pharmaceuticals, Inc., 61 U.S. 4805 (1993).

Faust, D., Ziskin, J., & Hiers, J. B., Jr. (1991). *Brain damage claims: Coping with neuropsychological evidence.* Marina del Rey, CA: Law and Psychology Press.

Frederick, R. I., & Foster, H. G. (1991). Multiple measures of malingering on a forced-choice test of cognitive ability. *Psychological Assessment, 3*(4), 596–602.

Gouvier, W. D., Cubic, B., Jones, G., & Brantley, P. (1992). Postconcussion symptoms and daily stress in normal and head-injured college populations. *Archives of Clinical Neuropsychology, 7*(3), 193–211.

Gouvier, W. D., Prestholdt, P. H., & Warner, M. S. (1988). A survey of common misperceptions about head injuries and recovery. *Archives of Clinical Neuropsychology, 3*, 331–343.

Gouvier, W. D., Uddo-Crane, M., & Brown, L. M. (1988). Base rates of postconcussional symptoms. *Archives of Clinical Neuropsychology, 3*, 273–278.

Grosz, H., & Zimmerman, J. (1965). Experimental analysis of hysterical blindness. *Archives of General Psychiatry, 13*, 225–260.

Guilmette, T. J., Hart, K. J., & Giuliano, A. J. (1993). Malingering detection: The use of a forced-choice method in identifying organic versus simulated memory impairment. *The Clinical Neuropsychologist, 7*, 59–69.

Hiscock, M., & Hiscock, C. K. (1989). Refining the forced-choice method of detection of malingering. *Journal of Clinical and Experimental Neuropsychology, 11*, 967–974.

Horne v. Marvin L. Goodson Logging Co., 83 N.C.APP. 96, 349 S.E.2D 293 (1986).

Iverson, G. L., Franzen, M. D., & McCracken, L. M. (1991). Evaluation of an objective assessment technique of the detection of malingered memory deficits. *Law and Human Behavior, 15*, 667–676.

Iverson, G. L., Franzen, M. D., & McCracken, L. M. (1994). Application of a forced-choice memory procedure designed to detect experimental malingering. *Archives of Clinical Neuropsychology, 9*, 437–450.

Kane, R. L., & Kay, G. C. (1992). Computerized assessment in neuropsychology: A review of tests and test batteries. *Neuropsychology Review, 3*(1). 1–117.

Krause, N. (1985). Common sense glossary of medical-legal terms. *Journal of Nurse-Midwifery, 30*(2), 122–124.

Kurlychek, R. T. (1984). The contributions of forensic neuropsychology. *American Journal of Forensic Psychology, 2*(4), 147–150.

Larrabee, G. J. (1990). Cautions in the use of neuropsychological evaluation in legal settings. *Neuropsychology, 4*, 239–247.

Lees-Haley, P. R., & Brown, R. (1993). Neuropsychological complaint base rates of 170 personal injury claimants. *Archives of Clinical Neuropsycholgy, 8*, 203–209.

Lezak, M. D. (1983). *Neuropsychological assessment* (2nd ed.). London: Oxford University Press.

Malloy, P. R. (1994). *Understanding frontal lobe function and dysfunction*, Presentation at the 14th Annual Conference of the National Academy of Neuropsychology, Orlando, FL.

Martin, R. C., Bolter, J. F., Todd, M. E., Govier, W. D., & Niccolls, R. (1993). Effects of sophistication and motivation on the detection of malingered memory performance using a computerized forced-choice task. *Journal of Clinical and Experimental Neuropsychology, 15*, 867–880.

McCaffrey, R. J., Williams, A. D., Fisher, J. M., & Laing, L. C. (1993). Forensic issues in mild head injury. *Journal of Head Trauma Rehabilitation*, *8*(3), 38–47.

Miller, E. (1986). Detecting hysterical sensory symptoms: An elaboration of the forced-choice technique. *British Journal of Clinical Psychology*, *25*, 231–232.

Niccolls, R., & Bolter, J. (1991). *Multi-Digit Memory Test*. San Luis Obispo, CA: Wang Neuropsychological Laboratories.

Nies, K. J., & Sweet, J. J. (1994). Neuropsychological assessment and malingering: A critical review of past and present strategies. *Archives of Clinical Neuropsychology*, *9*, 501–552.

Pankratz, L. (1979). Symptom validity testing and symptom retraining: Procedures for the assessment and treatment of functional sensory deficits. *Journal of Consulting and Clinical Psychology*, *47*(2), 409–410.

Pankratz, L. (1983). A new technique of the assessment and modification of feigned memory deficit. *Perceptual and Motor Skills*, *57*, 367–372.

Pankratz, L. (1988). Malingering on intellectual and neuropsychological measures. In R. Rogers (Ed.), *Clinical assessment of malingering and deception*. (pp. 169–192). New York: Guilford Press.

Pankratz, L., Binder, L., & Wilcox, L. (1987). Assessment of an exaggerated somatosensory deficit with symptom validity assessment. *Archives of Neurology*, *44*, 798.

Pankratz, L., Fausti, S. A., & Peed, S. (1975). A forced-choice technique to evaluate deafness in a hysterical or malingering patient. *Journal of Consulting and Clinical Psychology*, *43*, 421–422.

Prigatano, G. P., & Amin, K. (1993). The Digit Memory Test: Unequivocal cerebral dysfunction and suspected malingering. *Journal of Clinical and Experimental Neuropsychology*, *15*, 537–546.

Sattler, J. M. (1988). *Assessment of children* (3rd ed.). San Diego: Author.

Satz, P. (1988). Neuropsychological testimony: Some emerging concerns. *The Clinical Neuropsychologist*, *2*, 89–100.

Smith, A. (1968). The Symbol Modalities Test: A neuropsychological test for economic screening of learning and other cerebral disorders. *Learning Disabilities*, *3*, 83–91.

Theodore, L. H., & Mandelcorn, M. S. (1973). Hysterical blindness: A case report and study using a modern psychophysical technique. *Journal of Abnormal Psychology*, *82*, 552–553.

Wedding, D. (1991). Clinical judgement in forensics neuropsychology: A comment on the risks of claiming more than can be delivered. *Neuropsychology Review*, *2*, 233–239.

Willer, B., Johnson, W. E., Rempel, R. G., & Linn, R. (1993). A note concerning misconceptions of the general public about brain injury. *Archives of Clinical Neuropsychology*, *8*, 461–465.

Wong, J. L., Regennitter, R. P., & Barrios, F. (1994). Base rate and simulated symptoms of mild head injury among normals. *Archives of Clinical Neuropsychology*, *9*, 411–425.

Ziskin, J., & Faust, D. (1988). *Coping with psychiatric and psychological testimony* (Vols. I–III, 4th ed.). Marina del Rey, CA: Law and Psychology Press.

4

The Malingering of Memory Disorder

J. MICHAEL WILLIAMS

Forensic applications of the neuropsychological examination are a relatively recent development. Psychologists rarely served as experts in personal injury cases before clinical neuropsychology matured to its present situation. Most forensic psychology applications were in the areas of competency to stand trial and criminal responsibility. Clinical forensic neuropsychology also represents a singular area in which the examination actually assists in establishing the extent of neurological consequences of brain injuries. As the legal profession has learned to use neuropsychologists as effective experts in their litigation of cases, this role has come to significantly influence the atmosphere of private practice. Even if a case is not in active litigation at the time of examination, the neuropsychologist anticipates that litigation, or some sort of formal disability determination, is probably in the near future and designs the assessment accordingly.

The development and elaboration of forensic neuropsychology practice was essentially unforeseen by the field as it was maturing from infancy in the past two decades. Neuropsychologists were not generally prepared for it. As a practice setting, the legal environment was unfamiliar to most psychologists and neuropsychologists and their efforts to cope with it were naive. Neuropsychologists were surprised that the adversarial legal system could not incorporate the egalitarian and objective presentation of truth and uncertainty, part of a system of values they acquired as graduate students. An expert who expressed honest uncertainty on cross-examination was not invited to be an expert again. Neuropsychologists were, and still are, manipulated by the adversarial system through financial incentives to stand on one side of the fence or the other, to profess their allegiance to the plaintiff

J. MICHAEL WILLIAMS • Department of Clinical and Health Psychology, Allegheny University of the Health Sciences, Philadelphia, Pennsylvania 19102.

Detection of Malingering during Head Injury Litigation, edited by Reynolds. Plenum Press, New York, 1998.

or defense. They are further compelled to argue the case for the lawyers or they will not be recruited to serve again and they will suffer the financial loss associated with disconnection from the lucrative forensic referrals.

This accelerated development in such an unfamiliar and stressful environment has resulted in a number of problems for clinical neuropsychology. Among these are that neuropsychologists have become very conservative in their clinical practice. Cross-examination has made them cagey and defensive. Neuropsychologists are hesitant to adopt new tests and methods in their own field because they are afraid they will have to defend the methods someday in court. The usual confidence practitioners had in their tests has now become a type of dogmatic attachment to old methods just to maintain a sense of security. Of germane interest to this chapter, this conservative posture has resulted in strong beliefs among practitioners that the tests they use are essentially inviolate and are not affected by extraneous factors such as malingering. In fact, because neuropsychological methods have a relatively high degree of measurement error, these tests should, unfortunately, be affected by such factors to a greater extent than other assessments of personal injury, such as medical examinations. Other medical and allied professions that were involved in personal injury litigation have long recognized malingering as a highly significant problem that affects the validity of their assessments and must be examined in every case. It is only recently that malingering has been given the attention it deserves by neuropsychologists. Now, malingering detection is probably the most popular topic at professional meetings and it is fair to say that neuropsychologists are presently preoccupied with its accurate detection. The early investigations of malingering have focused on memory disorder, and this is the focus of the present chapter.

Memory disorder is the most common complaint following brain illness or injury (Schacter & Crovitz, 1977). Through exposure to various realistic and even fanciful presentations in the popular media of amnesia following a blow to the head, it is also the most common symptom known to anyone who might sustain a brain injury. Most people understand many of the basic features of poor memory; disorders such as aphasia and visual neglect are not common knowledge. As a consequence, memory disorder is probably the most common malingered disability when someone falsely claims personal injury following brain trauma or illness. This is the symptom most familiar to the malingerer and, hence, the symptom most often mimicked. The discrimination of true from factitious memory impairment is the foundation of the study of malingering in neuropsychology. Investigation of malingered memory impairment ranges from studies of memory itself to the use of memory procedures as symptom validity tests. This chapter will review the possible strategies that may be used to affect memory disorder following injury, strategies used to detect malingered memory disorder, and some proposals for new techniques to detect false memory impairment.

THE GENERAL CONDITION OF FACTITIOUS RESPONDING

The situation of a subject attempting to perform worse than actual ability is often simply described as *malingering*. However, such a simple application of this term is misleading. *Malingering* is usually applied to a situation in which the subject is consciously engaged in faking impairment; it implies that the subject has a clear intention and plan for faking. Situations in which the subject unconsciously exaggerates deficits, manifests hysterical symptoms or other psychological disorder that affects performance, are not adequately categorized as malingering.

For these reasons, the study of these extraneous factors might best be subsumed under a general heading of *factitious responding*, of which malingering is a subarea. The other subareas include the exacerbation of deficits that is the result of a psychological disorder in which the motivation is unconscious, such as hysteria, dependency, and psychological depression, and the simple exaggeration of symptoms accompanied by denial and suppression of this exaggeration as dishonest. These areas vary considerably in the degree to which conscious motivation is present. For example, patients with hysterical amnesia are, by definition, completely unaware of the psychological meaning of their memory disorder (Brady, 1966; Gorman, 1982; Perkin, 1994; Samuel, 1977). On the other hand, patients who are using their deficits to maintain dependent family relationships may have some conscious understanding of the role the impairment plays in their family adjustment (Stevens, 1986).

By expanding the area of investigation, the true diversity and complexity of each patient's situation is available for examination and interpretation. In allowing for the role of unconscious processes, the dishonesty inferences that are exclusively associated with malingering are dissociated from the concept of faking: It is possible to fake a poor performance without formulating a conscious and intentional plan (Braverman, 1978). This broader conceptualization is also consistent with most clinical situations in which we actually examine patients. Few are the patients who walk through the door with an intention to fake impairment who have carefully planned a strategy to accomplish this goal. Most are fundamentally honest people who are placed under extreme financial pressure to perform worse than they can actually perform, or they are people with psychological disorders for whom cognitive difficulties are a symptom.

This various blend of motivations and levels of conscious awareness has resulted in considerable confusion about the prevalence of factitious responding and the ability of clinicians to detect it. Most clinicians do not apparently believe that factitious responding is common (Bigler, 1990; Blakely & Harrington, 1993; Trueblood & Schmidt, 1993). This is probably the result of considering the prevalence of frank, dishonest malingering among one's own clinical referrals; such clear and intentional faking is unusual. However, if one includes the incidence of mild or moderate symptom exaggeration, psychological depression, and conversion reactions, then the prevalence of factitious responding must be judged to increase.

A TEST OF MEMORY OR A TEST OF FACTITIOUS RESPONSE STYLE?

In the consideration of extraneous influences such as malingering, one myth to dispel is that neuropsychological tests are always completely valid and, hence, always assess true ability; they are never significantly affected by extraneous factors, such as the psychological states of low motivation, inattention, and malingering. The numerous studies of psychological depression and malingering suggest that tests are very sensitive to these sources of systematic extraneous influence (Cullum, Heaton, & Grant, 1991; Snow, Tierney, Zorzitto, Fisher, & Reid, 1990). These factors can manifest themselves in such extreme fashion that a test of memory can be transformed into a test of psychological depression or malingering response style. The variance is so affected that the test now measures a completely different construct.

For most clinical neuropsychology practitioners this is a difficult validity problem to incorporate into their reasoning about tests and serves as a major impediment to accepting the influence of malingering on tests. These factors are sources of considerable uncertainty in clinical judgments. It is certainly easier to make inferences about function when tests are always reliable and measure the same constructs at each testing session.

Unfortunately, the extent of these influences is essentially unknown at the time of the testing. Most clinicians simply exclude them by observation and inference. If the patient does not appear depressed or obviously malingering, then it is inferred that such factors have not influenced the test scores. Given that these factors are impossible to incorporate systematically into the test scoring, the clinician is probably biased in concluding that they are probably not present and, hence, the test scores only represent ability levels. In the case of malingering, there is one other source of bias. Because malingering represents a dishonest activity, the reporting of its presence in a neuropsychological report is associated with social aversion and anxiety. Such an explanation for test findings represents an accusation of dishonest behavior and is only done when the testing situation is frankly extreme and the examiner has overwhelming evidence that the patient was malingering.

Another myth common among clinicians is that the patient's self-report has greater validity than memory test scores. As clinical reasoners are primed to infer pathology and deny the presence of malingering (Wedding & Faust, 1989), they are quick to question the validity of the tests they administer when they find negative results, rather than qualify the complaints of patients. If this is combined with a request to evaluate a patient for the plaintiff, then fertile ground is cultivated for a bias that negative test findings mean that the tests are not valid measures of the "subtle" cognitive impairment that presumably underlies the patient's complaints and the claims of personal injury. It is one of the unusual situations in which clinical reasoners do not engage in their usual practice of reifying the tests (Wedding & Faust, 1989). Any reasonable summary of the literature on memory self-report suggests that the patient's report of memory impairment is highly inaccurate in most circumstances and especially when the patient has sustained a brain injury (Allen & Ruff, 1990; Faust, 1995b, Gilbertson et al., 1992; Vander & Charles, 1993; Wong, Regennitter, & Barrios, 1994). It has also been established that there is a high base rate of complaints among the general population (Gouvier, Uddo-Crane, & Brown, 1988). The only reasonable conclusion is that test results should be trusted when there is a discrepancy. Yet, there is a search on among the practitioners in the forensic area to find the ideal measure of "subtle" disorders of memory and attention. Certainly the development of the PASAT represented an attempt to find a measure of sustained attention that would be so sensitive that it would reveal the underlying subtle attention deficits of patients with mild head injuries. This search has been largely futile. Now that the PASAT is properly normed (Brittain, LaMarche, Reeder, Roth, & Boll, 1991), correct inferences will be made regarding the impairment of sustained attention associated with mild head injury. This will probably result in fewer cases in which the patients' complaints are supported by low PASAT standard scores. Prior to normative studies of the test, clinicians were not anchored by any objective standard score and it was easy to modify the interpretation of PASAT raw scores to support the patients' complaints. It may be that the patients' complaints of attention disorder were invalid and not the tests of attention.

For these reasons, malingering is probably greatly unreported by clinical practitioners. More subtle manifestations of malingering are unnoticed or neglected. However, this conclusion must be qualified by the fact that the actual prevalence of malingering is impossible to determine so as to test the hypothesis that malingering is common and underreported. As no true malingerers will ever identify themselves, it is virtually impossible to know the incidence of the malingering in neuropsychology. Only in areas where there are highly valid malingering detection methods (e.g., Rickards & De, 1995) can such an incidence be accurately known.

TYPES OF FACTITIOUS RESPONDING

Although the term *malingering* is applied to cases in which the subjects intentionally attempt to perform worse than they can, there are other manifestations of factitious responding that include unconscious motivation and subtle attempts to exaggerate deficits. All of these manifestations involve similar patterns of performance on tests and similar detection methods. These types may be conveniently divided into three main types: malingering, hysterical and psychological disorders, and exaggeration of deficits.

Malingering refers to conscious and intentional faking of poor responses on tests. Patients who adopt an intentional faking strategy usually have an extremely clear secondary gain and often have virtually no genuine cognitive impairment (Franzen, Iverson, & McCracken, 1990; Nies & Sweet, 1994). Usually they are involved in litigation that includes unusual claims of personal injury and disability. These characterizations are the result of a process of elimination and inference. Patients with genuine cognitive impairment do not need to malinger to establish their claims of injury, or may only exaggerate symptoms. The true malingering patients must usually fake the entire level and type of impairment. As a consequence, their level of conscious awareness of their faking attempts is quite high. Such patients make active attempts to plan a strategy to appear impaired.

Patients who thus consciously malinger are probably not common (Braverman, 1978). Such patients recognize the dishonest, and even criminal nature of their behavior, and this is inconsistent with the motivation of most patients referred for evaluation. Because they usually have no clear idea of the patterns of impairment that should be present so as to mimic traumatic brain injury, their malingering is usually transparent. It also involves dishonest behavior with the risk of being caught. For these reasons, true malingerers are probably not the most common practitioners of factitious performances.

Hysterical disorders, including conversion reactions that include amnesia and dissociative reactions, are probably also less common. These involve unconscious processes and psychological disorders that are characterized by dissociations and symptoms of illness that factor into a neurotic condition. Dissociations involve unconscious denial of experiences that are anxiety-related, such as those associated with psychological trauma (Gilbertson et al., 1992). As a result, claims of amnesia are common. They may be dissociations of recent anxiety-provoking experience, to repression of all biographical memories and fugue states (Resnick, 1993; Schacter, 1986). One possible explanation for transient global amnesia includes hysterical dissociation (Stevens, 1986). Patients with these disorders are occasionally referred for evaluation by neuropsychologists. However, they are seldom involved in litigation and they are not usually motivated by tangible secondary gains; their motivations are psychological and they are often amnesic for specific, anxiety-related experiences.

The final general category of factitious responding includes patients who have sustained a traumatic brain injury or other neurological illness and who exaggerate the genuine neuropsychological impairment that is present or prolong genuine symptoms that were present soon after the injury but have now recovered. These patients are not properly malingering because they are usually not intentionally attempting to fake impairment. As they are often involved in litigation, their incentives are the same as those of a malingering patient but they are usually not consciously aware of the exaggeration, and have not formed a plan to perform worse than they actually can perform. This is the most common manifestation of factitious performance and the most difficult to detect because the patient has an accurate understanding of the symptoms and is simply manifesting them for a longer period of time.

One characteristic these types have in common is that they all involve subjects who are attempting to perform worse than they actually can perform. This common objective results in a common set of signs of factitious responding on the tests. Whenever individuals attempt to perform worse than their actual ability, they may engage in certain activities on memory tests that indicate they are attempting this. Such signs may serve as markers of factitious responding and malingering. The fact that one person is motivated by secondary gains and another by neurotic dependency should not result in different signs of factitious responding. From the point of view of performance, they both have a common task ahead of them and the signs of factitious responding should be apparent in both performances.

STRATEGIES OF MALINGERING ON MEMORY TESTS

Clues to the manner in which malingering and factitious responding will be manifested in test responses lie with the strategies that anyone might follow when responding to a memory test. How is it possible to do worse than one actually can on common memory assessment procedures and still appear convincing? The answer to this question represents the major task of the malingering subject. The way in which the malingering subject formulates a plan to accomplish this often suggests methods to detect its presence. The structure of conventional memory batteries may contain common features that vary in their sensitivity to strategies of malingering and factitious responding.

Most batteries include sets of verbal and visuo-spatial memory tasks in which information is presented and retention is assessed by direct recall or recognition procedures. Verbal content includes lists of words and short prose passages. Visuo-spatial content includes geometric figures that are shown to the subject and recall is tested by having the subject draw the figure later; recognition is assessed by requesting the subject to indicate the figure shown before when it is presented among a set of distractors. Finally, most memory batteries include a test of immediate recall, such as Digit Span. The following is a summary of methods that are possible given the structure of current memory test batteries.

Intentional Wrong Responding

With this approach, the subject knows the correct answer but chooses the incorrect one. This strategy is the obvious one to employ if one is making a conscious attempt to perform poorly. However, the subject must plan some approach to intentional wrong responding. If every response was incorrect, then the examiner could easily infer that the subject is malingering. To appear convincing, intentional wrong responding must be done with some model or understanding of how many errors will appear convincing and short of the number of errors that will appear absurd. Producing such a pattern on every test presented is probably a difficult task and success probably varies from test to test. On some tests, the error rate required to produce a convincing result is better understood from the description given by the examiner and the obvious structure of the tasks presented; on other tests, the structure of the test is not conducive to determining what error rate will result in a convincing pattern. For example, it is far easier to judge the correct error rate for a forced-choice recognition memory test than a memory test that relies on recall only. The former has set trials that are obviously summed to produce a raw score. The scoring of a recall task is far more difficult to ascertain from observation of the task itself. These discrepancies may be used to detect malingering. Presumably brain-injured and normal subjects who are behaving honestly will perform consistent with their level of ability and not with attempts to produce a convincing error rate (Wiggins & Brandt, 1988).

Inattention

A simple strategy to perform poorly on a variety of tests is to manifest distractibility and inattention. By not focusing attention on instructions or test content, the subject can presumably produce a poor performance and actually appear similar to many brain-injured patients who have impairment of attention and concentration. Of course, this strategy will not result in poor performance on every memory test, for many tests do not require a high degree of sustained attention. For example, a visuo-spatial recall memory test does not require the same degree of sustained attention as a verbal memory test using list-learning over multiple trials.

Slow Responses

Another general method one might use to perform poorly is to respond slowly. This will have a dramatic effect on timed tests or tests that have a specific timing of content presentation. Memory tests are not usually considered timed tests in the sense that scores on memory tests are not usually affected by how quickly a subject responds. However, slow responding on immediate recall tasks, such as Digit Span, probably results in lower scores. Using the computer-mediated version of the memory Assessment Scales (MAS), Beetar and Williams (1995) found that subjects instructed to malinger performed slowly on every task presented to them. Likewise, the assessment of response time improves the accuracy of symptom validity tests (Rose, Hall, Szalda, & Allen, 1995). Slow responses have a dramatic effect on tests that have time bonuses, such as the Block Design and Object Assembly subtests of the Wechsler Adult Intelligence Scale.

Haphazard Responses

This strategy is similar to intentional wrong responding in that the subject makes incorrect responses. However, these responses are made in the context of guessing and responding erratically. There is not a clear decision to make a specific error, the subject simply responds in haphazard fashion and makes a number of errors in the process. Malingering subjects can typically engage in this strategy on tasks that allow multiple responses. These include recognition memory tests, such as the Continuous Recognition Memory Test (Larrabee, 1992) and the Warrington Recognition Memory Test (Millis, 1994), and other tests that span numerous items, such as the Speech Sounds Perception Test and the Category Test, both subtests of the Halstead–Reitan Battery (Heaton, Smith, Lehman, & Vogt, 1978).

Systematic Random or Sequential Responding

Although random and haphazard responding appear the same, the difference indicated here is between a general, unplanned guessing strategy and one that is a conscious attempt to respond in a formal random fashion. As with haphazard responding, recognition tasks with many items are sensitive to this approach. Here, the systematic nature of the responding takes the form of choosing the option presented on one side of a recognition trial every third trial or some other pattern that is unrelated to whether the choice is correct or incorrect. Such strategies usually produce a random pattern of errors although the sequential nature of the approach is detectable by analyzing the subject's pattern of responses. The Category Test is a good example of a test that can be easily responded to by a systematic random strategy.

SYMPTOM VALIDITY TESTS THAT RELY ON MEMORY

It is remarkable that virtually all of the methods proposed as specific malingering, or "symptom validity" tests are recognition memory tests (Binder, 1992; Binder & Pankratz, 1987; Hiscock, Branham, & Hiscock, 1994). These tests usually incorporate one of two major strategies. The first malingering strategy is to present the subject with a task that is easy but appears difficult. The malingering subject will be presumably duped by this and perform worse than even severely brain-injured subjects. The best example of this is the Rey 15-Item Test (Arnett, Hammeke, & Schwartz, 1995; Lee, Loring, & Martin, 1992) and its variants. Here the subject is presented with five rows of three items. Row one contains the numbers 1, 2, and 3; row two, the Roman numerals I, II, and III; row three, a square, triangle, and circle; row four, the letters A, B, and C; and row five, letters a, b, and c. Although this test is a good example of the strategy, it has not served well as a malingering test (Millis & Kler, 1995; Schretlen, Brandt, Krafft, & Van Gorp, 1991; Simon, 1994). This is probably because it is so easy that all but the dullest malingering subjects perceive its true difficulty and respond in the normal range. It also suffers from a lack of norms and comparisons with brain-injured patients. Because it does not rely on worse-than-chance response levels, scores must be compared to a normative and validity standard. Although some rules of thumb have been proposed (Lee et al., 1992), it is currently unknown how many errors one must make to be correctly classified as a malingerer.

The second major strategy involves worse-than-chance responding in a recognition memory format (Binder, 1993). If a subject responds at a level worse than chance, the inference is made that the subject must have intentionally responded incorrectly on a large number of trials and engaged in malingering. Even the most impaired subject who can take the test will perform at chance level or better.

The reason that memory skill was chosen instead of some other cognitive ability that can be assessed using recognition procedures is probably the result of the strong association of memory assessment with recognition measures. Another reason may be that symptom validity tests must appear to be difficult without actually being so difficult that subjects make a large number of true errors. Memory tests can be conveniently tailored for difficulty by simply extending the delay between presentation and testing, or by simple manipulations of the test content, such as adding more items or making the items more complex.

Because worse-than-chance responding is all that is required in the design of these tests, it should be possible to design a symptom validity test that incorporates some other cognitive function. For example, a test could be constructed of simple and complex arithmetic problems that used a forced-choice recognition paradigm for indicating the answers to problems. Likewise, recognition of speech sounds, dichotically presented syllables or rhythmic patterns could be set into a forced-choice format and scored for chance levels (Gold, Lubinsky, & Shahar, 1981).

Malingering tests utilizing worse-than-chance methods had great promise when they were first developed. They did not require normative studies, they were efficient to administer, and performance worse than chance was pathognomonic of malingering. However, studies of these tests have revealed that they are probably not sufficiently specific when worse-than-chance responding is used as the criterion of malingering (Beetar & Williams, 1995; Binder, 1993; Frederick, Sarfaty, Johnston, & Powel, 1994; Guilmette, Hart, & Giuliano, 1993). Because so few malingerers perform worse than chance, scores result in far too many false-negative assignments. It is probably difficult to produce so many errors that one performs worse than chance. Many malingering subjects may also notice how easy these tests are to complete and realize that responding worse than chance will be perceived as too extreme by examiners (Cliffe, 1992). Indeed, the subject can perform perfectly on the test by remembering only the first digit of the pairs of digit strings presented in the task. Many of the clinical cases examined by the author using these tests have made spontaneous comments about the low test difficulty.

There are two directions to pursue in the development of these tests that might solve some of these validity problems. The first would be to use items that assess memory or some other cognitive ability that are much more difficult than the items embodied in most current symptom validity tests (Martin et al., 1993). In this way, malingering subjects will not "see through" the test and understand that a large number of errors will appear extreme.

The second would be to collect normative and validity data for the tests and use the combination of a standard score comparison and worse-than-chance responding to make inferences regarding the tests (Slick, Hopp, Strauss, Hunter, & Pinch, 1994). A standard score derived from normative subjects would allow for a statement of probability concerning the presence of malingering rather than the pathognomonic approach suggested by worse-than-chance responding alone. Such studies should include representative samples of unimpaired and brain-injured subjects.

EVIDENCE OF MALINGERING ON COMMON MEMORY TESTS

Although memory procedures are commonly the foundation of symptom validity tests, the study of malingering on conventional memory batteries has received less research attention. Although positive findings on symptom validity tests indicate motivation to malinger, they are not absolute proof that the subject malingered on other tests, such as the conventional memory battery that was administered to determine impairment. The area of malingering detection would move a great step forward if malingering and factitious responding could be determined by signs present in the responses to the clinical testing itself. This would allow for the inference that the subject malingered on the test used to make clinical judgments of impairment.

Benton and Spreen (Benton & Spreen, 1961; Spreen & Benton, 1963) examined malingering on the Benton Retention Test by asking volunteers to imagine they had sustained a traumatic brain injury with memory disorder. These subjects were compared with subjects with confirmed brain injury. They discovered that subjects simulating malingering performed worse than the brain-injured subjects and made unusual errors, such as the intrusion of figures that were not presented. However, the other errors made by malingering simulators were very similar to those made by the brain-injured subjects.

One of the first studies of this type (Brandt, Rubinsky, & Lassen, 1985) compared college students instructed to malinger with nonmalingering controls and patients with Huntington's disease or traumatic brain injury. A 20-item word list was used as the memory test. It included free recall and a forced-choice recognition procedure. The authors discovered two findings that have been replicated in one form or another in a number of studies conducted in recent years. The first was that few of the subjects asked to malinger actually performed worse than chance. A number of malingering subjects and patients performed at chance levels. The second major finding was that the groups differed only on the recognition component of the list-learning task. The recall task did not appear discriminating. Wiggins and Brandt (1988) examined autobiographical memory, implicit memory, and list-learning among amnesic patients, subjects instructed to malinger, and nonmalingering controls. Although malingering subjects correctly answered significantly fewer autobiographical memory questions, only the recognition component of the list-learning task was consistently discriminating.

Iverson, Franzen, and McCracken (Franzen et al., 1990; Iverson, Franzen, & McCracken, 1991, 1994) also compared volunteers feigning impairment, nonmalingering controls, and brain-injured subjects using a 21-item list-learning task. They also discovered that malingerers and amnesic subjects did not differ on recall components of the test but performed very differently on the forced-choice recognition component. They also found a high rate of worse-than-chance responding among malingering subjects (60%). This unusual and elevated rate may be the result of the subjects' perceiving the test used in this study as a more difficult test. Hence, fewer subjects saw it as such an obvious test of malingering.

Bernard (1990) used the Wechsler Memory Scale-Revised (WMS-R), the Auditory Verbal Learning Test, and the Rey Memory Test. He compared samples of undergraduate volunteers who were asked to malinger with those who were instructed to perform their best. The malingering subjects performed worse than controls on virtually all subtests of these tests. The best discriminating variable was the difference score between recall and recognition measures. Bernard (1991) used the Rey Auditory Verbal Learning Test (RAVLT) to examine serial position and other aspects of list-learning among groups of patients who had sustained traumatic brain injury, volunteers asked to malinger, and control subjects. A serial position effect was discovered: the malingerers reported fewer items from the first part of the RAVLT list.

Mittenberg, Azrin, Millsaps, and Heilbronner (1993) examined patterns of malingering on the WMS-R. They recruited 39 patients with brain injury and compared them with 39 normal volunteers asked to malinger on the test. The malingering subjects performed worse than the brain-injured subjects on every subtest of the WMS-R. The only consistent marker of malingering was the difference score between the Attention/Concentration Index and the Global Index. The malingerers performed badly on the Attention/Concentration Index as well as the other subtests. Brain-injured patients usually performed worse on consolidation measures from the WMS-R and relatively better on Attention/Concentration measures. Malingerers presumably do not know that subjects with amnesia actually do well on tests of immediate recall and sustained attention (Owens, 1995). This may explain the major result of this study and suggests a general procedure for developing malingering indices in the future.

Beetar and Williams (1995) compared subjects instructed to malinger and nonmalingering controls on the Memory Assessment Scales (MAS), a forced-choice symptom validity test similar in design to the Portland Digit Substitution Test (PDST), Rey's 15-Item Test, and Rey's Dot Counting Test (Hiscock et al., 1994; Palmer, Boone, Allman, & Castro, 1995). All of these tasks were computer mediated and this allowed for the accurate measurement of response times for each part of the examination. The authors discovered that malingering subjects performed much worse than control subjects on virtually every task presented to them. However, no malingering subject performed worse than chance on the symptom validity test. As the MAS has clear and equivalent recall and recognition components, it was possible to examine the hypothesis that recall and recognition components are dissociated among malingerers. This dissociation is derived from the findings of Brandt et al. (1985), Wiggins and Brandt (1988), and Bernard (1991). These studies strongly suggested that malingerers performed far worse on recognition tasks and that the contrast of recall and recognition might result in the best method to detect malingering using conventional memory tests. A valid, normative comparison of these is only possible with a few tests, including the MAS (Williams, 1992) and the California Verbal Learning Test (CVLT; Delis, 1987; Millis, Putnam, Adams, & Ricker, 1995). Beetar and Williams (1995) discovered a large dissociation between the recall and recognition components of the MAS subtests. Although the malingering subjects performed worse than the control subjects on recall tasks, they performed far worse than controls on recognition tasks. This stands in contrast to the performance of brain-injured subjects and normative subjects, who both typically have equivalent scores on these components.

A very compelling difference in response times were also discovered by Beetar and Williams (1995). The malingering subjects were dramatically slower in performing on every task making up the MAS and the symptom validity scales. They were slower in recalling individual words during the list-learning task, slower in reciting individual digits on the digit span task, slower in drawing figures on the visual recall tasks, and slower in making choices in the recognition components of the MAS. These slower times were effective in reducing scores on some tests and not others. For example, slow responding probably affected the score on digits span but scores derived from the recognition trials of the visuospatial memory tests were probably not affected by a delay in making a choice. Simple reaction time was also found to be highly discriminating in a study that compared it with the PASAT (Strauss, Spellacy, Hunter, & Berry, 1994). The malingering subjects performed much slower than brain-injured patients. This general finding of delayed responding is consistent with poststudy interviews of subjects instructed to malinger who mentioned this strategy as one method they used to perform worse than they actually can (Goebel, 1983; Iverson, 1995).

GENERAL METHODS FOR DATA ANALYSES AND THE CLINICAL UTILITY OF SYMPTOM VALIDITY TESTING

The early studies of malingering were apparently designed to find a reliable and valid method that would utilize worse-than-chance responding, such as the PDST (Binder, 1993). Such a method would represent an extremely specific measure of malingering. A high degree of specificity is crucial because of the social context of assessing malingering. A conclusion that a referred patient is malingering and behaving dishonestly has greater social consequences than a conclusion that the patient's memory is poor. If worse-than-chance responding was characteristic of every malingering subject and not characteristic of subjects responding honestly, then a very efficient and effective method of detecting malingering would have been quickly discovered and available to practitioners. An additional major advantage of such a method is that such a test does not need to be normed and can be easily created by any practitioner with a set of index cards and a marking pen.

Unfortunately the studies of forced-choice techniques that rely on worse-than-chance responding suggest that very few malingering subjects perform so badly that their response level falls below chance. Few studies found a rate of worse-than-chance responding greater than 5% of the sample asked to malinger. The high expectations for worse-than-chance responding were derived from case reports that became prominent in the early investigation of malingering (Binder & Pankratz, 1987; Pankratz, 1983). These cases probably represented exceptional examples of poor responding.

A number of studies have also used discriminant function analyses to assess the discriminative power of regression-ordered combinations of tests (Bernard, Houston, & Natoli, 1993; Bernard, McGrath, & Houston, 1993; Heaton et al., 1978; Iverson & Franzen, 1994; Millis et al., 1995; Millis & Putnam, 1994). The studies typically find a very high degree of discriminative power, some approaching 95% correct classification. These high classification rates are somewhat misleading. They simply suggest that the performance level of the malingering group is sufficiently different from the comparison groups. The studies usually do not reveal different patterns of performance by the use of discriminant functions. The classification rate increases with the distance in level of performance between the malingering subjects and the group or groups with which they are being compared. If the malingerer simply scores worse than normals and better than brain-injured subjects, then the discriminant functions will appear highly discriminating. The major difficulty with this method, as it is currently applied, is that investigators have relied almost exclusively on the conventional scoring of the tests used in the analyses. Particular discriminating features of malingering, such as a dissociation between recall and recognition, are often obscured by the numerous differences in level of performance on a number of tests and subtests. It is consequently unlikely that discrimination formulas that are created through essentially unguided empirical analyses will render consistent and valid clinical detection methods. The strength of discriminant function analysis will be in suggesting which measures may work as signs of malingering and suggesting alternative scoring methods for the conventional tests. Unfortunately, investigators using discriminant function analyses have taken a completely exploratory approach and expected the analyses to reveal the discriminating measures. If a hypothesis-testing approach were taken, investigators would discover the discriminating power of measures that have some theoretical foundation. For example, the recall and recognition dissociation could be examined using discriminant function analysis and its discriminating power could be determined. Unfortunately, many convention memory tests are not scored for this distinction. Discriminant function analysis will never find these unique discriminating signs if such conventional tests are used.

The investigation of symptom validity testing is moving toward normative studies and standard score comparisons of malingering, brain-injured, and control subjects. If these tests have a future role as an aid to clinical evaluation, it is in the direction of conventional standard scored comparisons rather than decision rules based on worse-than-chance responding. Normative studies require considerably greater effort in test development than simply comparing subjects asked to malinger or finding exceptional cases of malingering and giving the test to these subjects. It also results in a statement of probability regarding malingering rather than the definitive statement that results from methods that use worse-than-chance responding. Unfortunately, normative studies of symptom validity tests rely on level of performance only and many brain-injured subjects probably score at the level of the malingering subjects. As a consequence, the score levels of malingering subjects will probably not be distinguishable from the brain injured subjects. This suggests that even normative comparisons will not significantly enhance the validity of symptom validity tests. In the end, these tests may be used and interpreted only when worse-than-chance responding occurs with the understanding that use of the tests will result in numerous false-negative determinations and that most malingerers will not be detected.

PERFORMANCE CONTRAST ANALYSIS IN THE DETECTION OF MALINGERING

Indirect references to a general theoretical model for malingering detection have appeared in a number of studies and discussions of malingering and factitious responding. For example, some authors point out that subjects who try to malinger or engage in factitious responding will attempt to mimic memory disorder as they understand it, and this understanding may significantly differ from true amnesia (Nies & Sweet, 1994). These discrepancies between true amnesia and the possibly incorrect understanding of it by the malingerer may result in significant markers of factitious responding. For example, most people do not know that patients with organic memory disorder usually have immediate recall scores (e.g., Digit Span) that are within the average range and only do badly on consolidation measures. As a consequence, most people will perform poorly in both areas when they try to malinger.

Another major difference between everyday knowledge of impairment and true impairment lies with general levels of ability associated with various types and levels of brain injury. People in everyday life who try to malinger have virtually no knowledge of the level of memory test scores that characterize specific brain illnesses, such as traumatic brain injury and cerebral vascular accident. Even neuropsychologists who have such general knowledge would probably have great difficulty producing the correct number of raw score errors that would result in the standard score levels that are associated with the brain illness the neuropsychologist is trying to mimic.

A third general trend will be for people who feign impairment to produce idiosyncratic responses that are believed by them to represent impaired performance (Rawling & Brooks, 1990). This is a common observation of clinicians who observe malingering. For example, when responding to the Digit Span task, one patient evaluated in the author's laboratory accurately reported every second digit of the digit string. Although the patient apparently felt this indicated impaired performance, and in fact the patient would receive a low score, this pattern of responses indicates a high level of sustained attention and immediate recall. This kind of idiosyncratic and unusual response is derived from the limited knowledge of the cognitive sequelae of brain injury available to everyday people who try to feign such disorders. They may eventually serve as markers of malingering and factitious responding. Indeed, Rawling and Brooks (1990) systematically collected a number of these unique signs for the Wechsler Adult Intelligence Scale and Wechsler Memory Scale and formed a type of inventory scale. Unfortunately, many of the items are so specific that malingering subjects do not produce them at a sufficient base rate that they are discriminating (Milanovich, Axelrod, & Millis, 1996).

THE METHOD OF PERFORMANCE CONTRASTS

All of these methods rely on the comparison of a subject's performance to known patterns of genuinely normal and impaired performance. If a subject performs at the level and pattern characteristic of brain injury, then the presence of brain injury is inferred. If the subjects perform at the impaired level but makes unusual errors, then the presence of malingering is suggested. Worse-than-chance performance represents an unexpected level of performance, rather than pattern. That is, this level is so low it is uncharacteristic of subjects with brain injury and normals. All of the detection methods examined thus far rely on such contrasts and it is possible that a general model of malingering detection might be created by the synthesis of previous findings and the development of a general approach to making these contrasts. In this way, a composite methodology could be designed that combines the best of a number of effective methods.

These observations are also similar to the type of analysis conducted by individual clinicians when they make the determination of malingering. Most clinical cases of malingering involve a patient whose report of cognitive impairment or test results are so unusual that the clinician concludes the patient is fabricating a disorder. Usually the inconsistencies increase over the course of the evaluation to the point where some critical point is attained and the clinician is compelled to infer that the patient is malingering. This informal reasoning process essentially involves assigning a probability to malingering status based on the accumulated inconsistencies.

If inconsistencies represent a method of detecting malingering, then they can be systematically and empirically summarized to formulate a valid and reliable malingering scale. Scores on this scale would then represent the probability that a subject is malingering or engaged in some pattern of factitious responding. As such, it would represent the unique discrepancies characteristics of factitious responding and not those that might characterize unique neuropsychological syndromes or poor responding in general.

SOURCES OF INCONSISTENCIES

If a patient claims severe impairment or produces very low memory scores following a mild head injury, then this represents an inconsistency that contributes to an assessment of factitious responding or malingering. If a patient performs very badly on one verbal memory test and well on another, then this likewise represents a discrepancy that contributes to an inference of factitious responding. These are two examples of the types of inconsistencies used by clinicians to make judgments of malingering and may be incorporated into an empirical model of malingering detection.

There are three major areas in which discrepancies occur that might be used to construct a malingering index: (1) the relationship of injury severity to cognitive function, (2) the interrelationship of subtests, (3) the relationship of premorbid abilities to abilities measured after the injury. The first area involves the relationship of level and type of brain illness to cognitive impairment following such illnesses. In general, injury severity level, as measured by such factors as coma level at admission and extent of brain lesion observed using neuroimaging, should allow for general predictions of cognitive outcome. Of course, such relationships represent the foundation of clinical neuropsychology. However, although much is known regarding these relationships in general, there is probably insufficient knowledge to form an empirical regression model. For example, there is sufficient knowledge of the relationship between traumatic brain injury severity measures and cognitive function to conclude that an empirical regression model may be constructed. However, because so few studies used correlation or regression models and there are no meta-analyses of the studies examining severity measures, a regression model cannot be constructed.

The second area involves the interrelationship of tests and subtests themselves. Tests and subtests are intercorrelated and predict each other. Inconsistencies are expressed as scores that are sufficiently disparate that they violate the known relationships between the tests. An extreme example would be a subject who scored very high on the Vocabulary subtest of the Wechsler Adult Intelligence Scale and very low on the General Information subtest. These two subtests are moderately correlated and individual scores should not be far apart. The degree of deviation can be calculated and the results can contribute to a discrepancy measure that represents the probability that an extraneous influence has affected the scores. In fact, these kinds of discrepancies among tests are those that factor into clinical judgments about malingering.

The final major source of discrepancies involves the relationship of premorbid status and current test results. For example, a nonaphasic, brain-injured subject with a high level of education should still have good spelling, arithmetic, and other academic skills after sustaining the brain injury. Likewise, verbal tests and others that have at least moderate correlations with education should maintain that relationship among individual subjects. Again, clinicians have discovered these discrepancies and use them to construct an inference of malingering. The most common situation involves a patient with a mild head injury who performs very badly on a test of an ability that should maintain premorbid levels, such as spelling or reading.

These factors also interact in the same sense that regression models combine variables with predictive power. For example, a patient with a high education who suffers a severe injury may have poor academic skills measured after the injury that are attributable to the brain injury. Although high premorbid education results in a prediction of high academic skills, the injury severity level suggests low scores are likely, even to include academic areas.

Fortunately, these areas probably represent independent sources of predictive power. Although premorbid demographics may be related to the occurrence of brain injury, available sources suggest that premorbid status is unrelated to injury severity; coma level, neurological deficits, and extent of brain lesion are certainly the result of the circumstances of the brain trauma itself and are not correlated with extent of education or other premorbid factors. Likewise, the interrelationship of tests should not be affected by injury severity or premorbid status. As a consequence of this independent source of predictive power, the measurement of inconsistency may be independently computed from known empirical relationships within each of these areas. There have been no investigations that have combined these areas so the specific knowledge of their independent or redundant relationships are not sufficiently known at the present time to compute regression coefficients.

SOURCES OF INFORMATION CONCERNING THESE FACTORS

The conventional method used to estimate premorbid abilities utilizes demographic variables that are correlated with IQ scores. These are combined into a regression model that represents the best composite of predictor variables (Barona, Reynolds, & Chastain, 1984). These variables most prominently include education and occupation. Premorbid prediction models that use demographic variables have moderate predictive power and have associated multiple *R* values of approximately .6. There are as yet no studies that have specifically examined methods to predict premorbid memory ability. However, there are indications of the predictive power of demographics in the relationship of IQ to memory test scores (Wechsler, 1987; Williams, 1992). This low to moderate relationship suggests that demographic variables probably also predict memory scores in a similar fashion as they predict IQ scores. In addition, the few investigations that have computed simple correlations suggest that regression models including education and occupation should represent low to moderate predictive power.

Such a model could be used to construct a component of a performance contrast measure. This would be done by computing the expected memory score using the demographic regression model and then subtracting this score from the one acquired from administration of a memory test. This adjusted score would then be combined with the ones produced by regression models derived from the other domains.

The major qualification of expected memory scores predicted by premorbid factors are scores predicted by injury status. Such predictions represent the second major domain of performance contrast. Unfortunately, empirical studies of injury severity as a predictor of cognitive outcome that have used regression models are rare. Although a few studies have reported independent simple correlations between severity measures and outcome, only Williams, Gomes, Drudge, and Kessler (1984) explicitly combined severity measured and premorbid estimates as predictors of IQ and the Halstead Impairment Index. They found that a premorbid estimate of cognitive function derived from demographic variables predicted postinjury cognitive function as well as a coma level at admission, a major severity measure describing closed head injury.

The only methods available to construct a regression model based on injury severity are those derived from meta-analysis. The mean differences and variances in memory scores for groups of patients with different levels of severity can be used to compute a correlation coefficient representing the relationship (Mullen & Rosenthal, 1985). This correlation can then be used to predict memory scores from injury severity measures. Unfortunately, a meta-analysis of the cognitive outcome of closed head injury, or any other brain illness, has never been conducted. It is not possible to construct the model until this is accomplished. However, short of complete regression studies, a meta-analytic method represents a good first step. It also represents a composite of all of the available studies rather than a model derived from one or a few studies using regression.

Until the meta-analysis is completed, there are only suggestions derived from individual studies and narrative reviews that might be used to construct some approximation of the model. The models formulated by clinical reasoners must also conform to knowledge of the relationship derived from these studies. For example, a clinician evaluating a patient who has sustained a mild head injury has an expectation for a level of performance derived from studies of mild head injury and other facts about this disorder extracted from clinical lore and experience. These expectations are apparent in the statements expressed by clinicians when a patient attains scores that are inconsistent with the expectations; a patient with mild head injury and highly educated who scores low on tests of verbal intelligence is suspected of malingering. This occurs because mild head injury has not been shown typically associated with impairment of such abilities.

A performance contrast could be developed from a single study or a group, short of meta-analysis. Of course, such a contrast would have greater error than one derived from a complete empirical study. For example, a series of studies of mild head injury could be contrasted with a series examining moderate and severe injuries. A general expectation could be constructed and combined with the expectations derived from premorbid status.

The final area of performance contrast involves the prediction of performance levels based on the interrelationship of subtests making up the neuropsychological examination. Virtually all of these tests have statistically significant interrelationships that should be maintained in an individual profile even when the subject performs poorly. For example, the Vocabulary and General Information subtests of the WAIS-R are correlated approximately .8 (Wechsler, 1981). This suggests that if one score is known, the other is likely to be similar. Other tests have similar relationships that could be used to construct a performance contrast. Clearly these relationships are also used by clinicians when making the inference of malingering. If a patient does very poorly in an inconsistent fashion, then the clinician suspects malingering. For example, if a subject does very well on the Arithmetic subtest of the WAIS-R and very poor on the Digit Span subtests, then the clinician may suspect a malingered performance on the Digit Span. This presumably occurs because the subject does not know that the tests are correlated. Malingering subjects also do not know what constitutes a bad score on every test.

A performance contrast could be easily constructed from known relationships between the tests making up the neuropsychological examination. A number of studies have reported the intercorrelation of subtests of the WAIS-R, the Halstead–Reitan Battery, the Luria–Nebraska Battery, memory tests, and a variety of other subtests. These could be used to construct a comparison score that would represent the degree to which the subject's actual scores represent known relationships between these tests. Unfortunately, multivariate studies of these relationships have also not been completely conducted such that a single prediction for each subtest would be possible. This could only be done using the results of a factor analysis involving all of the most common instruments in one analysis. In this way, an estimated score for a single test could be computed by a linear combination of the weights corresponding to each factor. However, all of the required factor analyses have not been done. The performance contrasts must be constructed from the WAIS-R and the other batteries that have been factor analyzed and individual correlations must be used for the remaining tests and for relationships between test batteries. For example, the score on the Vocabulary subtest of the WAIS-R can be predicted by the corresponding linear composite of weights derived from the factor analysis of the WAIS-R subtests (Cohen, 1957).

Another approach might simply include the one or two subtests that have the highest correlation with the target subtest. A performance estimate could be derived from these that would probably approximate the predictive power of multivariate procedures.

SUMMARY AND FUTURE DIRECTIONS

A major, largely unforeseen development in the history of clinical neuropsychology was the prominent role practitioners now play in the determination of personal injury in cases of traumatic brain injury and other brain illness under litigation. The common tendency to reify tests and enhance their validity, which often does not have a public setting in which to be challenged, now comes directly into conflict with clients who try to fake a bad performance on tests; clinical neuropsychologists are confronted in a public manner with a threat to the validity of their tests and their own expertise. If a patient could malinger a bad performance and have such an undistinguished profile on the tests that the patient could not be detected, then the neuropsychological tests themselves have uncertain validity. Reactions to this situation and the general denial of the prevalence of malingering have generally subsided as forensic neuropsychology has matured. After all, why would neuropsychologists have less difficulty with malingering than any other expert in the forensic setting (Daniel & Resnick, 1987; Dush, Simons, Platt, Nation, & Ayres, 1994; Harris, 1979; Keltner, May, Johnson, & Post, 1985)? The study of malingering has moved beyond the controversies about whether clinicians are able and willing to detect it (Bigler, 1990; Faust, 1995a; Fast & Guilmette, 1990); the developing literature clearly suggests that clinicians using conventional strategies of interpretation cannot detect malingering and need some new systematic approach to the interpretation of conventional tests or new specialized symptom validity tests.

As long as a substantial number of malingering patients perform better than chance on the forced-choice symptom validity tests, they will not be the final answer to malingering determination. Although their sensitivity is likely poor, they will probably have some place in the assessment of malingering because of their specificity. Subjects who actually perform worse than chance are doing so poorly that they logically must be malingering. Unfortunately, the great majority of malingering subjects do not apparently perform worse than chance.

The future investigation of symptom validity tests should include a variety of methods in addition to the forced-choice, recognition procedures that have been used in the past. The contrast of recall and recognition methods should be developed as part of a specific symptom validity test. They should also be expanded to include other patterns of responding, such as consistency measures and response latency (Beetar & Williams, 1995; Frederick & Foster, 1991). Priming and implicit processes should also be examined and contrasted with declarative memory abilities (Horton, Smith, Barghout, & Connolly, 1992). They can also be expanded to include other cognitive functions, such as speech sounds discrimination (Aplin & Kane, 1985), sensory perception (Binder, 1992; Pankratz, Fausti, & Peed, 1975), and visuospatial memory (Frederick et al., 1994).

Future research should be directed toward discriminating types of factitious responding. It may be possible to distinguish malingering from unconscious exaggeration of deficits. These may also be distinguished from psychological depression, conversion hysteria, dissociative amnesia, and other disorders that are associated with attempts to perform worse than one actually can perform. If distinctive patterns are discovered, then this would considerably reduce the confusion and controversy in the definition of malingering itself.

A common clinical observation of malingerers is that they do not make subtle distinctions in the tests they attempt to fake (Nies & Sweet, 1994). They cannot discriminate which neurological functions were assessed as an attempt to simply detect malingering. Future studies should investigate the hypothesis that malingerers will fake on a variety of procedures, including physiological measures, and whether these are correlated. If such tests predict each other, then this allows for the use of the contrast between physiological measures, such as EMG and evoked potentials and their functional equivalents, as malingering detectors (Howard & Dorfman, 1986). For example, it is possible to absolutely determine if a subject is malingering an auditory acuity impairment by contrasting the typical functional auditory perception test with auditory evoked potentials (Musiek, Bornstein, & Rintelmann, 1995; Rickards & De, 1995; Sulkowski, Sliwinska, Kowalska, & Bazydlo, 1994). Malingerers may report hearing loss but the evoked potential study verifies that hearing occurs. If malingerers who report memory disorder also manifest faking on tests of auditory perception, then these highly accurate tests can be used to predict the presence of malingered memory disorder.

Another method that should be explored is the use of contrary malingering instructions in the introduction to the testing session. Such instructions include statements such as, "We have methods designed to assess whether you have given your complete and honest effort during the test session. These methods have an extremely high degree of accuracy. We can determine whether a test subject is attempting to perform worse than possible on the tests." If they work, such instructions will obviate the use of symptom validity tests or any elaborate malingering detection method: No one will attempt to fake bad!

The final area of promising new approaches involves the development of performance contrasts. This technique elaborates the concept of inconsistencies in the interrelationship of items and subtests, and injury severity and premorbid factors and subsequent test findings. If malingerers express any inconsistency or patterns that are contrary to normal and impaired abilities, then a general performance contrast method should detect them. Performance contrasts have been developed in rudimentary forms (Rawling & Brooks, 1990) and make up the foundation of clinical judgments of malingering. However, the future will bring a number of methods derived from multivariate procedures and the meta-analysis of studies of these factors.

The success of malingering detection rests on the answer to this question: Do malingerers produce a different pattern of performance on neuropsychological tests than brain-injured subjects? If they do not, then research studies will never find a method to discriminate them from brain-injured subjects using specialized or conventional tests. This may be the true state of malingering, and the lack of an underlying, valid difference between the groups may explain the general failure of symptom validity tests and the inability of clinicians to detect malingering. Because poor memory is an undeniable fact of life among people without brain injury, it may be possible to exaggerate the usual errors one experiences in everyday life and produce a convincing impairment of memory following a mild head injury. Of course, this conclusion is not yet proven and many areas that may render discriminating variables have yet to be examined. The great hope of this entire area of investigation is that there is some measure or construct in which the malingerer systematically performs in a manner different from brain-injured subjects. As virtually no malingering subjects have any idea of the unique features of true neuropsychological syndromes, measures of these unique features should be the foundation of performance contrasts between the malingering subject's performance and true memory disorder. Thus far, this general model of malingering detection is greatly understudied and should form the foundation of a number of new malingering detection methods.

REFERENCES

Allen, C. C., & Ruff, R. M. (1990). Self-rating versus neuropsychological performance of moderate versus severe head-injured patients. *Brain Injury*, *4*(1), 7–17.

Aplin, D. Y., & Kane, J. M. (1985). Variables affecting pure tone and speech audiometry in experimentally simulated hearing loss. *British Journal of Audiology*, *19*(3), 219–228.

Arnett, P.A., Hammeke, T. A., & Schwartz, L. (1995). Quantitative and qualitative performance on Rey's 15-Item Test in neurological patients and dissimulators. *The Clinical Neuropsychologist*, *9*(1), 17–26.

Barona, A., Reynolds, C. R., & Chastain, R. (1984). A demographically based index of premorbid intelligence for the WAIS–R. *Journal of Consulting and Clinical Psychology*, *52*(5), 885–887.

Beetar, J. T., & Williams, J. M. (1995). Malingering response styles on the Memory Assessment Scales and symptom validity tests. *Archives of Clinical Neuropsychology*, *10*(1), 57–72.

Benton, A., & Spreen, O. (1961). Visual memory test: The simulation of mental incompetence. *Archives of General Psychiatry*, *4*, 79–83.

Bernard, L. C. (1990). Prospects for faking believable memory deficits on neuropsychological tests and the use of incentives in simulation research. *Journal of Clinical and Experimental Neuropsychology*, *12*(5), 715–728.

Bernard, L. C. (1991). The detection of faked deficits on the Rey Auditory Verbal Learning Test: The effect of serial position. *Archives of Clinical Neuropsychology*, *6*(1–2), 81–88.

Bernard, L. C., Houston, W., & Natoli, L. (1993). Malingering on neuropsychological memory tests: Potential objective indicators. *Journal of Clinical Psychology*, *49*(1), 45–53.

Bernard, L. C., McGrath, M. J., & Houston, W. (1993). Discriminating between simulated malingering and closed head injury on the Wechsler Memory Scale–Revised. *Archives of Clinical Neuropsychology*, *8*(6), 539–551.

Bigler, E. D. (1990). Neuropsychology and malingering: Comment on Faust, Hart, and Guilmette (1988). *Journal of Consulting and Clinical Psychology*, *58*(2), 244–247.

Binder, L. M. (1992). Forced-choice testing provides evidence of malingering. *Archives of Physical Medicine and Rehabilitation*, *73*(4), 377–380.

Binder, L. M. (1993). Assessment of malingering after mild head trauma with the Portland Digit Recognition Test [published erratum appears in J Clin Exp Neuropsychol 1993 Nov; 15(6):852]. *Journal of Clinical and Experimental Neuropsychology*, *15*(2), 170–182.

Binder, L. M., & Pankratz, L. (1987). Neuropsychological evidence of a factitious memory complaint. *Journal of Clinical and Experimental Neuropsychology*, *9*(2), 167–171.

Blakely, T. J., & Harrington, D. E. (1993). Mild head injury is not always mild; implications for damage litigation. *Medicine, Science and the Law*, *33*(3), 231–242.

Brady, J. P. (1966). Hysteria versus malingering: A response to Grosz and Zimmerman. *Behaviour Research and Therapy*, *4*(4), 321–322.

Brandt, J., Rubinsky, E., & Lassen, G. (1985). Uncovering malingered amnesia. *Annals of the New York Academy of Sciences*, *444*(502), 502–503.

Braverman, M. (1978). Post-injury malingering is seldom a calculated ploy. *Occupational Health and Safety*, *47*(2), 36–40.

Brittain, J. L., LaMarche, J. A., Reeder, K. P., Roth, D. L., & Boll, T. J. (1991). Effects of age and IQ on Paced Auditory Serial Addition Task (PASAT) performance. *The Clinical Neuropsychologist, 5*, 163–175.

Cliffe, M. J. (1992). Symptom-validity testing of feigned sensory or memory deficits: A further elaboration for subjects who understand the rationale. *British Journal of Clinical Psychology, 31*(Pt. 2), 207–209.

Cohen, J. (1957). The factorial structure of the WAIS between early adulthood and old age. *Journal of Consulting Psychology, 21*, 283–290.

Cullum, C., Heaton, R., & Grant, I. (1991). Psychogenic factors influencing neuropsychological performance: Somatoform disorders, factitious disorders and malingering. In H. O. Doerr & A. S. Carlin (Eds.), *Forensic neuropsychology*. (pp. 36–72). New York: Guilford Press.

Daniel, A. E., & Resnick, P. J. (1987). Mutism, malingering, and competency to stand trial. *Bulletin of the American Academy of Psychiatry and the Law, 15*(3), 301–308.

Delis, D. (1987). *The California Verbal Learning Test*. San Antonio, TX: The Psychological Corporation.

Dush, D. M., Simons, L. E., Platt, M., Nation, P. C., & Ayres, S. Y. (1994). Psychological profiles distinguishing litigating and nonlitigating pain patients: Subtle, and not so subtle. *Journal of Personality Assessment, 62*(2), 299–313.

Faust, D. (1995a). The detection of deception. Special Issue: Malingering and conversion reactions. *Neurologic Clinics, 13*(2), 255–265.

Faust, D. (1995b). The detection of deception [Review]. *Neurologic Clinics, 13*(2), 255–265.

Faust, D., & Guilmette, T. J. (1990). To say it's not so doesn't prove that it isn't: Research on the detection of malingering. Reply to Bigler. *Journal of Consulting and Clinical Psychology, 58*(2), 248–250.

Franzen, M. D., Iverson, G. L., & McCracken, L. M. (1990). The detection of malingering in neuropsychological assessment. *Neuropsychology Review, 1*(3), 247–279.

Frederick, R. I., & Foster, H. G. (1991). Multiple measures of malingering on a forced-choice test of cognitive ability. *Psychological Assessment, 3*(4), 596–602.

Frederick, R. I., Sarfaty, S. D., Johnston, J. D., & Powel, J. (1994). Validation of a detector of response bias on a forced-choice test of nonverbal ability. *Neuropsychology, 8*(1), 118–125.

Gilbertson, A. D., Torem, M., Cohen, R., & Newman, I. (1992). Susceptibility of common self-report measures of dissociation to malingering. *Dissociation: Progress in the Dissociative Disorders, 5*(4), 216–220.

Goebel, R. A. (1983). Detection of faking on the Halstead–Reitan Neuropsychological Test Battery. *Journal of Clinical Psychology, 39*(5), 731–742.

Gold, S., Lubinsky, R., & Shahar, A. (1981). Speech discrimination scores at low sensation levels as a possible index of malingering. *Journal of Auditory Research, 21*(2), 137–141.

Gorman, W. F. (1982). Defining malingering [Review]. *Journal of Forensic Sciences, 27*(2), 401–407.

Gouvier, W. D., Uddo-Crane, M., & Brown, L. (1988). Base rates of post-concussion symptoms. *Archives of Clinical Neuropsychology, 3*, 273–278.

Guilmette, T. J., Hart, K. J., & Giuliano, A. J. (1993). Malingering detection: The use of a forced-choice method in identifying organic versus simulated memory impairment. *The Clinical Neuropsychologist, 7*(1), 59–69.

Harris, D. A. (1979). Detecting non-valid hearing tests in industry. *Journal of Occupational Medicine, 21*(12), 814–820.

Heaton, R. K., Smith, H. H., Lehman, R. A., & Vogt, A. T. (1978). Prospects for faking believable deficits on neuropsychological testing. *Journal of Consulting and Clinical Psychology, 46*(5), 892–900.

Hiscock, C. K., Branham, J. D., & Hiscock, M. (1994). Detection of feigned cognitive impairment: The two-alternative forced-choice method compared with selected conventional tests. *Journal of Psychopathology and Behavioral Assessment, 16*(2), 95–110.

Horton, K. D., Smith, S. A., Barghout, N. K., & Connolly, D. A. (1992). The use of indirect memory tests to assess malingered amnesia: A study of metamemory. *Journal of Experimental Psychology: General, 121*(3), 326–351.

Howard, J. E., & Dorfman, L. J. (1986). Evoked potentials in hysteria and malingering. *Journal of Clinical Neurophysiology, 3*(1), 39–49.

Iverson, G. L. (1995). Qualitative aspects of malingered memory deficits. *Brain Injury, 9*(1), 35–40.

Iverson, G. L., & Franzen, M. D. (1994). The Recognition Memory Test, Digit Span, and Knox Cube Test as markers of malingered memory impairment. *Assessment, 1*(4), 323–334.

Iverson, G. L., Franzen, M. D., & McCracken, L. M. (1991). Evaluation of an objective assessment technique for the detection of malingered memory deficits. *Law and Human Behavior, 15*(6), 667–676.

Iverson, G. L., Franzen, M. D., & McCracken, L. M. (1994). Application of a forced-choice memory procedure designed to detect experimental malingering. *Archives of Clinical Neuropsychology, 9*(5), 437–450.

Keltner, J. L., May, W. N., Johnson, C. A., & Post, R. B. (1985). The California syndrome. Functional visual complaints with potential economic impact. *Ophthalmology, 92*(3), 427–435.

Larrabee, G. J. (1992). On modifying recognition memory tests for detection of malingering. *Neuropsychology, 6*(1), 23–27.

Lee, G. P., Loring, D. W., & Martin, R. C. (1992). Rey's 15-Item Visual Memory Test for the detection of malingering: Normative observations on patients with neurological disorders. *Psychological Assessment, 4*(1), 43–46.

Martin, R. C., Bolter, J. F., Todd, M. E., & Gouvier, W. D. (1993). Effects of sophistication and motivation on the detection of malingered memory performance using a computerized forced-choice task. *Journal of Clinical and Experimental Neuropsychology, 15*(6), 867–880.

Milanovich, J. R., Axelrod, B. N., & Millis, S. R. (1996). Validation of the Simulation Index-Revised with a mixed clinical population. *Archives of Clinical Neuropsychology, 11*(1), 53–60.

Millis, S. R. (1994). Assessment of motivation and memory with the Recognition Memory Test after financially compensable mild head injury. *Journal of Clinical Psychology, 50*(4), 601–605.

Millis, S. R., & Kler, S. (1995). Limitations of the Rey Fifteen-Item Test in the detection of malingering. *The Clinical Neuropsychologist, 9*(3), 241–244.

Millis, S. R., & Putnam, S. J. (1994). The Recognition Memory Test in the assessment of memory impairment after financially compensable mild head injury: A replication. *Perceptual and Motor Skills, 79*(1, Pt. 2), 384–386.

Millis, S. R., Putnam, S. H., Adams, K. M., & Ricker, J. H. (1995). The California Verbal Learning Test in the detection of incomplete effort in neuropsychological evaluation. *Psychological Assessment, 7*(4), 241–244.

Mittenberg, W., Azrin, R., Millsaps, C., & Heilbronner, R. (1993). Identification of malingered head injury on the Wechsler Memory Scale–Revised. *Psychological Assessment, 5*(1), 34–40.

Mullen, B., & Rosenthal, R. (1985). *Basic meta-analysis. Procedures and programs.* Hillsdale, NJ: Erlbaum.

Musiek, F. E., Bornstein, S. P., & Rintelmann, W. F. (1995). Transient evoked otoacoustic emissions and pseudohypacusis. *Journal of the American Academy of Audiology, 6*(4), 293–301.

Nies, K. J., & Sweet, J. J. (1994). Neuropsychological assessment and malingering: A critical review of past and present strategies. *Archives of Clinical Neuropsychology, 9*(6), 501–552.

Owens, R. G. (1995). The psychological signatures of malingering: Assessing the legitimacy of claims. *American Journal of Forensic Psychology, 13*(1), 61–75.

Palmer, B. W., Boone, K. B., Allman, L., & Castro, D. B. (1995). Co-occurrence of brain lesions and cognitive deficit exaggeration. *The Clinical Neuropsychologist, 9*(1), 68–73.

Pankratz, L. (1983). A new technique for the assessment and modification of feigned memory deficit. *Perceptual and Motor Skills, 57*(2), 367–372.

Pankratz, L., Fausti, S. A., & Peed, S. (1975) A forced-choice technique to evaluate deafness in the hysterical or malingering patient. *Journal of Consulting and Clinical Psychology*, *43*(3), 421–422.

Perkin, G. D. (1994). Conversion hysteria/malingering. *Journal of Neurology, Neurosurgery and Psychiatry*, *57*(8), 1004–1005.

Rawling, P., & Brooks, N. (1990). Simulation Index: A method for detecting factitious errors on the WAIS-R and WMS. *Neuropsychology*, *4*, 223–238.

Resnick, P. J. (1993). Defrocking the fraud: The detection of malingering. *Israel Journal of Psychiatry and Related Sciences*, *30*(2), 93–101.

Rickards, F. W., & De, V. S. (1995). Exaggerated hearing loss in noise induced hearing loss compensation claims in Victoria. *Medical Journal of Australia*, *163*(7), 360–363.

Rose, F. E., Hall, S., Szalda, P., & Allen, D. (1995). Portland Digit Recognition Test–computerized: Measuring response latency improves the detection of malingering. *The Clinical Neuropsychologist*, *9*(2), 124–134.

Samuel, A. W. (1977). A review of malingering and hysteria in clinical practice [Review]. *Annals of the Royal College of Surgeons of England*, *59*(6), 511–513.

Schacter, D. L. (1986). On the relation between genuine and simulated amnesia. *Behavioral Sciences and the Law*, *4*(1) 4–64.

Schacter, D., & Crovitz, H. (1977). Memory function after closed head injury: A review of the quantitative research. *Cortex*, *13*, 105–176.

Schretlen, D., Brandt, J., Krafft, L., & Van Gorp, W. (1991). Some caveats in using the Rey 15-Item Memory Test to detect malingered amnesia. *Psychological Assessment*, *3*(4), 667–672.

Simon, M. J. (1994). The use of the Rey Memory Test to assess malingering in criminal defendants. *Journal of Clinical Psychology*, *50*(6), 913–917.

Slick, D., Hopp, G., Strauss, E., Hunter, M., & Pinch, D. (1994). Detecting dissimulation: Profiles of simulated malingerers, traumatic brain-injury patients, and normal controls on a revised version of Hiscock and Hiscock's Forced-Choice Memory Test. *Journal of Clinical and Experimental Neuropsychology*, *16*(3), 472–481.

Snow, W. G., Tierney, M. C., Zorzitto, M. L., Fisher, R. H., & Reid, D. W. (1990). The place of cooperation in the examination of neuropsychological impairment. *Archives of Clinical Neuropsychology*, *5*, 243–249.

Spreen, O., & Benton, A. (1963). Simulation of mental deficiency on a visual memory test. *American Journal of Mental Deficiency*, *67*, 909–913.

Stevens, H. (1986). Is it organic or is it functional: Is it hysteria or malingering? *Psychiatric Clinics of North America*, *9*(2), 241–254.

Strauss, E., Spellacy, F., Hunter, M., & Berry, T. (1994). Assessing believable deficits on measures of attention and information processing capacity. *Archives of Clinical Neuropsychology*, *9*(6), 483–490.

Sulkowski, W., Śliwinska, K. M., Kowalska, S., & Bazydlo, G. G. (1994). Electric response audiometry and compensational noise-induced hearing loss. *Otolaryngologia Polska*, *48*(4), 370–374.

Trueblood, W., & Schmidt, M. (1993). Malingering and other validity considerations in the neuropsychological evaluation of mild head injury. *Journal of Clinical and Experimental Neuropsychology*, *15*(4), 578–590.

Vander, K., & Charles, J. (1993). Client self-report: Assessment of accuracy. *Journal of Applied Rehabilitation Counseling*, *24*(30), 22–25.

Wechsler, D. (1981). *The Wechsler Adult Intelligence Scale*. San Antonio, TX: The Psychological Corporation.

Wechsler, D. (1987). *The Wechsler Memory Scale–Revised*. San Antonio, TX: The Psychological Corporation.

Wedding, D., & Faust, D. (1989). Clinical judgement and decision-making in neuropsychology. *Archives of Clinical Neuropsychology*, *4*, 233–265.

Wiggins, E. C., & Brandt, J. (1988). The detection of simulated amnesia. *Law and Human Behavior, 12*(1), 57–78.

Williams, J. M. (1992). *The Memory Assessment Scales*. Odessa, FL: Psychological Assessment Resources.

Williams, J. M., Gomes, F., Drudge, O., & Kessler, M. (1984). Predicting outcome from closed head injury by early assessment of trauma severity. *Journal of Neurosurgery, 61*, 581–585.

Wong, J. L., Regennitter, R. P., & Barrios, F. (1994). Base rate and simulated symptoms of mild head injury among normals. *Archives of Clinical Neuropsychology, 9*(5), 370–383.

5

Detecting Malingering on the Luria–Nebraska Neuropsychological Battery

CHARLES J. GOLDEN AND CHRISTINE A. GRIER

Malingering is a condition in which a patient consciously feigns symptoms of a physical or psychological disorder for the purposes of gain. This purpose may be conscious or unconscious in terms of the individuals' awareness of their own motivation. However, the attempts to falsify test responses are deliberate.

The incentive for deception usually involves the avoidance of criminal responsibility, the acquisition of monetary compensation through bad faith litigation or disability claims, retaliation for some perceived loss, or a need for recognition as to the seriousness of their problems. Individuals may deceive themselves as to their reason for deception, perhaps feeling that the deception is the only way in which "true" justice or the proper outcome may be achieved. Malingerers may feel quite justified in their behavior rather than regarding it as a deception or as a criminal act.

Malingering is especially complicated in that it may appear both in a pure form, where the client is truly intact, and in a mixed form, in which the client has a combination of real and feigned or exaggerated problems. Malingering must always be separated from exaggeration related to unconscious factors, an inability to cooperate for emotional or neurological reasons, or an inability to tolerate the stress of normal testing situations. This is especially important in brain injury as clients' judgment and reasoning may be quite impaired leading to bizarre behaviors that can cover up a real brain injury.

CHARLES J. GOLDEN AND CHRISTINE A. GRIER • Center for Psychological Services, Nova Southeastern University, Fort Lauderdale, Florida 33314.

Detection of Malingering during Head Injury Litigation, edited by Reynolds. Plenum Press, New York, 1998.

Neuropsychological tests are generally highly susceptible to malingering. If an individual is intact, the nature of a right or wrong answer may be very clear. In such cases, giving a wrong answer is easy and requires little sophistication or knowledge about the tests or about neuropsychology. Both a simple lack of motivation and a high level of apathy can also result from brain injury and can cause malingering-like profiles unintentionally: in the presence of deliberate deception, such lack of trying is simple to reproduce and complex to identify.

Initially, neuropsychological tests were not used for purposes of assessing for malingering. Neuropsychological tests were intended to assess premorbidly normal people who had acquired a brain injury. Such people were assumed to be motivated to do well except in circumstances where they were fatigued or unwilling to be tested, conditions that could easily be identified by the clinician without the use of additional instrumentation.

However, over time, neuropsychologists came to be used as expert witnesses in personal injury and criminal cases. These conditions produced the motivation to malinger and introduced the possibility of sophisticated malingering where the client was deliberately trying to affect test results in a negative manner. Failure to detect malingering on neuropsychological tests can result in unjust compensation and evasion from criminal prosecution, as well as other undeserved benefits. As a result of the increased use of neuropsychologists in the legal system, several instruments have been created to assess for malingering.

The Luria–Nebraska Neuropsychological Battery (LNNB) was originally developed at a time when malingering was not considered a major issue. Issues of fatigue, motivation, ability to cooperate, and the like were considered in the design of the original test, but not the issue of deliberate faking. Over the past two decades, however, users of the LNNB have faced the same challenges as users of other neuropsychological tests, and a variety of methods for detecting malingering have been developed.

INTRODUCTION TO THE LNNB

There are currently three forms of the LNNB. Forms I and II are very similar to one another, consisting of 12 basic clinical scales plus a series of scales derived for specific additional purposes. The test items are all scored as 0 (normal), 1 (borderline), or 2 (abnormal). Each scale of the test uses items that revolve around a basic theme: Motor, Tactile, Rhythm, Visual, Receptive, Expressive, Reading, Writing, Arithmetic, Memory, Intelligence, and Intermediate Memory.

The Motor scale consists of items that measure speed, coordination, copying, drawing, and the execution of motor acts from verbal instructions of varying complexity. The Rhythm scale includes items to detect the ability to discriminate tones and rhythmic patterns, and to reproduce specific tones and rhythmic patterns.

The Tactile scale evaluates tactile sensitivity (including two-point discrimination), finger agnosia, fingertip number writing, and stereognosis.

The Visual scale consists of a range of nonmotor visual items ranging from basic identification to spatial analysis, three-dimensional analysis, foreground–background discrimination, overlapping figures, and visual closure. The Receptive Language scale consists of items that test phonemic discrimination, following basic commands, and following complex commands. Expressive Language involves items that require repetition, pronunciation, verbal expressive sequences, and expressive–intellectual items that require the completion of sentences and the generation of speech on specific topics.

Three scales measure achievement-type skills. These include the Writing scale, which measures the ability to copy letters, generate letters on request, and write words and sentences. The evaluation includes both motor writing and spelling abilities. Reading includes the ability to recognize letters, generate the sounds for letters, reading nonsense syllables, and reading words and sentences. The Arithmetic scale evaluates the ability to read and write numbers, do simple calculations, and do simple algebraic problems.

The Memory scale examines short-term memory with and without interference. Items focus on verbal and nonverbal immediate memory. The Intermediate Memory scale attempts to look at delayed memory, asking the client questions about items within the test as a whole that must be retained or recognized over a 1- to 3-hour period of time. Finally, the Intelligence scale measures those basic skills as seen in tests like the WAIS and the Stanford–Binet. This includes vocabulary, similarities, metaphors, reasoning, verbal arithmetic, picture arrangement, absurdities, and generalizations.

In addition to these standard "clinical scales" the test items can be used to generate special-purpose scales (as is done with the Minnesota Multiphasic Personality Inventory). For the purposes of this chapter, the most important derived score is Pathognomonic, a scale derived to measure the acuteness and general functional seriousness of a brain injury. This scale, using items scattered across the test, is sensitive to a wide range of brain injury and difficult to fake in a "believable" brain injury profile.

All of the LNNB scores are reported as T scores with a mean of 50 and a standard deviation of 10. High scores are indicative of more dysfunction. An abnormal score for any individual is determined by the individual's critical level, a score determined by the person's age and education. The critical level can vary from about 50 to 70 depending on these background variables. For the purposes of this chapter, however, all scores have been adjusted so that all presented cases have a critical level of 60.

When test scores are profiled, each scale is assigned a summary number for graphing purposes which will be used throughout this chapter. The appropriate summary symbols for each scale are as follows: Motor (C1), Rhythm (C2), Tactile

(C3), Visual (C4), Receptive Language (C5), Expressive Language (C6), Writing (C7), Reading (C8), Arithmetic (C9), Memory (C10), Intelligence (C11), Intermediate Memory (C12), and Pathognomonic (PATH).

The latest form of the test (Form III) is a substantially revised version generated initially from a factor analysis of results from the original scales. New scales were identified that were more factorially pure and that showed better psychometric characteristics. In addition, areas not tested by Forms I and II were added to the test to make it more comprehensive, and overall procedures were streamlined to shorten the length of the test. In addition to covering all of the areas in the initial tests, Form III has added coverage for nonverbal sound interpretation, visual-intellectual skills, speeded repetition, reading comprehension, and spelling while also revising the memory scales and adding separate scales for visual and verbal memory.

Form III also uses a T-score system with a mean of 50 and a standard deviation of 10, but for this form low scores reflect poor performance. For consistency, only Form I and II cases are used in this chapter but special rules for Form III are noted when they differ from Forms I and II.

DETECTING MALINGERING

The major approaches suggested for detecting malingering with the LNNB include (1) the addition of other tests specifically designed to measure malingering, (2) the use of specific formulas or LNNB scores, (3) the use of forced-choice analysis on those portions of the LNNB where they are appropriate, (4) the internal consistency of the LNNB scores, (5) test–retest reliability of the LNNB for both scales and items, and (6) the relationship between LNNB scores and neurological and historical information. These will be examined individually in the next sections.

Using Additional Test Devices

One common technique used with the LNNB has been the addition of tests specifically aimed at malingering. As these tests are reviewed elsewhere, they are not reviewed here in detail but we will briefly review some techniques that appear promising and have been used with the LNNB in the past.

One new technology in detecting symptom exaggeration or malingering of memory deficits is termed *symptom validity testing* (SVT; Bernard, 1990). SVT is any multiple-trial, forced-choice task specifically designed to detect simulated cognitive or sensory impairment (Bickart, Meyer, & Connell, 1991).

According to Guilmette, Hart, and Giuliano (1993), symptom validity techniques typically involve the administration of forced-choice formats where subjects are asked to recognize a previously presented stimulus from among two stimuli. According to binomial probability theory, it is expected that even subjects with true memory disturbances will perform at chance level. Any performance below chance level suggests that the subjects may be attempting to feign neuropsychological deficits.

The most common symptom validity measure designed to be used as a clinical test for malingering is the Portland Digit Recognition Test (PDRT), which is a forced-choice recognition memory test (Binder, 1993). Because the patient is forced to choose between two options, binomial probability analysis holds that random responding should produce a score of 50%. Worse-than-chance responding over many trials is therefore interpreted as a systematic effort to respond incorrectly. However, probability analysis may be ineffective for detecting more sophisticated attempts to feign impairment.

Binder and Willis (1991) found that brain-damaged individuals who were not seeking financial compensation for injuries performed significantly better than mild head injury patients who were seeking compensation. In a separate study, Binder (1993) suggested that poor performances on the PDRT are associated with a motivation to exaggerate impairments for financial gain. The data also support the use of the PDRT as a valid test of exaggerated memory impairment.

Consistent with findings by Hiscock and Hiscock (1989), Binder (1993) also demonstrated that patients who were seeking financial compensation performed more poorly on PDRT items that appeared to be more difficult than patients not seeking compensation. It appears that an increase in perceived item difficulty may invite a person inclined to malinger to perform less well on tasks that appear hard than on tasks that appear easy. Data thus support the use of the PDRT as a valid test of exaggerated memory impairment.

The Hiscock Digit-Memory Test (HDMT) was developed as an alternative to the more obvious measures of motivation that are disguised as memory tests (Slick, Hopp, Strauss, Hunter, & Pinch, 1994). Hiscock and Hiscock (1989) attempted to increase face validity on the HDMT by increasing the length of time between presentation and recognition so as to increase perceived difficulty by the subject (Slick et al., 1994).

Slick, Hopp, and Strauss (1992) made two major modifications to the HDMT to produce the Victoria Revision, which was designed to be a more efficient means of detecting dissimulation or motivational problems (cited in Slick et al., 1994). Slick et al. (1994) found that all subjects feigning memory impairment performed significantly worse than brain injury patients, especially on the portion of the test that appeared to be more difficult.

Guilmette et al. (1993) found that a brain-injured group was able to perform the HDMT successfully at a cutoff rate of 90% correct. This led Guilmette and colleagues to suggest that the 50% hit rate is far too conservative and should be increased to approximately 90%, as 100% of the brain-injured subjects were correctly classified at this rate. Similarly, Prigatano and Amin (1993) found that even for patients with severe cerebral dysfunction, performance ranged between 95 and 100%. By contrast, the suspected malingerers performed at about 74% correct.

Martin, Bolter, Todd, Gouvier, and Niccolls (1993) devised a computerized forced-choice recognition memory test that was modeled after the HDMT to provide clinicians a convenient, standardized method for stimulus presentation and scoring. Martin et al. (1993) found that performances of brain-injured patients were almost identical to the control group and well above both groups of malingerers.

Gfeller, Cradock, and Falkenhain (1994) administered the Seashore Rhythm Test to three groups of undergraduate students. As expected, subjects simulating cognitive impairment performed significantly lower than those instructed to perform optimally. However, the subjects who were provided information regarding deficits commonly experienced after head injuries did not perform differently than those who were not provided such information (Gfeller et al., 1994).

Bernard (1990) was interested in examining the ability to fake believable memory impairments on several widely used neuropsychological tests of memory. The author, following guidelines put forth by Rogers (1988a), administered the WMS-R, the ROCFT, the RMT, and the AVLT to three groups: a control group, a malingering incentive group, and a malingering nonincentive group (cited in Bernard, 1990). Prior to testing the experimenter offered a $50 bonus to the two individuals from the malingering incentive group who provided the most convincing display of memory disturbance. The malingering groups both performed significantly worse on the memory tests than the control group, but the incentive group did not perform significantly different than the nonincentive group. A discriminant function analysis produced an accuracy rate of 77% on cross-validation. Malingerers were generally identified on the basis of poorer performance on recognition versus recall tasks.

Each of these tests is reasonably short and fits in well with the administration of the LNNB. It is recommended that these tests be integrated into the administration of the LNNB by giving them sometime during the middle of the test. In this way, additional attention will not be drawn to these tests during the administration.

Scores on the LNNB

As noted earlier, the LNNB was not designed with the detection of malingering (by the objective scores) as a goal. However, some formal and informal studies have attempted to evaluate scores or patterns that could identify malingerers.

Mensch and Woods (1986) administered the LNNB to 32 subjects with average and above-average IQs who were offered a small reward for appearing brain-injured. The researchers in this study sought to determine if the above average subjects were more capable of feigning brain injury on the LNNB.

In a multivariate analysis of the effects of sex, IQ, and instructions to feign injury or not on the LNNB, Mensch and Woods discovered that the only statistically significant factor in feigning brain injury was the instruction to feign or not. Therefore, subjects with above-average intellectual abilities were not more capable of feigning brain injury than subjects of average intellectual ability.

In addition, Mensch and Woods (1986) discovered that only 16% of the subjects instructed to feign brain injury on the LNNB produced deficits on the Pathognomonic scale, which according to Golden, Hammeke, and Purisch (1980) was devised "in order to bring together items that are highly indicative of brain damage and are rarely missed by patients with a thought disorder or patients with peripheral neurological involvement" (p. 63) (cited in Mensch & Woods, 1986). Therefore, the assertion can be made that the Pathognomonic Scale is sensitive to malingering subjects.

Golden (1992), in an unpublished study, compared two groups of 10 normal subjects asked to malinger. The first group of malingerers was told that their goal was to fool the examiner into believing they had a brain injury without being caught. They were given a basic history and a set of complaints to tell their examiner.

The second group was simply told to produce test results that would show they were brain-injured and were also given a basic history and a set of complaints. The examiners were unaware of the fact that the individuals were malingerers and believed them to be clinical referrals seen in the course of a neuropsychological clinical practice.

Golden found that the malingerers in the believable group were able to avoid detection by the examiners, but had difficulty faking the test. In an attempt to make their deficits believable, the malingers attempted to pass easy items but fail hard items. However, the construction of the LNNB makes most of the items seem easy. As a result, 7 of the 10 malingerers produced profiles judged clinically as normal. None of the 10 malingerers produced elevated scores on the Pathognomonic scale, and none produced lateralized differences between the right and left side of the body. The scales that most often showed elevations were Intermediate Memory, Memory, Arithmetic, and Intelligence (which also are the last scales to be administered).

In the group given instructions simply to prove they were brain-damaged (without admonitions of believability or fooling the tester), 6 of 10 produced abnormal profiles. In 4 of these 6 cases, the examiner picked up the malingering, reporting inconsistent motivation and cooperation as well as inconsistencies in test results.

Figure 1 shows the differences in mean scores between the two groups. The higher profile was produced by the second group (no instructions about believability). The lower profile was produced by the group concerned about believability. Using a cutoff of 60, only the second group produced any average

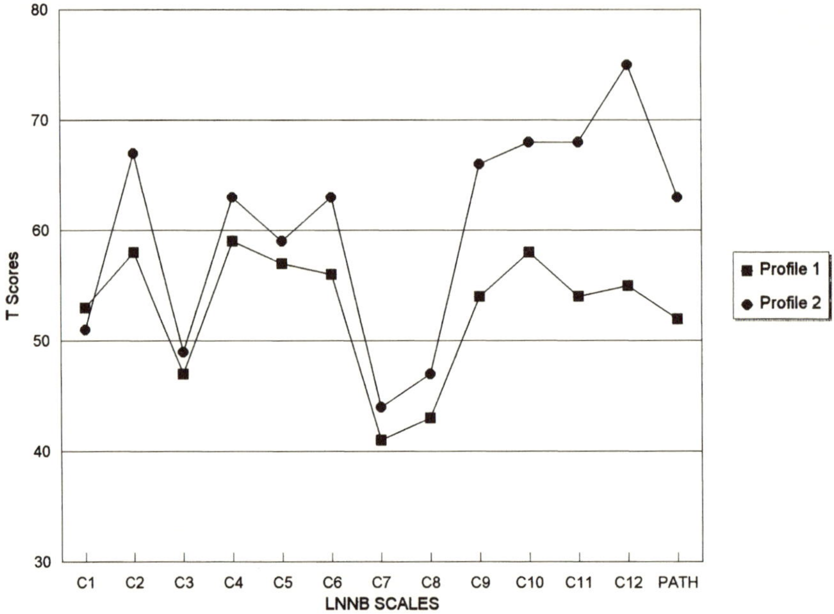

FIGURE 1. LNNB profiles of malingerers with instructions to ensure believability (squares) and those with instructions simply to fake (circles).

scores above that point. Other than elevations, however, the profiles are very similar.

Two of the cases produced brain-damaged profiles that were not identified, yielding elevations primarily on the same scales as the first malingering group. Of the four, one produced abnormal scores on the Pathognomonic scale. Thus, this group could be divided into several subgroups: a group unable to produce an abnormal profile, a group that exaggerated deficits so that their malingering was obvious, and a group that produced more believable deficits. Typical profiles from these three groups are shown in Figure 2.

An investigation of these three profiles again reveals many similarities between them. The normal profile is simply characterized by lower scores, with the client unable to identify which items to "miss." The believable profile differs in having slightly higher scores, enough to exceed the cutoff point (adjusted here to 60 in each case) but not enough to suggest malingering. Interviews with these subjects suggested that the approach taken by both groups was identical, with one set of subjects simply doing better but for no clear reason. It is suggested that these profiles are really the same, and simply represent two ends of a continuum such

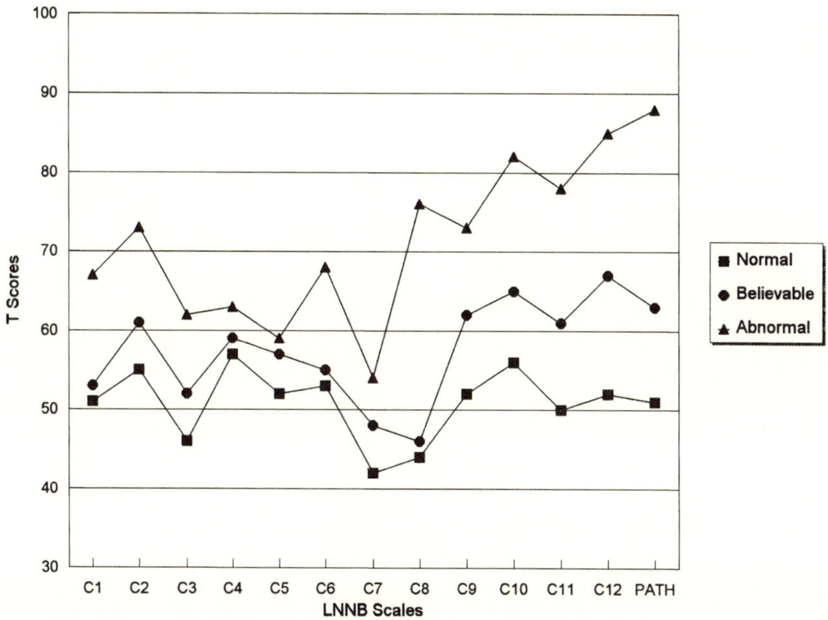

FIGURE 2. Average LNNB profiles of malingerers with normal profiles (squares), believable profiles (circles), and abnormal profiles (triangles).

that those that by chance fall into the brain-damaged range become more "believable" rather than by some clever strategy that allows the client to fake.

The last profile is characterized by scores that are inconsistent with the clients' history. They suggest a brain injury that is quite severe, almost on the level of a moderate dementia affecting even normally overlearned and resistant behaviors. The clients' behavior, demeanor, history, and ability to socially interact all contradicted this conclusion even in the absence of more detailed and finer analysis of the test results.

This last profile is also of interest in that it is commonly seen in actual brain-injured clients who choose to malinger. In most cases, these are patients with mild brain injury, most often to the anterior areas of the brain, whose real symptoms are mild and often denied by others. Such individuals may come to an examination ordered by an insurance company and they have decided that they must "prove" they are brain-injured. As a result, they produce an exaggerated and impossible profile that labels them as malingerers even though they may actually have a milder and more subtle (but real) condition.

The results suggest that believable faking on the LNNB may be difficult precisely because the items seem so easy on the surface. Although malingerers can choose to miss any and all items, they appear to produce either severely impaired and inconsistent deficits or relatively normal profiles. The pathognomonic score appears to be useful as one indicator of malingering as well, but one must recognize that some 10–20% of people with clear injuries will also have normal pathognomonic scores.

Several case examples will illustrate the use of this type of profile recognition.

Case 1. Case 1 shows the profile of a client with a mild head injury. The client was injured in a two-car head-on accident. There was a short period of unconsciousness (less than 5 minutes). The patient had walked away from the accident, and refused medical help. He eventually went to a physician for "whiplash" syndrome, but never complained about neuropsychologically related problems.

Despite improvement in his physical condition, on return to work he had numerous problems. He was unable to focus properly, his social relationships were disrupted, and the quality of his work declined precipitously. His home life demonstrated a similar pattern, with his wife becoming increasingly disgusted at what she considered his deliberate neglect of his family and his irritability. His children became increasingly afraid of him.

He was eventually referred to several neurologists, who declared him normal. A psychiatrist suggested he had PTSD and prescribed Ativan, which the patient took once and refused to take again. The patient was fired from work for poor performance and inability to cooperate with management. He hired a lawyer to sue his former employer (a government entity).

The lawyer had him referred to a vocational psychologist, who found that the client was perfectly able to work and that the firing had been unfair. The government's specialist found that he had faked problems at work so as to file the lawsuit. He was referred to a psychiatrist to be evaluated for malingering. The psychiatrist, on learning the history, suggested to the man he had a brain injury. The client and the lawyer seized on this suggestion, arguing now that the client was disabled and protected by the ADA.

Next, the client was referred for neuropsychological testing by the government. The client came to the examination against his will, having been ordered by the court. The client was by this time quite convinced that he had a brain injury. He was also relatively hostile to experts in general, believing they had given him a "runaround." Although he ostensibly cooperated with the LNNB, his performance and speech were much slower than when he was in a nontesting interview situation.

His profile reveals many elevated scores (all scores above 60 are abnormal in this and in all future examples). The profile as a whole is characteristic of a moderate to severe dementia or a severe brain injury. The clear discrepancy between the history and the test results, without any supporting neurological or neuroradiological evidence, pointed to this client as a malingerer. His claim for a brain injury was later denied.

Case 2. Case 2 was an unusual case that was directly suspected of malingering. A bus involved in an accident on a local street had been occupied by only one passenger (according to the driver). Within 7 days of the accident, however, eight claims for injuries had been made by people claiming to be passengers. This female claimed to have suffered orthopedic injuries as well as a head trauma that had rendered her unconscious for about 10 minutes. A physician hired by her lawyer diagnosed a postconcussion syndrome and brain contusion. The client claimed problems in executive functions, memory, and attention. She stated she could no longer remember the names of friends or how to do her job (a grocery store checkout clerk).

The client had been referred for a Halstead–Reitan by another psychologist, who found impaired scores on Category, TPT, Rhythm, Speech Sounds, and Finger Tapping. He concluded that she had suffered a significant diffuse brain injury.

As in the previous case, the client was ordered into testing by the court. She presented herself as neatly dressed and well organized. She was driven to the evaluation by her husband because she stated she had developed a fear of the roads. She was very interested in a description of the test procedures, asking many questions.

She was told that the test consisted of very simple procedures that should not offer any significant problems. As can be seen for the second case in Figure 3, she completed the test without any signs of difficulty. She had some problems with individual items, but the pattern of items missed had no clear explanation or consistency. The LNNB was interpreted as normal. Given the discrepancy between the LNNB and Halstead–Reitan, it was decided that she had likely malingered on the Halstead–Reitan. Several months later, when confronted with both the test results and the statement of the bus driver, she recanted her claims and ended by testifying against the lawyer and physician, who she said induced her to lie for some "easy money."

Case 3. Case 3 was injured in a work accident when he fell 3 feet from a ladder. There was no evidence that the client was unconscious, but he did have a large gash across the occipital region when he apparently landed on a sharp object of some kind. His behavior thereafter was reported to be sporadic, and memory and judgmental problems were identified. His wife complained that he had "changed" and his employer reported that he was unpredictable and inefficient at work despite a good prior work history.

Case 3 of Figure 3 shows his profile. He revealed mild impairment on six scales (including Pathognomonic). Moreover, the test results were consistent with his complaints and the reports from his family. The profile was consistent with a mild head injury and with the history reported by the client. It was concluded that his problems were real and likely chronic as he was tested 18 months postinjury.

Although this was a workmen's compensation case, which normally limits damages and awards, his accident was caused by an employee of another contrac-

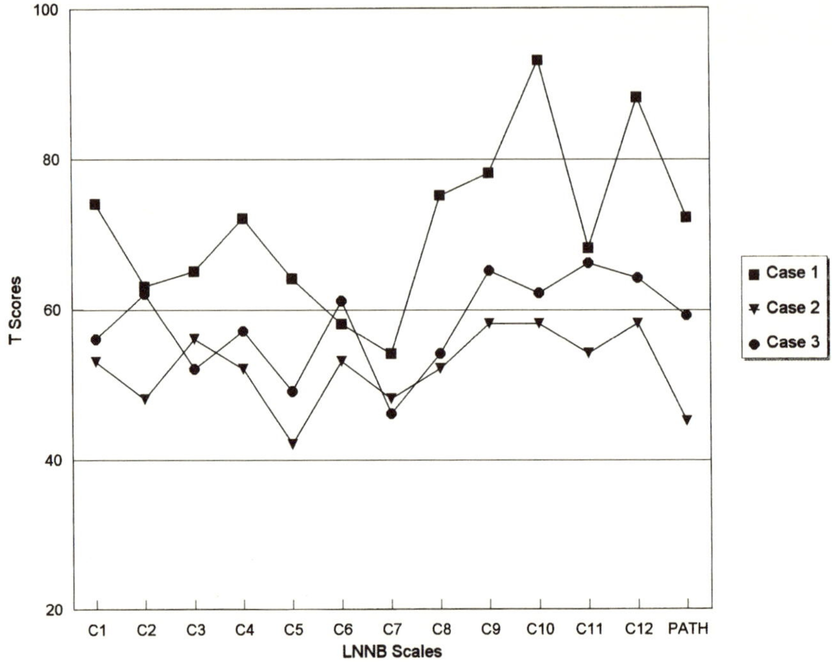

FIGURE 3. LNNB profiles from Case 1 (squares), Case 2 (triangles), and Case 3 (circles).

tor and thus he was free to sue that contractor. An out-of-court settlement awarded the client several million dollars for loss of wages, loss of enjoyment, and loss of consortium.

About 8 months after the client received the money, his "chronic" symptoms had disappeared and he had started his own business. Although he never revealed that he had faked the test results directly, he appeared to gloat over the "stupidity" of the medical establishment. It is highly likely that the symptoms were feigned in this case.

In reviewing the entire protocol, there were no indicators even after the fact that the client had malingered which were missed at the time. Whether out of luck or guile, the client had managed to fake this examination as well as several others. It can be speculated that giving the test a second time might have helped identify some discrepancies, but such a possibility is only speculation.

Forced-Choice Analysis of the LNNB

Several of the LNNB scales have items that are essentially forced choice ("yes/no" or similar answers) in nature. These items lend themselves to the same kind of chance analysis as seen in the Portland and other tests. These items can be found, for both Versions I and II, on

1. Scale 2 (Rhythm): Items 52–54 (all five trials on each item)
2. Scale 3 (Tactile): 66–69 (all four parts of these four items), 72, 73 (both parts of these two items)
3. Scale 5 (Receptive): 121, 122, 124–127 (all four parts separately), 129–131
4. Scale 9 (Arithmetic): 210 (each of three parts), 211 (each of two parts)

Overall, Forms I and II contain 52 items or subitems that meet the forced-choice criteria. By chance, we would expect all clients to achieve a score of 26. As noted in the previous literature regarding other tests, these scores can be effectively used to screen for some obvious forms of malingering.

In general, our initial work has suggested that scores below 70% indicate poor motivation or possible malingering. This is consistent with cutoffs from other similar tests. Our initial work with these criteria has suggested that they are effective. Less than 10% of confirmed brain injury clients tested to date have fallen into the malingering range. Normal controls instructed to malinger show more variation. As noted earlier, these clients fall within two groups: those generating normal profiles and those generating impaired profiles. Of nine malingerers generating impaired profiles on Forms I and II, seven would have been identified by the above malingering scales. As would be expected, all clients who generated normal profiles were not identified as malingerers.

The most recent form of the LNNB (Version III) is an expanded test that includes most of the items from Form II. It contains a subset of 36 items from the earlier version that appear on the forced-choice malingering scale. For Version III, these items can be found on:

1. Scale 4 (Nonverbal Auditory Processing): 3–6, 9, 10, 19–23
2. Scale 6 (Tactile Discrimination): 16, 20–30
3. Scale 15 (Complex Auditory Comprehension): 1–4, 8, 9, 12–17
4. Scale 22 (Arithmetic): 7

In all, there are 36 comparisons for these scales, with a chance response score of 18 expected. As with the earlier versions of the test, a cutoff point of 70% also appears appropriate. However, no specific studies have been done with Form III in this area except for extracting the same items from Forms I and II of the test.

In addition, Version III contains a forced-choice figural memory test (with 8 correct answers and 12 distractors) and a forced-choice verbal list learning memory test (with 12 correct answers and 14 distractors). Each of these tests offers forced-choice acquisition testing trials (80 possible comparisons for figural memory and 104 items for list memory) and delayed trials (20 items for figural and 26 for list learning). In both tests, a target list of words or shapes is studied for a fixed period of time by the examinee, who is then shown the response lists and must indicate whether the items on the response list were in the target list or not.

Work with clearly defined brain-injured clients suggests the need for a lower cutoff score as patients with substantial memory deficits can perform at near-chance levels. To misdiagnose less than 10% of confirmed brain injuries, a cutoff of 60% appears appropriate in an evaluation of 75 patients. So as not to identify individuals with the most severe memory disorders, a cutoff of 50% would be necessary. However, such cases can easily be separated on the basis of clinical observation. It is not clear what percentage of malingerers or individuals with poor motivation would be picked up by this cutoff, but scores below 60% certainly should raise a red flag.

These scales from the LNNB have several potential advantages over some of the other tests that have been proposed and are in use. First, the LNNB items are scattered through the test and not concentrated in one place. This means that the client is not as likely to be alert to the nature of the items and how they differ from others items in the test, preventing them from attending only to these items. Second, they cover a wide variety of skills and thus do not focus on any one set of abilities. In giving these items, however, the examiner must insist on an answer from the client for every item. The presence of too many unanswered questions would skew the results of the testing.

Internal Consistency of LNNB Items

There is extensive work on the internal relationship of LNNB items (see Golden, Hammeke, et al., 1982, for a summary of this work). The LNNB scales, although showing high internal consistency, measure a specific domain (such as motor skills) by combining motor skills with a variety of other skills. Thus, on the motor scale one will find:

1. Motor speed items
2. Motor spatial items
3. Visual motor items
4. Motor–speech interactions (complex and simple instructions)
5. Motor copying
6. Oral motor
7. Motor–impulse control items

A similar phenomenon is found on all of the scales. As a consequence, these are specific cross-scale item correlations that reflect the presence of a basic deficit. For example, an inability to follow complex directions in Receptive Speech will affect specific items on the Motor and other scales within the test as documented in the previous literature.

Malingerers, however, are not aware of these relationships and will consequently show poor performance in a specific area (e.g., memory) but not on other items scattered through the test that are highly correlated with the memory items. Such an analysis allows the clinician to identify inconsistencies suggesting malingering, poor motivation, or fluctuating arousal and attention. Combined with other evidence, this provides an excellent check on the profile. None of the malingerers with impaired profiles in the study cited above were able to produce internally consistent profiles. Two case examples illustrate these points.

Case 4. This case arose from a car accident in which the client was a passenger in the back seat. She claimed to have hit her head on a side post of the car and to have been unconscious. EMT at the scene, however, found her lucid and awake, and her behavior in the ER was judged to be normal. There were no bruises on her head. The patient complained of no problems at that time, but 2 months later a lawsuit was filed in which the client claimed memory problems, inability to follow instructions, and problems with intellectual skills.

Her profile overall was in the abnormal range. She showed elevations on Receptive Language, Memory, Intelligence, and Intermediate Memory. Her overall performance on the forced-choice items was within the normal range, except for those items on the Receptive Language scale, where she received a score of 5/12 (41.7%). In contrast, she scored 100% for forced-choice items on the Rhythm scale.

An analysis of her performance revealed several strong inconsistencies. Her higher intellectual skills and abstractions were quite poor on Intelligence, whereas these items were performed quite well on the latter half of the Expressive Language scale. Although she was unable to follow even two-part instructions on Receptive Language, she was able to follow and execute complex instructions on the Motor and Visual scales without difficulty. Despite her memory being abysmal on the Memory and Intermediate Memory scales, she was able to retain instructions over prolonged periods of time on Tactile and Rhythm without any impairment.

These inconsistencies clearly pointed to malingering. In this case, the client lost her suit without admitting that she had malingered. It is of interest that she was able to return to work without difficulty within 1 month of the jury decision.

Case 5. This case (see Figure 4) shows a malingering profile that the authors have encountered several times. This woman had been driving her car and was sideswiped by a truck owned by a major corporation. Although her car received considerable damage, she was protected by an air bag and reported no problems at the scene. She refused to go to a hospital, and was picked up at the scene by her husband.

Nine months after the accident the client filed a lawsuit complaining of brain injury. This apparently arose out of conversations with a therapist she was seeing for recurrent nightmares and fear of driving that developed after the accident. The therapist was an MSW social worker who was initially treating the patient for posttraumatic stress.

The therapist became increasingly concerned over time with complaints by the patient of memory loss. She reportedly had difficulty remembering friends and had forgotten how to do her job as a billing clerk. She would lose things easily and

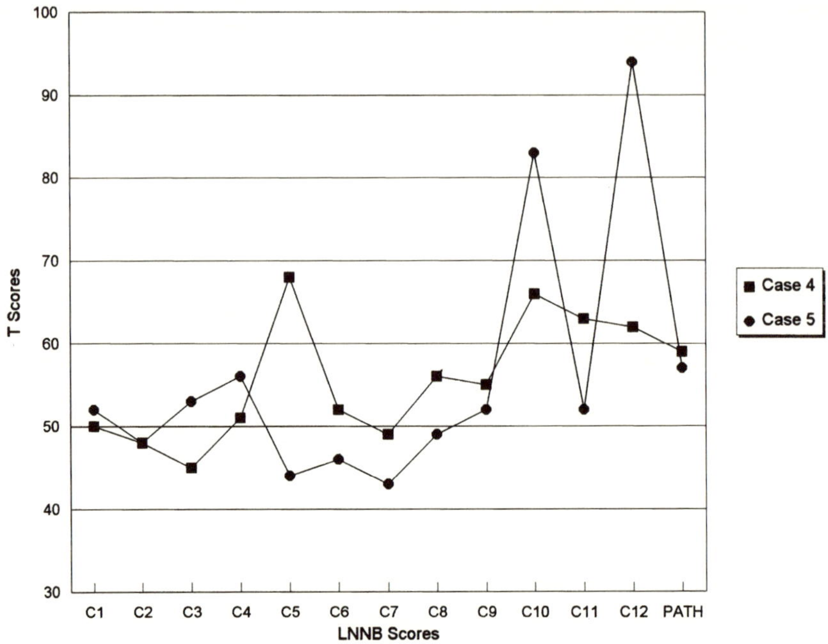

FIGURE 4. LNNB profiles for Case 4 (squares) and Case 5 (circles).

forget appointments. The therapy failed to produce any improvement, eventually leading to a suggestion by the therapist that the client may have suffered a brain injury.

Although the client initially rejected this idea, over the course of a month she became convinced that her problems were organic rather than psychological. Her husband hired a lawyer to file suit claiming severe memory problems arising from brain injury. She was seen for a WAIS-R and WMS-R by a clinical psychologist, who found that she had normal intelligence but that both visual and verbal memory scores were less than 60.

The client was referred by the insurance company for an LNNB. She produced the second profile seen in Figure 4, showing normal scores with the exception of substantial elevations on Memory and Intermediate (Delayed) Memory. Although such a combination of elevations is possible, it is unlikely in most injuries of this type where short-term memory scores are generally much more intact than delayed memory. This is not the case in this profile.

What is more obvious, however, is that in all of the items with complex instructions that require significant memory and those that require sustained memory, the client showed no problems at all. She did not require any repetition of instructions, nor show changes in performance that might relate to such severe memory problems. Her performance on the forced-choice malingering items, however, was normal.

The unusual scores and the inconsistency of the item patterns point to malingering, although it was our opinion that this was more unconscious rather than conscious, set off by the suggestion of the therapist. The client's claims for brain injury were denied, but she did receive some compensation for the PTSD.

Test–Retest Reliability

Neuropsychological tests differ widely in their test–retest reliability. This is because many more complex tests rely on the novelty of the testing situation as an aspect of evaluation. The LNNB, which focuses on more basic skills, does not rely on novelty significantly. As a result, test–retest reliabilities are higher than average and, in general, relatively short test–retest intervals of 1 month or less can be used. In addition, the reliance of the test on more basic skills minimizes variations in test scores substantially over sessions unless there is some change in the client.

Generally, retest scores are expected to be within 10 T score points of previous testing. In the cases of suspected malingerers seen by the authors, these discrepancies have been much greater, although the direction of change is not predictable. However, those who did poorly continue to do poorly but on different scales and items, although in some cases we have seen performance improve to normal levels. Two or more scales that differ by more than 10 points on retest would be considered suspicious. Four or more scales that differ without a change in the client's condition are generally indicative of malingering.

Case 6. This individual was a passenger on a trolley that was hit by a car. Although he was not considered injured by paramedics at the scene, he saw a doctor the next day and was diagnosed as having both a pain syndrome and a "severe brain contusion." The client filed suit against the city, operators of the trolley. Results of testing by the client's chosen psychologist revealed severe impairment with a Halstead Impairment Index of 1.0 when the client was tested 15 months after the accident.

The case referred for a second opinion 23 months after the accident. The client was brought to the testing by an associate of his lawyer, who waited for him throughout the diagnostic process. The client's profile is shown in Figure 5, with the results generally consistent with those of the Halstead. However, because of the history and the absence of independent medical evidence confirming such a brain injury, it was decided to request a second evaluation. This was granted by the court 29 months postinjury.

Figure 5 shows the results of the second testing. Eight of the thirteen scales showed differences of more than 10 T score points, although both profiles would be considered substantially elevated. More detailed analysis of items shows some

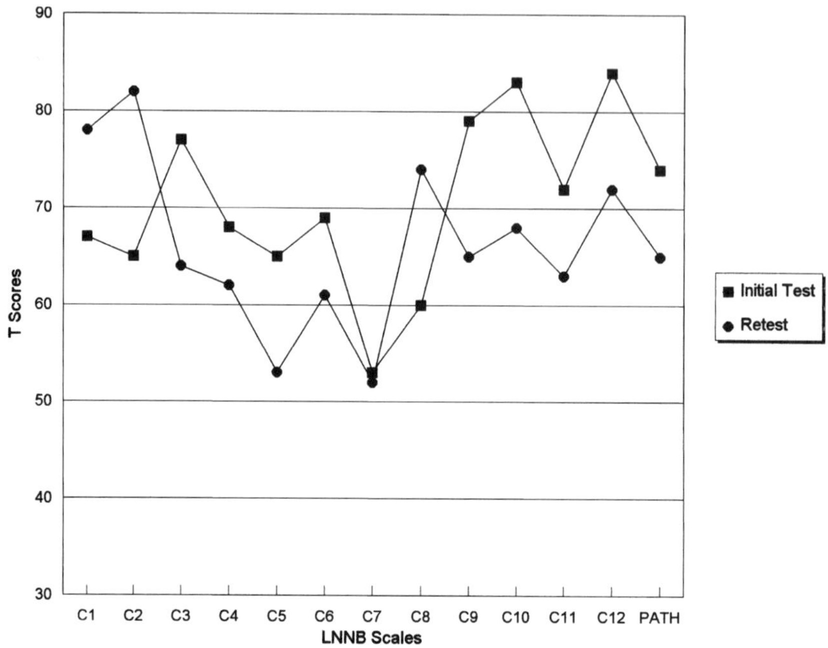

FIGURE 5. Test (squares) and retest (circles) LNNB profiles for Case 6.

significant differences as to which items were performed poorly. As there was no evidence of a change in the client's condition, it was concluded that this was a malingered profile. This was substantiated as well by a 48% accuracy rate on the forced-choice items along with the inconsistent history and neurological results.

Case 7. Case 7 was studied as part of a research project to evaluate test–retest consistency in severely impaired clients. This university student had been hit by a car while walking along a road. He suffered not only the effects of the direct trauma, but also substantial edema and hypoxia exacerbated by the time elapsed before getting him to a hospital. He had been struck at night by a hit-and-run driver who apparently left him to die. He was found by chance by a passing jogger.

The victim revealed severe left hemiplegia along with left-sided weakness, moderate aphasia, poor spatial skills, poor attention and concentration, mild loss of reading, writing, and arithmetic, and substantial memory impairment. He showed slow improvement over a 7-year course of treatment but remained substantially impaired. The two testings in Figure 6 occurred 3 months apart.

As can be seen, the two profiles are nearly identical. All of the scores are within 6 T score points, and the pattern of the test results has remained consistent. Item patterns are consistent as well. The patient achieved a score of 64% on forced-choice items. Overall, this pattern is clearly consistent with a serious injury.

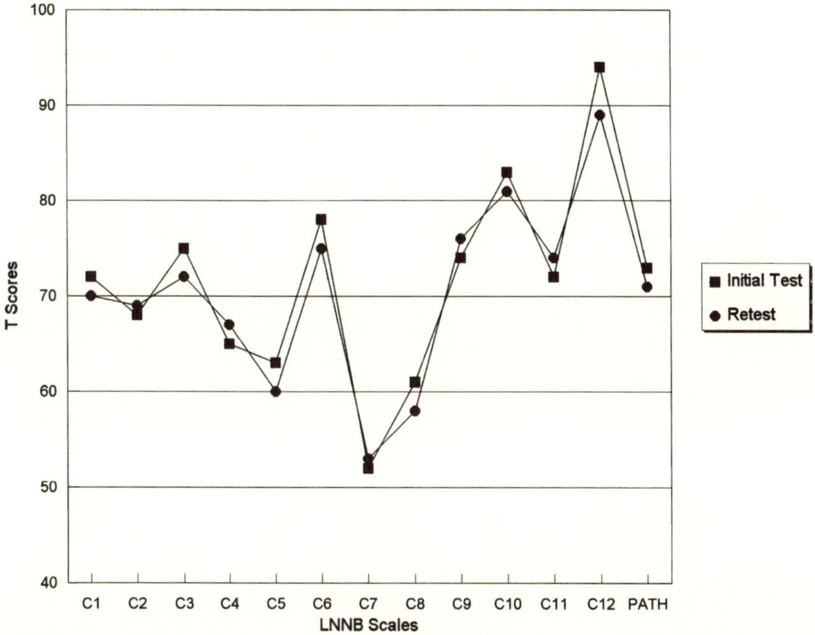

FIGURE 6. Test (squares) and retest (circles) LNNB profiles for a case of severe brain injury.

Case 8. Case 8 represents test–retest results of a case of mild head injury. This client was injured in an automobile accident. He was unconscious for about 30 minutes. He demonstrated good recovery but continued to have problems with memory and judgment, along with signs of emotional lability.

The client was tested 5 years postinjury, with the two testings separated by 123 days. As can be seen in Figure 7, the client's profiles are very similar with no scores differing by more than 8 points. The largest differences seem to be related to a problem on the second testing in sustained concentration which mildly affected the memory scores. The profiles as a whole show consistency between the two testings, and item analysis shows consistent deficits. The score on the forced-choice items was 84%.

Case 9. Case 9 represents a woman who fell from a second-floor balcony and landed on her head. She was unconscious for less than an hour, but demonstrated confusion and memory problems. She showed reasonable recovery through 30 days of rehabilitation. She continued to show agitation and was treated with low doses of Haldol initially, which was increased over time to deal with the agitation.

A lawsuit was subsequently filed, claiming behavior problems, memory loss, and considerable cognitive confusion. Her first testing with the LNNB, 18 months after the accident, revealed a profile characterized by inattention, inconsistent

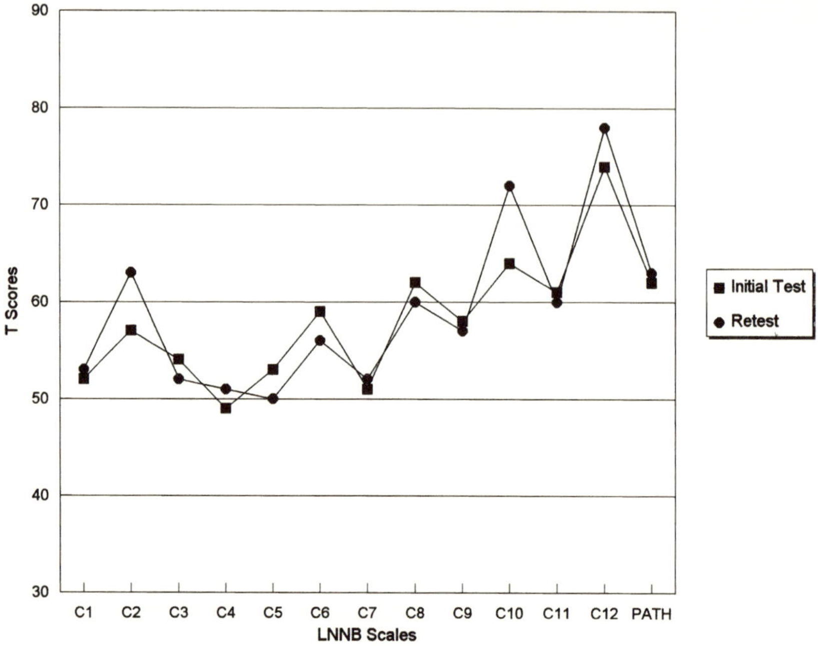

FIGURE 7. Test (squares) and retest (circles) LNNB profiles for a case of mild brain injury.

motivation, and deficits overall that seemed to suggest a much more severe head injury than reflected in the records. Item analysis did not clearly suggest malingering, but the score on the forced-choice items was low (62%). Because of these issues, a second testing was suggested.

The second testing was much improved over the first. The client showed improvement on every scale in the test battery, with every improvement exceeding 10 points. The resulting profile was more consistent, with scores on the forced-choice items exceeding 80%. However, the question remained as to whether this change suggested malingering by the client.

Evaluation indicated that the client had seen a new psychiatrist between the testings who had changed her medication. It was hypothesized that the client's change did not reflect malingering, but that the earlier results had been a function of her medication. This was consistent with the observation that this second testing showed no signs of malingering from any of the perspectives presented here. To confirm this conclusion, a third testing took place 6 months later.

As seen in Figure 8, the third profile is for all practical purposes identical to the second profile. All scores are within 10 T score points and the overall pattern is

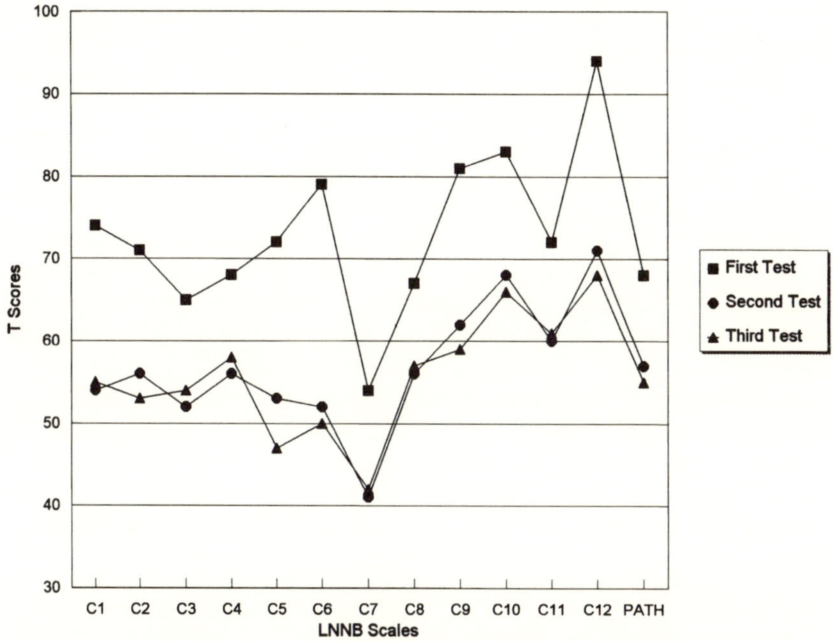

FIGURE 8. Sequential testing for a woman with mixed brain injury and malingering. The profiles reflect the initial testing (squares), a second testing (circles), and the final testing (triangles).

identical to the earlier testing. This confirmed the earlier conclusion that the second profile was a valid profile, whereas the first was invalid and distorted by medication effects. It should be noted that similar changes can of course be seen in recovering patients, or even in chronic patients where performance is decreased by an acute event. Such events may include illness, psychological instability, poor nutrition, or other psychological or biological events that may impact performance in a negative manner.

Item Consistency

Item consistency is similar to scale test–retest consistency but looks at the item level. All LNNB items are scored 0, 1, or 2 on Forms I and II. (For Form III, scores may go as high as 7.) Across retestings, there is a high degree of agreement across items in normal and brain-injured individuals whose conditions are stable. An analysis of normal and brain-injured retesting item profiles (Golden, Berg, & Graber, 1982; Plaisted & Golden, 1982) shows perfect item agreement in at least 90% of nonmalingering retest clients.

As a result, retest agreements of less than 90% are considered quite suspicious and are indicators of either a significant change in the patients' condition or malingering. Because of the complexity of the LNNB in terms of item variety and scoring, this is an area that is almost impossible to fake when an individual is deliberately trying to give a faked profile. It is a less effective measure when the individual tries to fake only one area (e.g., Memory or Motor skills) but such faking can be picked up with the other methods described here.

Case 10. This 35-year-old man fell off the back row of the football stadium bleachers at a high school football game, falling about 10 feet and breaking his left leg in three places. In addition to this injury, he claimed a head injury from hitting his head on a supporting strut of the bleachers. He was conscious and quite irritable at the scene. CT scan was normal and there was no evidence of a blow to the skull. The client claimed he was unable to return to work even after his leg had healed.

An evaluation by a psychologist yielded a conclusion of severe brain damage based on a WAIS, WMS-R, WRAT, and Rey Figure. The client showed a claimed IQ drop of over 20 points, along with memory performance consistent with dementia. He was referred by the school district for a second opinion. On the first

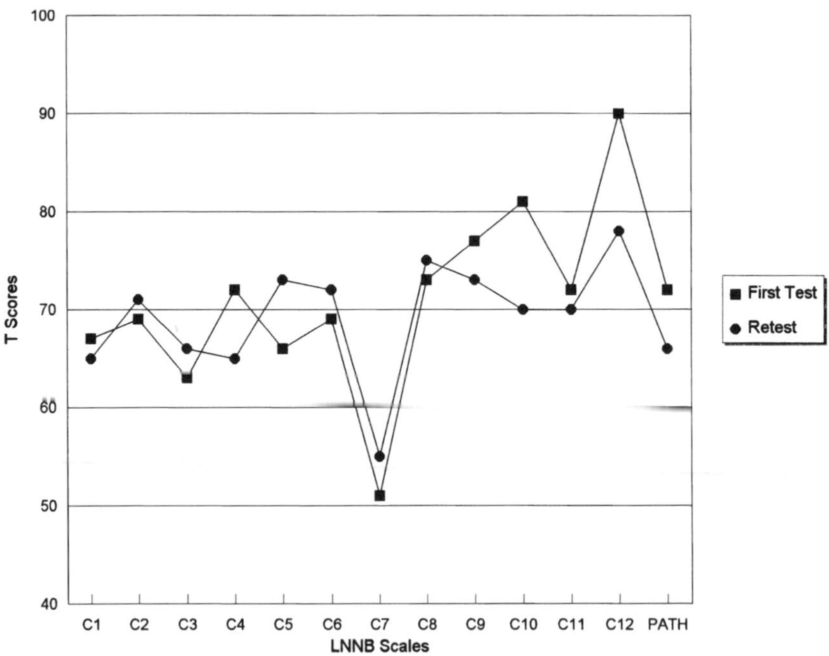

FIGURE 9. Test (squares) and retest (circles) LNNB profiles in a case of malingering.

testing, he performed very poorly as seen in Figure 9. He scored in the brain-damaged range on every scale except Reading (Scale 7). His score on the forced-choice items was a very poor 52%, something seen legitimately only in the most demented subjects tested in our studies.

As a consequence, a retest was suggested and arranged. As can be seen, the second profile differs from the first quite a bit but only two scales differ by more than 10 points. This suggests malingering, but is borderline and not as definitive as was expected. However, an evaluation of item agreement was quite clear: His scores agreed on only 73% of the items, well under the 90% cutoff. In addition, he again did poorly on the forced-choice items (58%). The evidence taken together pointed clearly toward malingering. This case was later settled for a nominal amount.

Case 11. This young woman had been injured as a passenger when two cars collided in a rural area late at night. The exact details are unclear, as the accident was not discovered for over 8 hours and the drivers of both cars were killed. The woman was wearing a seat belt, which may have saved her life. When found, she was conscious but confused. She was crying hysterically, probably at the realization that her husband (the driver) was dead. She had bruises on her knees, but no other signs of injury despite the severity of the accident and the totaling of the two cars.

At first, her problems were treated as PTSD rather than as a brain injury. A lawsuit was filed on her behalf for the death of her husband and her injuries, but that suit did not contend any brain injury. The therapy went slowly and made no progress. The woman continued to show memory problems, anxiety, delusional activity, hysteria, poor judgment, inability to return to work, and depression. This was all attributed to PTSD.

Two years after the accident a new lawyer was given the case. This lawyer was familiar with brain injury cases and noted the many similarities between her case and cases of frontal lobe damage. He sent her for an LNNB. The results are shown in Figure 10. She reveals elevations on Memory, Intermediate Memory, Expressive Language, Intelligence, Arithmetic, and Visual, a pattern consistent with a moderate brain injury in the frontal areas of the brain.

However, there were aspects of the case that brought the results into question. First, there was no clear history of any trauma to the head. Second, the defense contended that the problems were solely the result of PTSD and were unrelated to any organic problem. Third, the presence of depression and its effect on the results were raised as well. Lastly, the defendant alleged that the client was malingering solely for monetary gain and revenge.

In light of these concerns, a second testing was requested and completed. The results are shown in Figure 10. As seen, the overall profiles are extremely similar. Most impressively, however, the client showed identical answers on 97.4% of the questions. Combined with normal performance on the forced-choice items, these

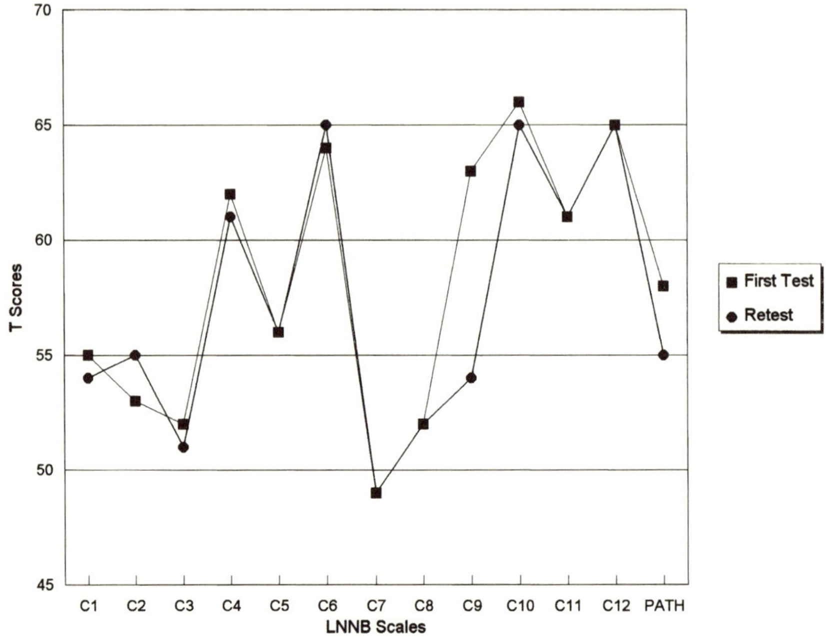

FIGURE 10. Test (squares) and retest (circles) LNNB profiles in a misdiagnosed case of a woman with a real brain injury.

findings clearly point to the reliability and accuracy of the profile as well as the presence of brain dysfunction despite the absence of a clear unequivocal history.

Consistency with History and Neurological Test Results

This is a major check for any neuropsychological test procedure. Although the association between neuropsychological findings and neurological and historical findings is not precisely one to one, there are well-documented relationships and an extensive literature that allow for a highly sophisticated examination of the consistency of these sources of information. This is a complex process that requires the highest level of training in neuropsychology. Several previous cases have illustrated these principles well but they can be further illustrated in several additional cases.

Case 12. This 29-year-old woman claimed brain damage from a bus–car accident in which she had been a passenger on the bus. The claimant said her head hit the seat in front of her, causing brain dysfunction. She was suing the bus company for negligent driving and failure to supervise their employees. (Ironically, the driver turned out to have a brain tumor causing unilateral neglect, which was likely the cause of the accident.) The client was quite angry and did very poorly across the test, despite the fact that she had driven herself to the appointment and was quite coherent in relating her history and the events of the accident. The results, seen in Figure 11, suggest a severe injury. Such findings are clearly inconsistent with the client's presentation, history, and negative neurological results. Her score on the forced-choice malingering items was also quite poor (53%).

When confronted with these findings, she eventually admitted to deliberately missing items in an effort to "punish" the bus company because it had treated her badly and failed to apologize. It became evident that her own needs were more for the bus company to admit an error rather than win a faked lawsuit. We were able to intervene with the company and the patient settled for attorney's fees, some lost wages, a public apology, and a lifetime transit pass. She was later able to return to a productive life as well as ride the bus.

Case 13. This woman had been working in an enclosed Midwestern office building when spraying for weeds was done outside the building. Because of an error by the contractor, poison was left open near the air intake for the AC/heating system, causing fumes to be drawn into the building. About 6% of the people in the

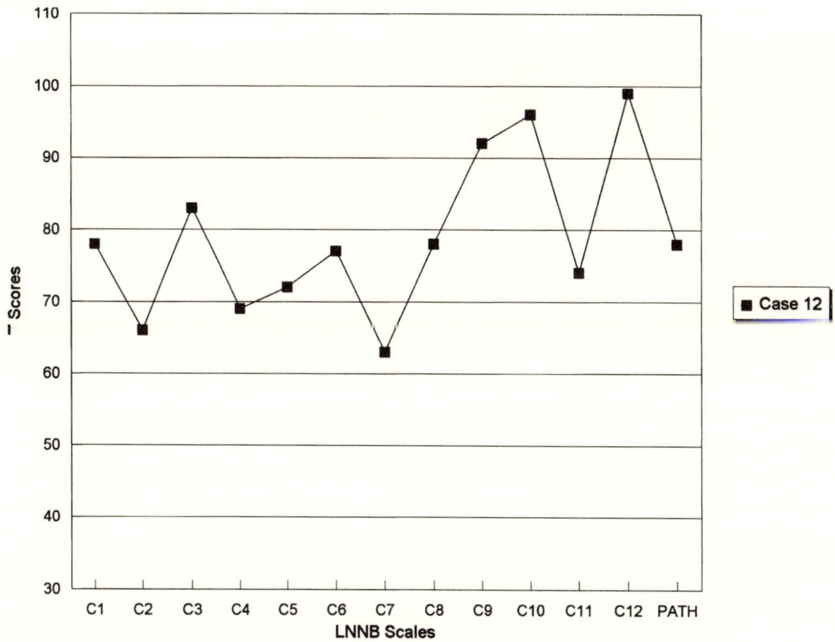

FIGURE 11. LNNB profile for Case 12.

building suffered nausea, headaches, dizziness, confusion, and disorientation. At first, all were treated and released, being told that nothing was wrong with them. In a small minority, symptoms persisted and even worsened over time, being exacerbated by medical opinions that the patients were fine.

This case showed a continued decline in memory and cognitive functions, increased irritability, and increasing sensitivity to all chemicals. Within 1 year, she was totally incapacitated. Neurological results, including MRI and SPECT, were normal. The client nonetheless continued to decline, becoming increasingly sensitive to chemicals until she was barely able to leave her home without having a serious physical reaction.

The client was tested four times over the course of 4 years. These testings are summarized in Figure 12. At first, she showed extremely impaired results, completely inconsistent with the neurological findings. Her score on the forced-choice items was 55%. She was interpreted as being a malingerer at that point, given the severity of the discrepancy as well as the somewhat hysterical attitude of the client. She denied this, and was sent to another psychologist for testing, producing the

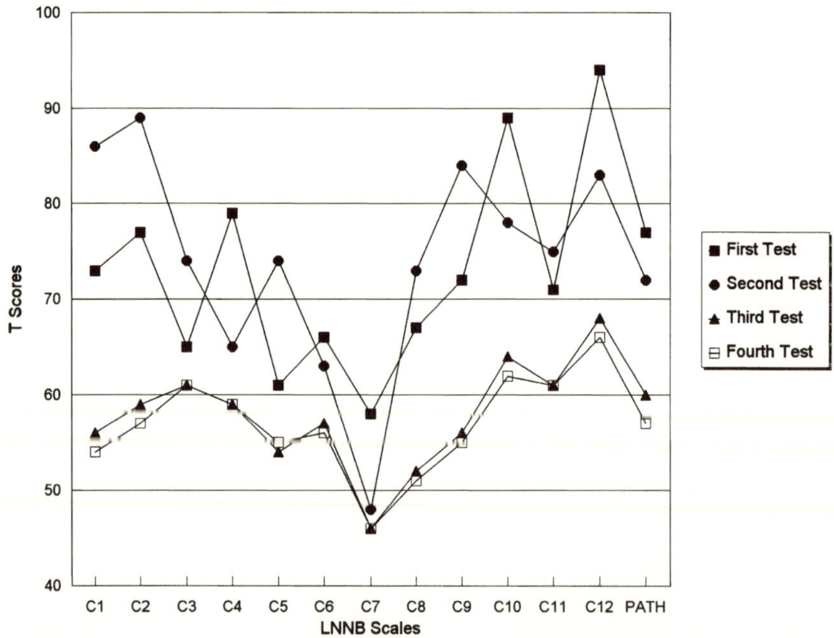

FIGURE 12. Four sequential LNNB testings for Case 12 with mixed malingering and brain injury. The initial testing (squares), a second testing (circles), a third testing (triangles), and a final testing (open squares).

second profile. This is also a severe profile with a poor performance on the forced-choice items (57%). Many of the scales differed by more than 10 T score points, and item agreement was a poor 83%. On this basis, it was concluded that the client did not have a real neuropsychological disorder.

The client and her attorney protested these conclusions and she was sent for further evaluation. At this time, it was suggested that the client's anger and hysteria might be interfering with her test performance, so it was suggested she enter into therapy along with medication to address the behavioral and emotional aspects of her problems. This included addressing her anger, her sense that people were out to get her, her depression, her worsening phobias, and her behavioral deficits.

Over a period of 1 year, the client was slowly able to show improvement in her depression, anger, and behavior, and began to act more reasonably. Despite this, she continued to show mild memory problems and mild problems with higher-level skills. At this time, she was tested again, yielding a profile that, although still impaired, suggested a milder injury more consistent with the known etiology. On this testing, the client achieved a score of 87% on the forced-choice items. This testing appeared much more reasonable, but there were still lingering questions given the previous history.

As a result, a final and fourth testing was completed 8 months later. This profile, seen in Figure 12, was almost identical to the earlier testing, with scores never varying by more than 10 points and the overall item agreement was 93%. The forced-choice item score was 87%. This profile clearly suggested that these final deficits were reliable and likely represented mild deficits secondary to her exposure.

This client illustrates a case in which initial testing clearly shows the presence of malingering or lack of cooperation, but which subsequently is shown to reflect real brain damage. This relates to the poor judgment of clients who feel the need to prove their deficits. In such cases, therapy can be useful in minimizing these signs of deception and eventually generating a meaningful profile.

DISCUSSION

The increasing utilization of neuropsychological findings in civil and criminal court proceedings has raised the issue of the importance of accurately detecting false performances on neuropsychological assessment devices. Unfortunately, clinical psychologists and neuropsychologists are limited to the patient's self-report regarding psychological and physical impairments, which thus has a profound impact on the clinician's diagnostic decision. Therefore, the clinician is responsible for being particularly aware of a patient's potential incentive for poor performance.

On the other hand, charges of malingering are very serious and cannot be made lightly. Despite the vast advances in our understanding of the brain, in neurodiagnostic testing, and in general medical and psychological sophistication, there remain many gray areas, especially when dealing with mild brain injuries or in working with patients whose premorbid problems place them at risk so that the effects of a legitimate brain injury are amplified.

Thus, any decision regarding malingering must be based on a sophisticated analysis of many sources of information. A thorough psychosocial history may provide the answers to the question of a patient's true motivation. Some potential indicators for malingering behavior include, but are not limited to: monetary compensation in civil tort cases, exoneration from criminal responsibility, psychiatric disturbance, referral by an attorney, suspicious patterns of responding on neuropsychological tests, inconsistent deficits with radiological, electrophysiological, or magnetic imaging results, and invalid or suspicious responding on certain MMPI-2 scales (i.e., high L, high F scores).

When using the LNNB, it is strongly recommended that one use both the within-test "malingering" scales as well as some of the independent tests that have been developed for malingering before such a diagnosis can be made. In actual practice, administration of the LNNB should give the clinician a good idea of whether malingering is actively suspected. If it is not, there is little reason for additional testing. If the results or other information suggest malingering, it is strongly suggested that additional testing be done even if that requires another session with the client. (However, we do not recommend any session in which only malingering tests are administered.)

In cases where large substantial decisions are made on the test results, we will often try to get a repeat testing. As noted above, this can be a powerful check on clients whose variable performance may be the result of malingering or poor motivation or may just be an odd pattern of deficits.

On the other side, we must look for predisposing conditions that would make a person susceptible to an injury. For example, a client who has learning deficits and hyperactivity may be ill equipped to deal with the impact of a minor brain injury. Individuals with minimal cognitive skills may be much more greatly impacted by a small loss than an individual who has more resources on which to draw. We must be careful to note preinjury individual differences which can have a profound effect on the expression of an injury.

In addition, we must separate between overt malingering for gain and the inability or unwillingness to cooperate because of a brain injury or an emotional condition. An individual severely traumatized in a crash may develop an inability to tolerate stress, either as a result of a frontal or subcortical brain injury or as an emotional reaction to the accident itself. Such individuals may produce profiles that are both inconsistent and amotivated, suggesting malingering without any overt malingering being present. The presence of a purely emotional condition that interferes with testing cannot be mistaken for malingering. Only when all of this information is integrated can such a valid conclusion be reached.

In the case of some frontal lobe clients, we may see unexplained variation in behavior depending on their current emotional and stress levels. Unable to control themselves or inhibit emotional reactions, such patients may vary greatly from day to day in their behavior depending on the "emotional" load they bring into a session. Observations of such patients over time may be necessary to truly define such clients if neurological or neuroradiological results are equivocal. In these cases, history and correlation with outside behavior play a very large role in assessing the meaning of such deficits. In such cases, however, there is generally an absence of intellectual loss. When claims of intellectual loss are made in the absence of supporting evidence, this will more strongly suggest malingering or some nonneurological emotional condition.

In addition, we must be aware that individuals will real brain injury may choose to malinger. Sometimes this is out of misguided greed, sometimes because they simply don't wish to cooperate, and sometimes because they think they are being clever. Just as we once debated whether schizophrenics were "organic" or "nonorganic" as if a dichotomy existed, we are not debating whether clients are malingerers or nonmalingerers. In both cases there is no clear dichotomy: Clients can belong to both groups at the same time.

Proper testing for malingering with the LNNB involves all of the methods used here, as well as the use of further methods as they are developed. The ultimate decision, however, must never rely solely on statistics but on an intricate analysis that weaves these methods together and balances them as demanded by the client's specific individual situation. Although the LNNB was not designed specifically to determine malingering, its design lends itself to an effective discrimination of those with malingering or emotional problems that affect test results. It is hoped that future research will further refine and improve on these methods.

REFERENCES

Bernard, L. C. (1990). Prospects for faking believable memory deficits on neuropsychological tests and the use of incentives in simulation research. *Journal of Clinical and Experimental Neuropsychology, 12*(5), 715–728.

Bernard L. C. (1991). The detection of faked deficits on the Rey Auditory Verbal Learning Test: The effect of serial position. *Archives of Clinical Neuropsychology, 6*, 81–88.

Bickart, W. T., Meyer, R. G., & Connell, D. K. (1991). The symptom validity technique as a measure of feigned short-term memory deficit. *American Journal of Forensic Psychology, 9*(2), 3–11.

Binder, L. M. (1993). Assessment of malingering after mild head trauma with the Portland Digit Recognition test. *Journal of Clinical and Experimental Neuropsychology, 15*(2), 170–182.

Binder, L. M., & Willis, S. C. (1991). Assessment of motivation after financially compensable minor head trauma. *Psychological Assessment: A Journal of Consulting and Clinical Psychology, 3*, 175–181.

Gfeller, J. K., Cradock, M. M., & Falkenhain, M. A. (1994, November). *Detecting feigned neuropsychological impairment with the Seashore Rhythm Test.* Poster presented at the Annual Conference of the National Academy of Neuropsychology, Orlando, FL.

Golden, C. J. (1992). [Performance of feigned malingerers on the Luria–Nebraska Neuropsychological Battery]. Unpublished raw data.

Golden, C. J., Berg, R. A., & Graber, B. (1982). Test–retest reliability of the Luria–Nebraska Neuropsychological Battery in stable, chronically impaired patients. *Journal of Consulting and Clinical Psychology*, *50*, 452–454.

Golden, C. J., Hammeke, T. A., Purisch, A. D., Berg, R. A., Moses, J. A., Jr., Newlin, D. B., Wilkening, G. N., & Puente, A. E. (1982). *Item interpretation of the Luria–Nebraska Neuropsychological Battery*. Lincoln: University of Nebraska Press.

Guilmette, T. J., Hart, K. J., & Giuliano, A. J. (1993). Malingering detection: The use of a forced-choice method in identifying organic versus simulated memory impairment. *The Clinical Neuropsychologist*, *7*(1), 59–69.

Hiscock, M., & Hiscock, C. K. (1989). Refining the forced choice method for the detection of malingering. *Journal of Clinical and Experimental Neuropsychology*, *11*, 967–974.

Martin, R. C., Bolter, J. F., Todd, M. E., Gouvier, W. D., & Niccolls, S. (1993). Effects of sophistication and motivation on the detection of malingered memory performance using a computerized forced-choice test. *Journal of Clinical and Experimental Neuropsychology*, *15*(6), 867–880.

Mensch, A. J., & Woods, D. J. (1986). Patterns of feigning brain damage on the LNNB. *The International Journal of Clinical Neuropsychology*, *8*(2), 59–63.

Plaisted, J. R., & Golden, C. J. (1982). Test–retest reliability of the clinical, factor, and localization scales of the Luria–Nebraska Neuropsychological Battery. *International Journal of Neuroscience*, *17*, 163–167.

Prigatano, G. P., & Amin, K. (1993). Digit Memory Test: Unequivocal cerebral dysfunction and suspected malingering. *Journal of Clinical and Experimental Neuropsychology*, *15*(4), 537–546.

Slick, D., Hopp, G., Strauss, E., Hunter, M., & Pinch, D. (1994). Detecting dissimulation: Profiles of simulated malingerers, traumatic brain-injury patients, and normal controls on a revised version of Hiscock and Hiscock's forced-choice memory test. *Journal of Clinical and Experimental Neuropsychology*, *16*(3), 472–481.

6

Detection of Malingering and Invalid Test Results Using the Halstead–Reitan Battery

RALPH M. REITAN AND DEBORAH WOLFSON

The problem of malingering, dissimulation, or even the nondeliberate production of invalid performances cuts at the core of the scientific basis of clinical practice in neuropsychology. The *Diagnostic and Statistical Manual of Mental Disorders* (DSM-IV) (American Psychiatric Association, 1994) cautions that malingering should be strongly suspected if an examination is done in a medicolegal context (e.g., the client was referred by an attorney for an evaluation). Binder (1990), in his review of forensic cases, stated that malingering should be considered a possibility whenever the test results may be related to an opportunity for financial gain.

The obvious need for a valid index of malingering or dissimulation has led to many studies, most of which used normal subjects instructed to pretend that they were brain-injured while taking neuropsychological tests (for a review of this literature see Franzen, Iverson, & McCracken, 1990; Nies & Sweet, 1994; and this volume). Although a number of investigations reported statistically significant differences between feigned malingerers and groups not suspected of malingering, there are two major problems plaguing these research efforts.

First, it is naive to assume that normal subjects instructed to fake the type of deficits that would result from a head injury would actually be able to simulate the neuropsychological impairment caused by brain damage. The subjects—who are usually normal, unimpaired, and relatively young—typically know very little

---

RALPH M. REITAN and DEBORAH WOLFSON • Reitan Neuropsychology Laboratory, Tucson, Arizona 85713.

Detection of Malingering during Head Injury Litigation, edited by Reynolds. Plenum Press, New York, 1998.

about the behaviors they are instructed to simulate (e.g., neuropsychological deficits). In addition, normal subjects pretending to be brain-damaged share none of the stresses, anxieties, guilt, depression, and desperation experienced by many litigants whose future financial stability may depend on the outcome of the neuropsychological examination.

Many plaintiffs may not even realize that they are not putting forth their best possible effort when taking the tests. In such cases, the real-life situation is far different from the laboratory, and laboratory results are open to serious question. As few subjects ever reveal that they have malingered, no one has been able to assemble a representative group large enough to perform even the first valid comparison of malingerers and nonmalingerers. How can the unique characteristics of malingerers be identified if we cannot compose an appropriate group to study?

The second major problem of current research studies is that the results attain at best only certain levels of statistical significance. The investigation of malingering requires methods that "diagnose" *each* subject correctly, rather than methods that yield only a probability statement about the likelihood that intergroup differences are the result of chance! Guesswork based on probability is not an adequate solution to the problem of identifying the individual subject who is malingering. As with neurosurgeons diagnosing brain tumors, the validity of the procedure narrows down to the individual case.

Because intergroup overlap occurs in essentially all distributions of scaled psychological performances, this problem might at first seem to be beyond solution. The difficulty derives primarily from the wide range of performances represented by the normal probability distribution, and is further complicated by the realization that an intelligent malingerer might perform better than a less able nonmalingerer. We can hardly presume that anyone scoring below a specified point on the curve is necessarily a malingerer.

Nevertheless, as reviewed in many of the chapters in this volume, neuropsychologists have devised a number of ingenious techniques and approaches to identify malingerers. Depending on the scores that are generated, each of these approaches may yield strong presumptive evidence of malingering in certain subjects. There is no assurance, however, that all instances of invalid test results are detected.

RESEARCH REPORTS BASED ON THE HALSTEAD–REITAN BATTERY

Research studies of malingering, dissimulation, and production of invalid test results (knowingly or unknowingly, deliberately or as a result of complex, interacting, and essentially unidentified forces) have only occasionally utilized test batteries designed to evaluate an individual's broad range of adaptive abilities. The approach customarily has been to administer a single test or to examine a single set of performances based on a presumption that the distributions of malingerers and nonmalingerers would be essentially nonoverlapping, or at most, minimally overlapping.

If malingering is viewed in the broader context of invalid test results, the nature of the problem as it relates to cerebral damage or dysfunction can be clarified. The psychologist's task may be to differentiate between valid and invalid indications of brain impairment rather than to evaluate the sincerity of the subject's motivation when taking the tests. Presumably, malingerers would not produce test results that reflected the genuine effects of brain damage, and this would reveal the invalidity of the malingerer's test results.

Individual tests are usually interpreted in terms of how well they are performed, and the method generally used to detect malingering is to identify scores that are lower than expected. Considering the range of performances among nonmalingerers, this simplistic model would be difficult to apply with any degree of accuracy. A battery of tests, however, would produce scores that allow comparisons of the individual's performances across a range of tests. Thus, a subject's scores could be compared with each other (an intraindividual approach) as well as with normative data (an interindividual approach). If the test battery was both sensitive and specific for brain injury, there might be a useful and valid basis for separating legitimate indications of brain damage from simulated scores.

In one sense, these considerations are reminiscent of the history and background from which current clinical procedures for neuropsychological assessment developed. Many neuropsychologists can remember the search to find a test of "brain damage" and the debates (and arguments) concerning which test was most effective. It appears that the approach to identifying malingerers is currently at a similar primitive stage. The field now views the prior attempts to develop the ultimate test for brain damage as simplistic and misguided, and recognizes that such a unidimensional approach would never have led to a scientific understanding of the complexity of the behaviors subserved by the brain.

The discipline of clinical neuropsychology has a great debt to Ward Halstead, who approached the problem of neuropsychological assessment from the scientific study of the effects of brain disease and damage. This approach was implemented by subdividing the broad conglomerate of factors called "brain damage" into more discrete independent variables whose behavioral correlates could in turn be differentially identified by using a range of neuropsychological tests.

The problem with using a procedure that investigates the intrinsic nature of malingering is that true malingerers, in contrast to brain-damaged individuals, are difficult to identify. Without a group of documented malingerers to study, there is obviously no prospect of identifying independent variables among group members that might form a basis for differential correlation with neuropsychological test scores, nor can any proposed indexes or scores be properly evaluated for their validity in differentiating malingerers from nonmalingerers.

Structural damage to the brain, along with its detailed characteristics, is a type of variable that in many cases can be reliably documented. Malingering is an independent variable that can be classified as a behavioral or psychological aberration, and such behavior disorders (e.g., depression, anxiety disorders, acute panic attacks, bipolar disorder, acute stress disorder, borderline personality disorder, and conduct disorder) can be defined only in approximate terms represented by generalities (see DSM-IV).

Although few neuropsychologists would claim to know the detailed characteristics of malingerers as defined by objective evidence, many neuropsychologists believe they can reliably recognize the neuropsychological manifestations of cerebral injury or damage. In practice, the clinical procedure is to identify those individuals who demonstrate genuine signs of cerebral impairment. If a subject does not demonstrate such signs, he or she must be classified as non-brain-damaged (and allocated to some other category, of which malingering is one possibility).

The procedure described above was followed in a study by Goebel (1983). In contrast to the many research investigations that used single tests, Goebel used the Halstead–Reitan Battery (HRB) to identify protocols that genuinely reflected brain damage and to differentiate the legitimate protocols from the test results produced by normal subjects instructed to fake the effects of brain damage. Goebel composed three groups: (1) 52 subjects with documented cerebral disease or damage, (2) 50 volunteer subjects presumed to not have brain damage, and (3) 152 volunteer college students also believed to be nonimpaired. The non-brain-damaged subjects were divided into four subgroups: one group of controls and three groups instructed to pretend that they had either right, left, or diffuse cerebral damage. The subjects were not given any specific information about the known effects of brain damage; instead, they were instructed only to alter their normal performances as if they had actually sustained brain damage and to attempt to produce believable and realistic test results.

The HRB was individually administered by two technicians trained and supervised by Goebel. Although the technicians were not informed of any subject's classification, they felt that it was "fairly easy" to detect fakers on the basis of the behavioral observations they made during the testing.

Goebel analyzed the results both statistically and through clinical evaluation of protocols. In each case, the brian-damaged subjects were differentiated at a highly significant level from the volunteers pretending to be brain-damaged. Each analysis showed that 97 or 98% of the "pretenders" were unable to simulate successfully the effects of brain damage. The brain-damaged subjects were classified with a somewhat lower accuracy rate; about 79% were identified correctly on the basis of clinical evaluation and a slightly higher percentage were correctly classified using discriminant functions as a basis for predicting group membership.

Considering the practical problems inherent in this type of research, it is not surprising that several aspects of Goebel's study have been criticized (Faust, Ziskin, & Hiers, 1991). In Goebel's study the majority of the brain-damaged patients were male, and gender distributions were not perfectly equivalent in the subgroups of non-brain-damaged subjects. Goebel cautioned against uncritical generalizations based on the findings, pointing out that normal subjects instructed to fake brain damage do not necessarily perform the same as true malingerers. During the postexperiment debriefing, many subjects reported feeling that they did not know enough about brain damage to be able to simulate the behavioral correlates effectively, and were uncomfortable in attempting to do so.

Finally, in terms of the results based on clinical interpretations, Goebel's study must be viewed as having an *N* of 1. The judgments were made only by the author, and it is unknown whether comparable classifications would have been made by other judges. Despite these possible problems, the results strongly suggest that the data produced by the subjects provided a basis for a rather striking differentiation between brain-damaged subjects and volunteers pretending to be brain-damaged.

Heaton, Smith, Lehman, and Vogt (1978) conducted a study using the WAIS, the HRB, and the MMPI to compare brain-damaged subjects and normal volunteers instructed to feign brain damage. The test results were analyzed both clinically and statistically. In this study, the volunteer malingerers were paid to participate and were offered a bonus if they faked successfully. In addition, these "malingerers" were told to imagine that their everyday functioning was greatly impaired by the head injury, that their earning power had been substantially reduced, and that they deserved all of the money the courts would award. They were encouraged to fake the most severe disabilities possible without revealing that they were faking. They were also given information about the circumstances that might occur with sustaining a head injury, such as hospitalization, duration of coma, skull fractures, posttraumatic seizures, and various aspects of the medical treatment and examinations.

A review of the mean test results reveals that the head-injured group generally scored in the normal range on WAIS variables. The absolute mean values of the Verbal subtests were generally higher than the means of the Performance subtests, and Digit Symbol had the lowest mean among the 11 subtests. Mean scores on the HRB tests were routinely in the brain-damaged range, and several MMPI scales had elevated means. The means were more variable for the volunteer malingerers than for the brain-damaged subjects.

Our review indicated that the relationships among scores were not in line with expectations based on our own experience with patients who have sustained a traumatic brain injury or other type of cerebral damage. For example, the Category

Test and especially the TPT were performed well for a group that made nearly twice as many errors as the average brain-damaged group on the Speech-sounds Perception Test. The malingering group had a remarkably slow finger tapping speed, an unusually high number of errors on the tactile finger localization test, and an extreme number of errors on the tests of bilateral simultaneous sensory stimulation. In fact, the volunteer malingerers demonstrated highly unusual relationships among performances on the HRB tests, which in its own right provided a basis for questioning the validity of the data. The MMPI results of the malingering group were also markedly deviant: 7 of the 10 clinical scales had mean scores exceeding 70 (and 3 of these 7 scales had means above 80).

It is not surprising that discriminant functions based on the neuropsychological tests results correctly classified 100% of the subjects included in the study and the MMPI scores classified 94% correctly. Although the technicians who administered the tests were led to believe that all subjects in both groups were scheduled for routine clinical testing, they commented on the subjects' effort expended when taking the tests and questioned the validity of the test scores for 7 of the 16 volunteer malingerers.

At this point one would be inclined to conclude that the test results of the Heaton et al. (1978) study provided a reliable basis for differentiating between the head-injured patients and the volunteer malingerers. Blind clinical evaluations by 10 judges, however, resulted in poor differentiation of the groups. The judges' unimpressive diagnostic accuracy ranged from chance level to about 20% better than chance. It is difficult to avoid concluding that the accuracy could have been improved if the judges had used an approach that evaluated the interrelationships of test results rather than an approach that reviewed tests essentially as independent measures. One of the major advantages of using a test battery is that it yields scores whose interrelationships can provide critical interpretive information. However, many neuropsychologists view a test battery only as a collection of tests that individually measure various psychological functions. It should be noted that we have no direct knowledge of the bases of interpretation used by the judges in this study.

The competent neuropsychologist must have a base of knowledge that enables him or her to differentiate between the legitimate types of brain disease and damage and simulated brain damage. Fortunately, this information has been known for many years (Hom & Reitan, 1982, 1984; Reitan, 1964; Reitan & Fitzhugh, 1971; Reitan & Wolfson, 1993). Familiarity with these research findings and experience applying them to individual subjects helps the neuropsychologist recognize the relatively unique relationships among test scores in traumatic brain injury and differentiate them from other categories of brain damage, normal performances, and simulated malingering.

Mittenberg, Rotholc, Russell, and Heilbronner (1996) also studied groups of nonlitigating head-injured subjects and volunteer malingerers. Analyses were first based on 40 subjects in each group, and a stepwise discriminate function, using data from 10 variables, correctly classified 88.75% of the subjects. The error rate was fairly similar in the two groups. The function was cross-validated on a second set of two groups, each based on 40 similar subjects, and 83.75% of these subjects were correctly classified. When the 10 predictor variables were applied to the total samples, the overall hit rate was 88.75%, with 83.75% being true positives and 93.8% being true negatives.

Mittenberg et al. found that this procedure was effective when applied to other groups, including those reported by Heaton et al. (1978) as well as to several individual cases. These results were viewed as a basis for suggesting that the discriminant function reported in this study may be useful in clinical practice. As with the data reported by Heaton et al., the mean scores for the groups used by Mittenberg and his colleagues suggest that volunteer malingerers perform certain tests very poorly, whereas groups with traumatic brain damage do better than expected on some tests.

Trueblood and Schmidt (1993) attempted to assess the validity of a number of possible indicators of malingering by evaluating the performances of persons who scored significantly below chance on symptom validity testing (8 persons from a sample of 106 consecutive cases) plus 8 persons who passed symptom validity testing but whose neuropsychological test results were considered improbable and were therefore of questionable validity. The HRB, the WAIS-R, and other tests were administered. Eight control subjects were selected from the sample by matching gender, age, and education with each group of 8 possible malingerers. Comparisons of the scores indicated that the controls and both groups of possible malingerers differed significantly ($p<.05$) on the General Neuropsychological Deficit Scale (GNDS), fingertip number writing perception, and Digit Span. California Verbal Learning Test Recognition, finger agnosia, and Speech-sounds Perception Test scores differed from the controls for only one of the groups of possible malingerers. The other 8 scores tested as possible indications of malingering were not significant.

It must be recognized that the significance of these findings depends on the presumption that all members of the target groups were validly identified by symptom validity testing or by test results that were considered to be improbable, and that the test results of the controls were not influenced by malingering, lack of effort, or other reasons for invalidity. The authors recognized that the validity of neuropsychological test data represents a complex problem that cannot be resolved simply by making a determination of malingering versus not malingering.

Other studies of malingering have focused on measures such as the Booklet Category Test, but because these altered versions of HRB tests have never been fully evaluated in terms of their significance regarding the many aspects of brain lesions (e.g., type, location, duration, and rate of progression) as has been done with the tests routinely included in the HRB, we have not included them in this review.

It is clear from the above studies that used the HRB (and from studies of malingering reported in the literature generally) that the current methods used to identify malingering show considerable promise, but none is yet able to correctly "diagnose" *every* malingerer. Instead, the procedures currently used to identify malingerers are essentially able only to offer statements about chance probabilities based on intergroup differences.

USE OF INTRAINDIVIDUAL TEST SCORES TO IDENTIFY INVALID TEST RESULTS

The task of identifying individual malingerers or dissimulators on the basis of psychological testing is no different in principle from diagnostic testing that evaluates the full range of psychiatric and neurological conditions. Psychologists have depended principally on level of performance to draw conclusions about a subject's neuropsychological functioning. Some psychiatric and neurological conditions are presumed to be associated with impaired performances, but in many cases psychiatric and neurological subjects perform within the normal range. Considering the broad range of performances found in the general population, it is unlikely that valid diagnostic conclusions could be inferred in individual cases using this method alone.

Many years ago, Reitan (1967) published a description of the systematic use of different approaches to interpret neuropsychological test data, and demonstrated with individual case illustrations how to use these various approaches in a complementary manner to draw inferences about neuropsychological diagnoses. The subject's level of performance was useful, but not uncommonly some test scores were in the normal range and some scores were impaired. This fact by itself represented the basis for a second approach to evaluation of test scores.

For example, if a subject performed poorly on tests that were sensitive to brain damage and performed relatively well on tests that were not sensitive, a comparison of these performances might have diagnostic significance. This method, probably used first by Babcock (1930), was utilized by a number of other psychologists, including Hunt (1943) and Wechsler (1955). This approach to interpretation used intraindividual test scores (comparing the subject with him- or herself on various tests) as contrasted with evaluating interindividual test scores (comparing the subject's scores with the rest of the population). Modifications of this procedure, especially in clinical neuropsychology, compared a subject's performance on the same test on each side of the body to make inferences about the status of the two cerebral hemispheres. It is helpful to use the subject as his or her own control because the wide range of variability, commonly seen in the general population, is largely controlled.

Although most tests designed to detect malingering have been based on the subject's level of performance on a single examination, with evaluation oriented toward normative standards, intraindividual comparison of test scores is also recognized as a useful complementary approach. The basic procedure of this approach is to review a subject's test scores and determine whether there are inconsistencies in performances that exceed the limits of probability.

The Case of Albert Johnson

This approach to interpretation is illustrated by the case of Albert Johnson, a 54-year-old man who was involved in a moving vehicle accident and sustained multiple injuries, particularly to his face, chest, and abdomen. The testing was done by a technician under the direction of an experienced clinical neuropsychologist hired by Albert's attorney. The purpose of the examination was to determine whether Albert demonstrated any impairment that might be attributed to the head injury. Before the testing began Albert was advised to perform as well as he could on every test and to ask for more information if any procedure was not clear to him. The examiner believed that Albert put forth his best effort during the examination and that a valid set of test results had been obtained.

At this point the reader should review Albert's test results to determine whether there are any significant indications of impairment. Also analyze the findings for any inconsistencies in adequacy of performance that might imply that Albert was malingering or not putting forth adequate effort when performing a task. (See Figures 1 and 2.)

Albert earned a Verbal IQ of 104, a score slightly above the average level. His Performance IQ of 85 was 19 points lower, falling in the Low Average range. His lowest scaled score on the Verbal subtests was 9; his highest scaled score on the Performance subtests was only 7. These results suggest that Albert was consistently less able on the Performance subtests than the Verbal subtests.

Albert's GNDS score of 26 was a borderline value, falling just above the cutoff point of 25/26. The Left Neuropsychological Deficit Scale (LNDS) score of 4 was significantly less than the Right Neuropsychological Deficit Scale (RNDS) score of 10, indicating that Albert might have very mild impairment of brain functions, with the right hemisphere more dysfunctional than the left hemisphere.

Three of the other four HRB measures that are most sensitive to brain damage had scores in the impaired range: Impairment Index, 0.7; Category Test, 90 errors; and Localization component of the Tactual Performance Test (TPT), 3. Note, though, that Albert performed extremely well on Part B of the Trail Making Test, completing the task in just 36 sec.

Albert also tended to perform somewhat poorly on other measures of central processing. Although he did relatively well on the Memory component of the TPT

The Halstead–Reitan Neuropsychological Test Battery for Adults

Name: Albert Johnson — Age: 54

Gender: M — Education: 11 — Handedness: (RH) 7 LH 0

Neuropsychological Deficit Scale (NDS) Summary

General NDS

Level of Performance	14
Pathognomonic Signs	2
Patterns	3
Right/Left Differences	7
Total GNDS Score	26
Left NDS	4
Right NDS	10

WAIS-R

VIQ	104
PIQ	85
FSIQ	95

Verbal Subtests		Performance Subtests	
Information	9	Digit Symbol	6
Comprehension	9	Picture Completion	6
Arithmetic	12	Block Design	7
Similarities	9	Picture Arrangement	6
Digit Span	12	Object Assembly	6
Vocabulary	12		

Minnesota Multiphasic Personality Inventory (MMPI)

		Hs	72
		D	80
		Hy	62
L	73	PD	55
F	55	MF	43
K	55	Pa	44
		Pt	52
		Sc	56
		Ma	43
		SI	62

Strength of Grip

Dominant hand	(R)	50.5	kg
Non-dominant hand	(L)	49.0	kg

Name Writing

Dominant hand	(R)	4	sec
Non-dominant hand	(L)	16	sec

Aphasia Screening Test: No dysphasia, but note drawing of the key.

Category Test (Booklet version)

Number of errors: 90

Tactual Performance Test

Dominant hand	(R)	8.8	Total Time	23.0
Non-dominant hand	(L)	9.0	Memory	8
Both hands		5.2	Localization	3

Seashore Rhythm Test

Number correct: 23 — 9

Speech-sounds Perception Test

Number of errors: 14

Finger Tapping Test

Dominant hand	(R)	56	56
Non-dominant hand	(L)	55	

Impairment Index 0.7

Trail Making Test

Part A	26	sec	0	error(s)
Part B	36	sec	0	error(s)

Bilateral Simultaneous Sensory Stimulation

RH	0	LH	0	Both:	RH	0	LH	0
RH	0	LF	0	Both:	RH	0	LF	0
LH	0	RF	0	Both:	LH	0	RF	0
RE	0	LE	0	Both:	RE	0	LE	0
RV	0	LV	0	Both:	RV	0	LV	0
	0		0			0		0
	0		0			0		0

Tactile Finger Recognition

RH 1 ___ 2 ___ 3 ___ 4 ___ 5 ___ RH 0 / 20

LH 1 ___ 2 ___ 3 ___ 4 ___ 5 ___ LH 0 / 20

Finger-Tip Number Writing

RH 1 ___ 2 ___ 3 ___ 4 ___ 5 ___ RH 0 / 20

LH 1 ___ 2 ___ 3 ___ 4 ___ 5 ___ LH 0 / 20

Tactile Form Recognition Test

Dominant hand	(R)	12	sec	0	error(s)
Non-dominant hand	(L)	9	sec	0	error(s)

FIGURE 1. Test results for Albert Johnson.

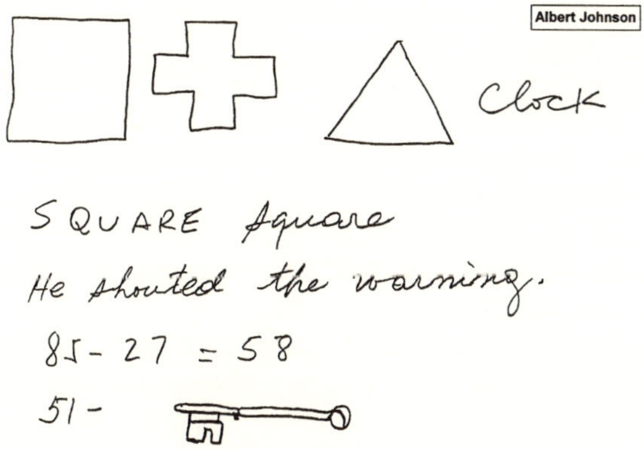

FIGURE 2. Test results for Albert Johnson.

(8), his Total Time score of 23.0 min was clearly in the impaired range. His scores on the Rhythm Test (23 correct) and the Speech-sounds Perception Test (14 errors) were also in the impaired range.

Albert's finger tapping speed and grip strength were adequate bilaterally, and there were no significant sensory-perceptual deficits. These data provide a basis for presuming that the relatively long TPT trials were related to higher-level rather than lower-level deficits. The test results up to this point reveal that Albert performed poorly on a number of tests, with the overall findings indicating mild generalized neuropsychological impairment.

Although the RNDS score (10) was considerably higher than the LNDS score (4), clinical evaluation of the lateralized findings suggested that the cerebral dysfunction was approximately equivalent for each hemisphere. On the TPT Albert was slow with his left hand as compared with his right hand. Although he drew most of the Aphasia Screening Test figures quite well, the mistakes he made reproducing the key are characteristic of persons with right-hemisphere dysfunction.

There were several indications of left-hemisphere impairment: somewhat slow finger tapping speed and grip strength with the right upper extremity as compared with the left upper extremity (even though the level of performance was adequate on both sides) and a slightly slower response time with the right hand than the left on the Tactile Form Recognition Test. In terms of overall assessment, the lateralizing indicators were not particularly strong or entirely convincing, but they were fairly characteristic of the type of impairment demonstrated by persons with a closed head injury. The rest of the test results were also consistent with this interpretation.

Albert's MMPI profile revealed various types of neurotic complaints with elements of depression. Although elevated scores on the neurotic triad are not diagnostic of a brain injury, such configurations are not uncommon among head-injured subjects (Reitan, 1955).

These findings led the neuropsychologist hired by the plaintiff's attorney to conclude that Albert exhibited mild to moderate brain damage, manifested by impairment of frontal reasoning processes (based particularly on the Category Test score of 90 errors). This conclusion was in turn based on a presumption that the Category test is a "frontal lobe" test; the neuropsychologist was not aware of the scientific study demonstrating that the Category Test has essentially no specificity for frontal damage (Reitan & Wolfson, 1995a).

This neuropsychologist also concluded that Albert had motoric and auditory processing deficits implicating the parietal and temporal areas. (It is somewhat difficult to infer the psychologist's basis for this conclusion. He perhaps incorrectly presumed that the Rhythm Test score of 23 implicated the right temporal area [see Reitan & Wolfson, 1989], and with regard to motor deficits, had noted that finger tapping and grip strength were only slightly better with the right hand than the left hand, whereas TPT performance was comparatively poor with the left hand) (see the summary sheet for details).

The neuropsychologist judged that the right-hemisphere dysfunction was greater than the left-hemisphere impairment, and attributed this to a possible contra-coup effect because the patient was reportedly struck on the left side of the head. The depression and anxiety demonstrated on the MMPI were attributed to Albert's physical injury as well as his cognitive deficits. Finally, because the injury occurred 14 months before the neuropsychological examination, the neuropsychologist concluded that Albert's cognitive impairment was most likely to be permanent.

Although it is understandable how a conclusion of brain damage might be inferred from these test results, experienced neuropsychologists would note one particular finding that would cast considerable doubt on this interpretation. Albert completed Part B of the Trail Making Test in only 36 sec—an extremely good score even for persons of high intelligence and excellent neuropsychological abilities. The neuropsychologist who interpreted the test results observed that Albert had performed relatively well on certain tests, and remarked that this was to be expected even in cases of mild to moderate brain injury. In fact, the neuropsychologist claimed that Albert's good performances supported his contention that Albert was making his best effort to do well on the tests.

If the neuropsychologist had referred to the Manual for Administration of the Trail Making Test, it would have been clear that not a single subject out of a sample of 200 brain-damaged subjects was able to complete Part B in less than 46 sec, and only 4 of these 200 subjects had scores of 69 sec or less. Only 2 of the 84 non-brain-damaged control subjects were able to complete Trails B in 36 sec or less.

If Albert could complete Trails B in 36 sec, it is reasonable to conclude that his poor performances, particularly on the Category Test, were unlikely to represent his best effort. Even if a subject decides to do poorly on an examination to support a claim of brain injury, he or she must still expend some effort to perform reasonably well on at least some of the tests so as to make the overall performance appear credible. The malingerer's problem is to produce a credible performance while still performing more poorly, at least on some tests, than represents his actual ability level—all without benefit of knowledge of normative data. When the subject has no knowledge of normative data, his or her ability to produce a set of test results that credibly reflect brain impairment is naturally limited. As in Albert's case, it is likely that a malingerer will have one or more test scores that are entirely incongruous with the other test results and previous examinations.

It must also be recognized that even though internal inconsistencies in a set of test results may cast doubt on the validity of the subject's performances, there is no guarantee that the inconsistencies will reach the level of detection in every case. One of the basic limitations of using a method that identifies inconsistencies among test results on a single examination is that the only way to evaluate a subject's performance on each test is to compare the subject's score to normative standards (performances by the rest of the population). Most subjects demonstrate some variability in performance on a battery of tests, and the ability to identify which disparities are essentially impossible often depends heavily on the neuropsychologist's experience and clinical judgment.

This approach to identifying malingering could be criticized for being opportunistic in selecting which particular tests to compare. In Albert's case we selected his good score of 36 sec on Trails B to compare with his score of 90 errors on the Category Test. We did not mention that Albert was able to complete 80 trials on tests of tactile finger localization and fingertip number writing without making a single error. The inexperienced neuropsychologist might consider perfect scores on finger localization and fingertip number writing more remarkable than a score of 36 sec on Trails B, but the experienced neuropsychologist would know that a subject is more likely to demonstrate no errors on the 80 sensory-perceptual trials than to complete Trails B in 36 sec.

If the defense attorney were to question the consistency of Albert's test results, the plaintiff's neuropsychologist could respond by comparing each test score against every other test score. Such a comparison would almost certainly reveal much more consistency than inconsistency, as many of Albert's scores reflected at least a mild degree of impairment. If the defense's neuropsychologist claimed that Albert's scores were inconsistent, he or she could easily be accused of focusing on selected test scores rather than performing an overall evaluation of the consistency of performances. Although the testifying neuropsychologist might protest and point out that there were gross inconsistencies in Albert's performances, the protest would still be based on clinical experience rather than documented evidence.

In conclusion, although it might be quite possible for an experienced neuropsychologist to correctly identify the invalidity of a subject's test protocol on the basis of inconsistencies among scores, there appear to be significant barriers to using this method in a fully convincing manner.

IDENTIFYING INVALID TEST RESULTS BY COMPARING TWO OR MORE TESTINGS

As noted above, most of the psychometric approaches used to detect malingering have evaluated test scores based on a single examination, with the results interpreted in terms of adequacy (or level) of performance. This method, which compares the subject's test scores with the rest of the population, has the disadvantage of battling the normal probability curve. Because malingerers are not the only subjects who perform poorly on neuropsychological tests, the level-of-performance approach has a serious inherent problem. Obviously, 50% of the normal population fall below the average level of performance, and severely impaired individuals often produce legitimately poor scores. Severe cognitive impairment may be associated with a degree of confusion that produces scores well below a chance level. Of course, malingerers may earn relatively good scores on a test even though they are not expending their best effort and are performing below their optimal level. A level-of-performance approach would completely fail to identify such malingerers.

In a prior section of this chapter we illustrated the implicit value as well as the problems in identifying malingerers by using an approach based on an evaluation of intraindividual (as compared with interindividual) test scores. In some cases (such as Albert Johnson's), a subject's performance on one test as compared with other tests may be a dependable basis for questioning the validity of the entire set of test scores. There is no assurance, though, that this approach would identify every person who was malingering. As we pointed out, there are additional problems concerning the use of clinical judgment in implementing this method.

However, intraindividual test score comparisons are not limited to comparing different tests administered at the same time. Another useful approach is to compare the subject's scores on the same test administered on two different occasions. This method also uses intraindividual comparisons of test scores (using the subject as his or her own control), and avoids the problems implicit in interindividual evaluations. We have been using this approach since the late 1970s to evaluate the validity of test scores produced by persons involved in litigation. We have frequently observed remarkable, and seemingly unbelievable, changes in test scores on the two examinations. These observations support the contention that subjects who are malingering or not putting forth their best possible effort (as might occur in persons involved in litigation) respond less consistently than subjects who are not adversely influenced by circumstantial factors.

For example, a subject may not remember the response he or she gave on the first testing to an item on the Information or Vocabulary subtest of the Wechsler Scale, and on the second testing give a response that is inferior (or perhaps superior) to the answer given on the first testing. Alternatively, persons without ulterior influences on their performances might be presumed to show less variability on the two testings because each response represented their best possible effort. Thus, test–retest comparisons can be performed by comparing the score produced on the same test administered on two different occasions and by comparing and analyzing responses to individual test items.

Cullum, Heaton, and Grant (1991), researchers who used three cases to illustrate this approach, stated that they believed that this was a previously unstudied method for detecting invalid test results. These authors compared subjects' performances on an extensive battery of tests on serial examinations and found highly variable performances that exceeded the presumed range for normal or neurologically stable subjects. Cullum et al. stated that "examination of performance reliability across testings may be a powerful means by which the neuropsychologist can detect patients who are not consistently putting forth adequate effort on the examination" (p. 168).

We have used this method for nearly 15 years and have often constructed charts to use during trial to illustrate the inconsistency of a plaintiff's responses. Information presented in this manner is quite understandable and convincing to jurors. For example, if a subject is able on the first testing to name the capital of Italy and on the second examination has no idea of the correct response, an explanation would seem to be necessary. If some type of traumatic event occurred that affected the litigant's memory, the explanation might be obvious. Another possibility is that the litigant was not expressing his or her best effort on the second examination, particularly if the pattern of knowing and then not knowing the correct answer was displayed in a number of instances. We will present two cases in which we were involved to illustrate this approach of detecting malingering or dissimulation. (The names of the subjects have been changed to protect their anonymity.)

THE CASE OF THE MALINGERING TRUCK DRIVER

Name:	John Sterling	Gender:	Male
Age:	54	Handedness:	Right
Education:	10	Occupation:	Truck driver

Background and History

John Sterling was driving his employer's truck when he struck a pothole and bounced upward, striking his head on the top of the truck cab. He was wearing a hard hat, and although he did not lose consciousness after the incident, he had many complaints, including constant headaches and pain in his neck, both arms, upper back, lower back, and left leg. He reported that the pain increased with any physical activity and when he became fatigued. He also complained of numbness and weakness in his arms, poor balance and coordination, spots in front of his eyes, difficulty focusing his eyes, pain in his right eye, and a cold sensation in his upper eyelids when they come in contact with his lower lids during blinking. He also reported experiencing episodes of dizziness.

John stated that occasionally his mind "goes blank" and he becomes entirely confused. He also reported that since the accident he has problems with memory and concentration and he feels that he has sustained some sort of brain damage. He notes that his problems appear particularly when he experiences any amount of stress. On such occasions he becomes so impaired that he cannot perform even simple tasks, such as signing his name or paying for groceries. He says that since the accident he has not been able to balance his checkbook, has tended to buy things that he does not need, and has loaned money to people who are unlikely to repay him. He estimated that he has lost approximately $20,000 because of these unnecessary purchases and poor loans. He says that he becomes confused trying to follow a conversation and has serious difficulty recalling any events. According to John, all of these problems postdate the accident, and he feels that the head injury is entirely responsible.

Medical examinations performed since the accident revealed cervical strain and cervical radiculopathy and polyneuropathy. An MRI showed a protruding cervical disk.

A review of John's previous illnesses and injuries revealed that about 23 years ago he was struck by an overhead door and sustained neck injuries that required physical therapy and traction. Six years later he was involved in another incident in which he was struck on the side of his head but appeared to recover quickly. About 3 years ago the arm of a crane struck him on the top of his head, resulting in headaches, neck pain, numbness and weakness in his arms, and pain in his lower back and left leg. Current x-rays revealed an old cervical fracture, a repaired intervertebral disk, and a fusion of the spinal column. John said that he recovered well from all of these injuries, and denied having any cognitive problems prior to the current head injury.

John left school at the age of 16, after completing the 10th grade. He said that he never liked school, hated to be confined indoors, and attended school only because it was required by law. He served in the Navy for 4 years and received an honorable discharge. He has worked for the same company for more than 30 years, driving a truck and operating a crane, but has been completely unable to work since the current injury.

John lives in a rural area, and in the past he has spent a considerable amount of time training and boarding horses. He says that he has always enjoyed working with horses, and did this so well that his income from training horses had equaled or surpassed his income as a truck driver. However, he says that his problems with balance and coordination since the injury have prevented him from working with horses, and he misses the activity more than anything else. Because of his impairment he has had to hire a man to care for the horses he currently owns and boards. Prior to the accident he enjoyed many outdoor activities, such as hunting, fishing, trap shooting, swimming, and horseback riding, but he is no longer able to engage in these activities. When he was asked whether he was bored with his present life, he replied, "How can you be bored when your brain is so dormant?" He believes that his cognitive impairment is more of a problem than his pain, and he says that he feels "incompetent and dumb."

Neuropsychological Evaluations

Testing I (10 Months Postinjury)

John Sterling's first neuropsychological evaluation was done 10 months after his injury. His attorney referred him for the examination, which was done by a nationally known clinical neuropsychologist.

Subject's Behavior during Testing. In his report, the neuropsychologist indicated that it was apparent during the testing that John's emotional status was somewhat fragile. He noted that John became visibly upset when tasks were difficult for him and that he complained of dizziness several times during the session.

The Neuropsychological Examination. An extensive number of psychological tests were administered, including the Boston Naming Test, the Symbol Digit Modalities Test, 8 subtests from the WAIS-R, the Sentence Repetition Test of the Multilingual Aphasia Examination, the Story Recall Test, the Sentence Building Test, the Hooper Visual Organization Test, Parts A and B of the Trail Making Test, the Visual Search Test, the Rey Complex Figure Test, the Bender Gestalt Test, the Rule Governed Drawings, and the Symptom Check List-90.

John was also given tests to complete at home, including the Gates–MacGintie Reading Test, the Raven Progressive Matrices, selected subtests of the Stanford–Binet Intelligence Test, and a single page of arithmetic problems involving addition, subtraction, multiplication, finding an average of four numbers, and solving two problems of the type included in the Wechsler Arithmetic subtest.

Report of Neuropsychological Findings on Testing I

The neuropsychologist concluded that John had an average intellectual endowment, even though his actual level of performance on intelligence measures was consistently well below average. The test results were interpreted as indicating a pronounced attention disorder, severe impairment of verbal memory, severe impairment of visual memory, tendencies toward perseveration, and diminished mental flexibility. The neuropsychologist concluded that John was mentally incapacitated and unfit for any kind of competitive employment. He believed that his prospects for rehabilitation or for learning a new trade were limited, and that he needed help in handling finances and personal affairs. In addition, he reported that information should be presented to John in "small units" to facilitate comprehension.

In his report, the neuropsychologist stated that John's pattern of deficits was characteristic of traumatic brain damage. He noted the injuries that occurred prior to the current accident and stated that they may have left some minor residuals, but felt that they probably did not compromise John's mental functioning significantly. He wrote the following conclusion: "As he presented at the time of my examination, he was clearly unable to hold a job in the competitive market and as such was very much disabled relative to his on-the-job function the day of the accident. It is, therefore, my opinion that his cognitive disabilities are in all probability due to the current industrial accident."

Testing II (8 Months after Testing I and 18 Months Postinjury)

John Sterling was reexamined 8 months later by a board-certified clinical psychologist. The referral came from a therapist at a pain center where John was being evaluated. The second examination included essentially the same tests as the first examination.

During the clinical interview John reiterated his complaints. He indicated that he has not been able to go back to work since the accident, but because the injury was work-related his company has been paying him $1400 per month. He reported that he has not had any income from training and boarding horses because he has not been able to do this kind of work since the injury.

Report of Neuropsychological Findings on Testing II

This psychologist felt that John's effort during the testing was questionable. More significantly, on many of the tests John performed much worse on Testing II than on Testing I. For example, his score on the WAIS-R Information subtest decreased from 9 to 3, and he scored at least somewhat lower on each of the other subtests. It was not possible for us to compare performances on all of the tests that were given at both examinations because many of the responses on the first examination were recorded illegibly.

The psychologist noted that John had many more complaints than would usually be warranted by a mild head injury. He also remarked that John performed very poorly on the tests, and that the deterioration since the first examination suggested that "the current evaluation cannot be relied upon." This psychologist concluded that John's poorer performance on the second examination was inconsistent with the pattern expected in head injury.

Testing III (8 Months after Testing II and 26 Months Postinjury)

John Sterling was reexamined 8 months later. The clinical psychologist who performed the third examination administered only a few tests and depended mainly on a clinical interview to evaluate the patient.

John's complaints were again very extensive, and essentially similar to his previous difficulties. He claimed that he was completely disabled and unable to perform any kind of work.

Results of Testing III. In a comparison of the test results on the three examinations, John performed much better on some tests and considerably worse on others. Up to this point, there was a progressive deterioration of performance on certain Wechsler subtests, whereas on other tests the level of performance was inconsistent. In general, John performed very poorly on the third examination. For example, he earned the following scores on the WMS-R: Verbal Memory, 64; Visual Memory, 52; General Memory, less than 50; Attention/Concentration, not given; and Delayed Recall, 53.

Report of Neuropsychological Findings on Testing III

The psychologist who conducted the third neuropsychological examination concluded that John had probably sustained some impairment of cognitive functions, but suggested that other factors, including medication, emotional status, and a tendency to focus on his pain and suffering, might also be affecting his current performance. There was no suggestion in the psychologist's report, though, that the test results were not entirely valid; in fact, the psychologist interpreted John's poor performances as indications of his neuropsychological impairment.

In summary, the three neuropsychological evaluations indicated that (1)John sustained significant and severe neuropsychological deficits that were in all probability attributable to the closed head injury, (2) John performed worse on the second examination than on the first, but there was a question about whether the scores were valid, and (3) John demonstrated significant neuropsychological impairment that could be attributed to his prior head injuries (without differentiation of the influence of each head injury) as well as to other factors such as medication and emotional status.

Testing IV (7 Months after Testing III and 33 Months Postinjury)

This situation led the defense attorney to request a comprehensive neuropsychological examination from another well-known clinical neuropsychologist. In his report this neuropsychologist listed John's multiple complaints, reviewed the results of the previous neuropsychological examinations, and noted the inconsistency in the three sets of test results.

Results of Testing IV. In addition to a clinical interview, this neuropsychologist administered a number of tests that had been given in previous examinations and included the Portland Digit Recognition Test (PDRT) (Binder, 1993) to determine whether John was malingering.

Report of Neuropsychological Findings on Testing IV

This neuropsychologist compared the results obtained on his examination with John's performances on the same tests in previous examinations. The scores on the fourth examination were somewhat better than the scores on the second examination, but still considerably worse than the results on the first examination. Although John did not do well on any of the tests in this examination, he performed extremely poorly on some of the tests compared with other tests.

The PDRT was administered to determine whether John was malingering. In this test the subject merely has to recognize a five-digit number, selecting from two alternatives. Although the PDRT is presented as a memory test, it actually requires intact motivation. Using a 5-sec delay before responding, John correctly answered 5 of 18 items. With a 15-sec delay he was correct on 7 of 18 items. Thus, he performed quite poorly, responding correctly on only 12 of 36 items. If he had been guessing on each item, he should have achieved close to a 50% level of correct responses. Statistical analysis of chance deviations from a 50% correct response rate indicates that John's results reached a probability of only .03, strongly suggesting that he was "faking bad."

The neuropsychologist stated in his report that he believed that John had not put forth a maximal effort on the tests, and concluded that it was not possible to determine whether any psychological impairment had occurred as a result of the current injury.

Final Evaluation. At this point the defense attorney contacted Ralph Reitan and asked him to evaluate John Sterling's entire file. A review of the test results from the four examinations revealed considerable variability in level of performance as well as in responses to individual items. Reitan notified the defense attorney that it appeared that John was malingering, and advised him to search for additional evidence to determine whether this was true. The attorney hired a private detective to videotape John as he went about his everyday activities. John, who did not know that he was under surveillance, demonstrated none of the difficulties (such as staggering and loss of balance) that he claimed to be experiencing as a result of the accident. In fact, the videotape showed John riding and training his horses and showing no signs of impairment. John's lawyer immediately resigned from the case after he saw the videotape. John was unable to find another lawyer willing to represent him, and the lawsuit was dropped.

THE CASE OF THE NEUROTIC SECRETARY

Name:	Katherine Gilmore	Gender:	Female
Age:	39	Handedness:	Right
Education:	17	Occupation:	Clerical Worker

This case illustrates an instance in which it was necessary to weigh evidence of possible brain impairment against evidence of emotional disturbances to reach an understanding of the client's complaints and symptoms. In addition, an analysis of the test data casts considerable doubt on the validity of the scores.

Background and History

Katherine Gilmore instituted a lawsuit against a large company, alleging that she had sustained memory loss and impairment, toxic encephalopathy, urinary infections, acquired immune dysfunction with chemical hypersensitivity, headaches, and pulmonary infections, and has been rendered sick, sore, nervous, neurotic, hysterical, and distressed as a result of exposure to carbon monoxide gas and sulfide gas fumes in her home over a period of approximately 3 months.

Neuropsychological Evaluations

One of the authors (Reitan) was asked to review the results of Katherine Gilmore's examination performed at the neuropsychology laboratory of a major medical center. These test results are presented on the following pages.

Without any knowledge of the patient's history or complaints, Reitan reviewed the test results and wrote the following brief conclusion: "Essentially normal test results. There are no significant indications of brain damage or dysfunction, but there are significant indications of emotional and personality problems."

Reitan communicated these conclusions to the attorney who had hired him, and at that time learned that the attorney represented the defendant. The attorney told Reitan that the plaintiff had secured opinions from experts who attributed all of Katherine's problems to the toxic exposure. Reitan was then asked to review all of the plaintiff's medical and neuropsychological records.

We will briefly discuss the HRB results before considering these additional medical records and Katherine's history information. The only test scores on the HRB that might be interpreted as showing any degree of impairment were on the Category Test (53 errors), Part B of the Trail Making Test (110 sec), and finger tapping speed (RH, 49; LH, 40). The only lateralizing effect in the entire battery having any possible significance was the mildly slow finger tapping speed with the left hand. It must be remembered, however, that women tend to tap somewhat slower than men.

Katherine's IQ values also tended to be lower than expected based on her education, but considering her many good scores on neuropsychological tests, the somewhat low IQ scores would not appear to be attributable to brain damage. Recognizing that normal subjects not uncommonly have a few test scores that are not as good as they might be, Katherine's overall results were within the normal range.

The MMPI profile suggested that Katherine had significant emotional problems. The defense attorney had not thoroughly investigated the plaintiff's history, and was not aware of her prior psychiatric difficulties. Reitan recommended that a comprehensive investigation be done to document any emotional problems the plaintiff might have had prior to the exposure to gas fumes.

The neuropsychologist at the medical center where the tests were administered interpreted the results in a very guarded manner, noting that (1) the emotional difficulties were more prominent than the neuropsychological deficits and (2) there were some mild indications of neuropsychological impairment, but it seemed likely that these findings were more likely to be related to depression and life-adjustment problems than to toxic exposure.

A review of Katherine's medical records based on evaluations performed after the toxic exposure did not reveal any significant findings. Results of several pulmonary function evaluations and the clinical neurological examinations were normal. A psychiatric evaluation was performed, but was based on only a single office visit, and the psychiatrist did not draw any definite conclusions.

One expert, an osteopathic physician who had a Ph.D. in toxicology, evaluated Katherine at her attorney's request. On the basis of the plaintiff's history and his examination, this physician concluded that "[Katherine Gilmore] has suffered brain damage similar to 'painter's solvent encephalopathy, lead encephalopathy, or encephalopathy from a variety of other chemicals,' and is completely unable to perform most usual activities of a person of the same age and training. Her learning abilities are impaired. It is certain from her background and work experience that she was in the superior range prior to her poisoning. Something is drastically wrong with Katherine Gilmore, and the history indicates that it is a sequelae [sic] of the carbon monoxide gas leak in her home."

Because of these conclusions, the toxicologist-physician referred Katherine to a psychologist for further evaluation. This psychologist and a colleague saw the plaintiff for four sessions over a period of 19 months and administered a considerable number of psychological tests. The defense attorney was initially given only an interpretive report of the examination, but he was eventually able to secure the raw-score data sheets for the tests. These documents turned out to be relatively useless, because the data of the examination, and sometimes even the patient's name, was not written on the data sheet. A review of the forms indicated that most of the test scores were in the normal range, but these two psychologists reported that Katherine had sustained significant mental, cognitive, and emotional problems secondary to toxic exposure.

During the 19-month period that Katherine was evaluated by these two psychologists, she was also examined at her own request by another clinical psychologist. This psychologist provided a letter summarizing his conclusions, and noted that the plaintiff's Wechsler Memory Scale Quotient of only 67 raised questions about her degree of cooperation (on the first evaluation Katherine earned a WMS score of 103). The psychologist believed that Katherine had significant emotional problems, but found no evidence that she had suffered adverse effects from toxic fumes.

Finally, a government agency to which Katherine had applied for assistance referred her to still another clinical psychologist for an evaluation. This psychologist conducted a clinical interview and administered the WAIS-R, the Trail Making Test, the Booklet Category Test, and the MMPI. His conclusion was that Katherine had impaired cognitive functioning, including severe problems of attention, concentration, and memory; periods of disorientation and confusion; difficulty with expressive language; and deterioration of cognitive functions during the interval following previous examinations. All of these deficits were attributed to toxic encephalopathy secondary to toxic exposure.

Reitan's recommendation to research the plaintiff's history in detail for evidence of emotional problems prior to the toxic exposure proved fruitful. The plaintiff had joined the Navy about 19 years before the toxic exposure episode, and while in the Navy had undergone numerous evaluations and hospitalizations for emotional and behavior problems. The Navy record was replete with reports of Katherine's many interpersonal conflicts, complaints, histrionic and egocentric behavior, and manipulative behavior (which all seemed quite similar to her postexposure complaints). She received a diagnosis of "emotionally unstable personality with passive aggressive features and characterized by impulsivity, low morale, poor judgment, naivete, and lability." It was decided that Katherine was most likely to become an increasingly chronic administrative nuisance, and she was discharged from the Navy. As might be expected, an investigation of VA Medical Centers and other hospitals in the areas in which she had lived uncovered many other psychiatric records.

At this point, the history information described a woman who (1) had demonstrated emotional instability over a number of years, (2) had allegedly experienced several months of exposure to carbon monoxide and sulfide gas fumes from a leaking furnace with resulting neuropsychological and emotional deficits, and (3) was described by some experts as having serious impairment resulting from toxic exposure and by other experts as having longstanding and continual emotional problems but no evidence of neuropsychological impairment of the type that might result from toxic exposure.

The defense lawyer felt that the scientific status and respectability of his experts would carry the case in his favor. The plaintiff's lawyer felt that the defense's "ivory tower" experts would not prevail against his experts, who had devoted their lives to clinical practice, had gained their knowledge working in the trenches, and knew from experience the kinds of problems endured by the "little" person who has been abused by the system. He believed that a jury, composed of persons who themselves had experienced the stress of trying to buck the system, would understand the plight of his client. The outcome of the trial appeared to rest on the jury's reaction to one set of experts versus another. What could be done to expose the truth?

Katherine had no medical evidence of impairment, nor was any such evidence expected to be produced. The case rested entirely on the neuropsychological findings. Which side did the neuropsychological findings support? Experts for the defense reached one conclusion; experts for the plaintiff had entirely different opinions. Were the neuropsychological findings that indicated brain impairment valid? Were they credible? How can this question be answered?

An evaluation of the consistency of the plaintiff's responses and performances often provides relevant information. It must be recognized that on successive examinations the tests are the same, the subject is the same, and the only variable should be the time of testing. If the subject has not improved or deteriorated (and the nature of the presumed disorder is undoubtedly relevant in this regard), the time of testing should not affect the results. If the subject makes his or her best effort on each examination, there should not be any significant changes in test results. However, if a subject does not put forth his or her best effort on an examination, it may be quite difficult to reproduce a comparable and credible diminished effort on a later evaluation.

Some litigants seem to feel a need to document on successive examinations their disability or impairment. Thus, on subsequent evaluations they perform more poorly instead of demonstrating the recovery pattern that would normally be expected considering the nature of the presumed impairing condition. When an individual sustains an insult to the brain, it is expected that the major deficits will be demonstrated soon after the insult and that the test scores will improve over time and correspond with clinical improvement following the insult. When there are striking deviations from this pattern (i.e., poorer performances on later examinations), the validity and value of the test results must be questioned.

In Katherine's case, we would expect to see better scores on successive administrations of the same tests, for two reasons: (1) positive practice effects based on the experience of having previously taken the tests and (2) gradual improvement over time as the plaintiff recovers from the brain insult. Poorer performances on subsequent testings therefore present a strong basis for questioning the plaintiff's effort and motivation, and in turn, the validity of any interpretations based on the test scores.

Because Katherine had been examined several times with the same instruments, there was an opportunity to compare the consistency of her scores over time, and this comparison revealed gross inconsistencies. For example, Katherine had taken the WMS on two occasions. On the first examination she earned a Memory Quotient of 103; a few months later she earned a score of only 67. On the first administration of the Booklet Category Test Katherine did quite well, making only 23 errors. However, when she was given the same test 6 months later, she made 77 errors!

The verbal subtests of the Wechsler Scale are particularly helpful in determining the consistency of a subject's performances. It is unlikely, for example, that the subject would know the capital of Italy on one testing and have no idea of the correct answer on the next testing. Some of the WAIS-R subtests were administered to Katherine two or three times, and the results were analyzed to determine their consistency.

A review of Katherine's responses reveals that she initially knew the capital of Italy, the continent on which the Sahara Desert was located, and the number of senators in the U.S. Senate. On subsequent examinations she did not know the answers to these questions and many others that she had initially answered correctly. Items showing improved responses on later testings might be a result of learning the information between testings, but it is also possible—and probably more likely—that the plaintiff was not putting forth her best effort on subsequent testings and did not remember (either deliberately or through lack of effort) how she had responded to items on the first testing. Comparative data of this kind, showing consistent failures after initial success and success after initial failure, have strong face validity for documenting that a subject's test scores did not reflect an optimal effort to do well and were not a reliable basis for neuropsychological interpretation.

Outcome

This case came to trial, and the plaintiff's experts presented their evidence to show that Katherine Gilmore was significantly impaired. The defense's case was based on Katherine's longstanding emotional problems and her extensive history of maladaptive behavior. The defense attorney emphasized especially that the test results were insufficient to reach any conclusions except that Katherine's responses had been grossly inconsistent from one testing to the next.

The jury's verdict was for the defendants. After the trial, the 12 members of the jury waited for an opportunity to discuss the case with the defense lawyers. All of the jurors thought that the case was fascinating. One man said he would have paid $200 for an opportunity to learn what he had learned in this case. The jurors recognized that the plaintiff was a sick woman, but it was clear to them that her problem was a longstanding emotional disturbance and not the result of exposure to toxic fumes.

These examples make clear that some litigants fail to produce consistent test results on consecutive examinations and that the test results cannot always be accepted as valid indications of the subjects' best abilities. Selected examples of this kind obviously do not provide information of how often these cases occur, nor do they provide a rigorous, standardized method for evaluating test–retest inconsistencies. Recognizing the need for a standard procedure, the next section describes a method for detecting invalid test results based on comparisons of results of two examinations of the same subjects, together with comparisons of results obtained from a group of head-injured litigants who were suing to recover damages and a group of head-injured persons who were not involved in litigation.

RESEARCH RESULTS: DEVELOPMENT OF SPECIFIC QUANTITATIVE PROCEDURES FOR DETECTING INVALIDITY OF NEUROPSYCHOLOGICAL TEST RESULTS

Few if any subjects admit that they have malingered. Although convincing evidence that a subject has malingered is discovered and actually documented in only a small number of cases, reasons often abound for suspecting that a subject has malingered or failed to put for the best possible effort. Because a group of proved malingerers has never been available for study (and if they were, one would have to question the validity of the results they produced!), how can the manifestations of malingering be discerned? Where would we be today in our understanding of the effects of brain damage if we had never studied a single group of persons with unequivocally established brain damage? The problem of malingering or dissimulation is even more complex, because it is entirely possible that many people, given the stresses and circumstances under which they are tested, may not even realize that they are not putting forth their best possible effort during a neuropsychological examination.

Considering the nature of the problem, and realizing that a focal point of interest often centers on the test result of litigants, we decided that practical and pertinent information might be discerned by comparing the neuropsychological test results of head-injured litigants with the performances of head-injured nonlitigants. Because many litigants are tested more than once before their case is finally settled, appropriate data are often available. We also had data from a research project involving serial testing of subjects who had never been involved in litigation because second-party liability was not an issue.

Our hypothesis was that there would be a significant advantage in comparing the subject's test results obtained on two testings rather than comparing the subject's scores with the rest of the population. If the subject performed to the best of his or her ability on both examinations, one would presume that the scores on the second testing would be at least comparable or possibly better (because of practice effects). If the subject was not putting forth his or her best effort, the scores on the two testings would be more variable, and perhaps even worse on the second testing, because of the need to "prove" one's impairment to others, such as insurance investigators or a jury.

We conducted three studies (Reitan & Wolfson, 1995b, 1996, 1997) that compared the test results of two groups of adult head-injured subjects. One group was involved in litigation related to the head injury; the other group was not. The same groups were used in all three studies.

Study 1: Consistency of Test Scores

Subjects

The nonlitigation group was composed of 17 males and 3 females who had sustained a head injury but were not involved in litigation. All of these subjects had volunteered to participate in a research project. The litigation group consisted of 14 males and 6 females, all of whom were involved in litigation to recover damages allegedly resulting from a head injury. It was impossible to compare accurately the severity of the head injuries in the two groups, primarily because the records of the litigation group varied and the diagnostic procedures had been performed in various locations. This made it difficult to obtain detailed and consistent records.

Neither group of subjects had been included in any systematic cognitive rehabilitation program, although a few subjects in the litigation group had received sporadic training to improve attention, concentration, memory, or other cognitive functions.

The mean age was 29.65 years ($SD = 14.91$) for the nonlitigants and 41.85 years ($SD = 10.19$) for the litigants. The mean education was 12.30 years ($SD = 2.23$) for the nonlitigants and 13.95 years ($SD = 2.84$) for the litigants. Comparisons of the distributions to evaluate age and education differences yielded t ratios of 3.02 ($p < .01$) and 2.05 ($p = .05$), respectively. Because of the differences in age and education distributions between the two groups and the inadequate comparative information about the severity of the subjects' head injuries, no direct comparisons were made of mean achievement (or error) scores on the various tests. Statistical analyses were based only on intraindividual difference scores that compared each subject's test scores obtained on two examinations.

The mean time between the two examinations was 12.00 months for the nonlitigants and 14.45 months for the litigants. The intergroup difference was not statistically significant ($p < .20$). However, the nonlitigants were initially tested soon after the head injury was sustained, whereas the litigants were initially tested at variable times following head injury.

An intergroup difference that may have been of significance derives from the fact that all of the nonlitigants were examined on a strict schedule (they were initially tested within a few weeks of the injury and retested 12 months later), whereas the litigants were initially tested at varying intervals following their head injuries. Thus, the nonlitigation group may have had a greater potential for demonstrating spontaneous recovery.

Another factor that may have had an influence on the results of this study was that all of the nonlitigants were tested by technicians who had been trained by and were directly responsible to one of the authors (R.M.R.). These technicians were schooled in precise and objective test administration. Subjects in the litigation group had usually been tested by opposing representatives of an adversarial procedure, hired by either the plaintiff or the defense. In 12 cases, Testing I was done by the plaintiff's psychologist and Testing II was performed by the defense psychologist; in 5 cases, Testing I and Testing II were done by different psychologists hired by the plaintiff; in 2 cases, Testing I was done for clinical purposes and Testing II was done by the plaintiff's psychologist; and in 1 case, Testing I was done by the plaintiff's psychologist and Testing II was performed by a neutral psychologist.

One might presume that examiner bias, if it existed, would be in the direction of finding less impairment by the defense psychologist, leading to a trend for better scores on the second testing.

Method

This study used intraindividual differences in test scores on the two testings for comparison of the two groups.

Procedure

Study I focused on tests that traditionally have been demonstrated to be relatively insensitive to brain damage (taken from the Wechsler Scale) and tests that have been shown to be particularly sensitive to brain damage (taken from the Wechsler Scale and the HRB). The postulate was that head-injured subjects involved in litigation would perform more poorly on the second examination than on the first, and head-injured subjects not in litigation would show improvement on the second examination (as a result of positive practice effects as well as spontaneous recovery). Thus, in accordance with the principle demonstrated by Reitan and Wolfson (1988) in their study of spontaneous recovery after head injury, we expected the greatest degree of improvement to occur on the tests that are most sensitive to brain damage.

The tests believed to be less sensitive measures were the Information, Comprehension, Arithmetic, Similarities, and Vocabulary subtests from either the WAIS or the WAIS-R. The more sensitive measures were the Picture Arrangement, Block Design,and Digit Symbol subtests from either the WAIS or WAIS-R, and the Category Test, Part B of the Trail Making Test, and the Localization component of the Tactual Performance Test (TPT–Localization) from the HRB.

Mean scores and standard deviations were calculated for each variable in each group. Mean changes between Testing I and Testing II were compared in each group by evaluating difference score distributions for each variable using *t* tests.

Only the tests that achieved a probability level of .025 or less were used to compute the Retest Consistency Index. Six tests reached the specified level of significance in differentiating the two groups: Comprehension, Picture Arrangement, Digit Symbol, the Category Test, Part B of the Trail Making Test, and TPT–Localization. Difference scores on these tests for the combined litigation and nonlitigation groups were transformed to a five-point scale to reflect the degree of inconsistency (a score of 5 indicated the greatest degree of inconsistency; a score of 1 reflected the least degree of inconsistency). Using *t* ratios, means for the two groups were compared for the total of the scaled scores for the six most sensitive tests (the Retest Consistency Index) as well as for the individual tests.

The distributions, based on the 5-point scale, were compared for the litigation group and the nonlitigation group, and a cutoff point that best differentiated the two groups was determined for the Retest Consistency Index.

Results

Table 1 presents means, standard deviations, *t* ratios comparing results of the first and second testings within each group, probability levels, and the proportion of subjects in each group that earned better scores on the second testing.

The nonlitigation group had improved mean values on each of the 11 tests, and on each test, more than 50% of these subjects had improved scores on Testing II. The improvement was statistically significant, however, only for Picture Arrangement, Digit Symbol, the Category Test, Part B of the Trail Making Test, and TPT–Localization. Conversely, on Testing II the litigation group had poorer means on each of the 11 tests. Less than 50% of the subjects in the litigation group showed improvement on the second examination, with the changes reaching significance at less than the .05 level on Similarities, Vocabulary, Picture Arrangement, Digit Symbol, the Category Test, and Part B of the Trail Making Test.

Although it was apparent that the general direction of change on Testing II was different for the two groups on every variable, the significance of intergroup differences was tested directly by comparing difference score distributions for the two groups on Testing I and Testing II. Mean difference scores between Testing I

TABLE 1. Means and Standard Deviations on Testings I and II for Nonlitigation and Litigation Groups; Comparisons of Testing I and II for Each Group; Percentage of Each Group Showing Improved Scores on Testing II; and Comparison of Difference Score Distributions, Based on Testing I and II, for the Two Groups

Group			Inf	Comp	Arith	Simil	Vocab	PA	BD	Digit Symbol	Category	Trails B	TPT-Loc
Nonlitigation	Testing I	M	10.20	10.45	9.10	11.60	10.10	9.00	11.40	8.75	45.95	109.00	3.25
		SD	3.27	3.65	4.91	4.22	3.57	3.31	3.68	3.42	27.88	63.91	1.65
	Testing II	M	10.45	11.30	9.95	11.70	10.20	11.00	11.70	12.05	35.90	89.40	4.35
		SD	3.27	3.80	4.48	4.66	3.93	3.77	3.60	3.50	27.45	53.76	2.52
		t	1.05	1.93	1.47	0.27	0.37	3.20	0.75	3.89	3.47	2.51	2.34
		$p <$	.40	.10	.20	.90	.80	.005	.50	.001	.001	.025	.05
	% improving on Testing II		55	62.5	60	55	52.5	72.5	62.5	100	80	72.5	77.5
Litigation	Testing I	M	9.75	9.65	8.10	9.25	10.20	9.00	7.55	7.15	65.80	118.25	2.60
		SD	2.07	2.70	2.77	2.84	2.42	2.38	2.16	2.25	27.13	64.55	1.90
	Testing II	M	8.85	8.70	7.65	8.35	9.20	7.50	7.15	5.20	80.20	153.50	1.75
		SD	2.50	2.39	3.30	2.62	2.14	2.74	2.80	1.58	33.57	79.94	1.25
		t	1.69	1.58	0.68	2.20	2.21	2.24	0.79	4.45	2.66	2.14	1.95
		$p <$	.20	.20	.50	.05	.05	.05	.50	.001	.02	.05	.10
	% improving on Testing II		40	40	37.5	32.5	30	30	45	22.5	30	27.5	30

and Testing II for each group and the significance of differences in the two groups are presented in Table 2.

As shown in Table 2, the probability levels on each test were equivalent to or less than the probability levels presented in Table 1 for the groups individually. This reflects the fact that the direction of change (better versus poorer scores on Testing II) was different for the two groups on each variable, consistently leading to larger inter- than intragroup differences.

The next step was to develop a five-point scale for converting difference scores to scaled scores. We included only those measures that yielded probability estimates of .025 or less and on which the two groups showed clearly significant differences. The six tests that met these criteria (see Table 2) were Comprehension, Picture Arrangement, Digit Symbol, the Category Test, Part B of the Trail Making Test, and TPT–Localization. Distributions of difference scores for the combined groups were tallied, and a score of 5 was assigned to the eight subjects (20% of the combined groups) who had the most inconsistent retest scores. A score of 4 was assigned to the next 20%, and so on, to a score of 1 for the most consistent subjects. (Some tied scores made it impossible to do this perfectly, but the 20% categorization was followed as closely as possible). Table 3 presents the chart for converting difference scores to scaled scores.

Difference scores between Testing I and Testing II for individual subjects were computed so that negative values corresponded with a poorer performance on the second examination, regardless of whether the test score represented an achievement score or an error score.

Finally, the distributions on this five-point scale were compared in the litigation and nonlitigation groups for each of the six tests that contribute to the Retest Consistency Index. As shown in Table 4, these scores were greater on each of the six measures for the litigation group than for the nonlitigation group, and the differences between the groups were statistically significant in each comparison. Nevertheless, there was a substantial degree of intergroup overlap in several of the distributions for individual tests. The Retest Consistency Index, which is the sum of the scaled scores for the six tests, was clearly a more stable measure than scores for any of the individual tests, as indicated by a t ratio (8.55) that was much larger than the t ratios for the individual tests.

An analysis of the Retest Consistency Index for the combined groups indicated that a cutoff score of 16/17 yielded the best separation of the two groups. Ninety percent of the litigants had a Retest Consistency Index of 17 or higher, and 95% of the nonlitigants had a Retest Consistency Index of 16 or less.

Conclusions

The results of this study clearly indicated that head-injured subjects involved in litigation tended to demonstrate much less consistent scores on retesting than head-injured subjects not in litigation. The Retest Consistency Index, a new

TABLE 2. Mean Difference Scores Based on Testing I and Testing II, *t* Tests Comparing the Difference Score Distributions for the Nonlitigation and Litigation Groups, and Probability Levels

Group		Inf	Comp	Arith	Simil	Vocab	PA	BD	Digit Symbol	Category	Trails B	TPT-Loc
Nonlitigation	Mean of differences	−0.25	0.85	0.85	0.10	0.10	2.00	0.30	3.30	10.05	19.60	1.10
Litigation	Mean of differences	−0.90	−0.95	−0.45	−1.10	−1.00	−1.50	−0.40	−1.95	−12.65	−34.65	−.85
	t	1.98	2.40	1.51	2.26	2.12	3.80	1.09	8.61	3.73	3.10	2.67
	$p<$	.10	.025	.20	.05	.05	.001	.30	.001	.001	.005	.02

TABLE 3. Scaled Score Conversion Table Based on Difference Scores for the Six Variables that Reached Significance Levels beyond a Probability of .025

Scaled Score	Comp	PA	Digit Symbol	Category	Trails B	TPT-Localization
	Difference scores (minus values equal poorer performances on Testing II)					
1	3 or more	4 or more	4 or more	16 or more	34 or more	2 or more
2	1 and 2	2 and 3	1, 2, and 3	4 to 15	8 to 33	1
3	0	0 and 1	0	3 to −3	7 to −7	0
4	−1	−1 and −2	−1 and −2	−2 to −16	−8 to −47	−1
5	−2 or less	−3 or less	−3 or less	−17 or less	−48 or less	−2 or less

measure based on six tests, differentially classified 90% of the litigants and 95% of the nonlitigants. Differentiation of the two groups was achieved at highly significant levels.

These results, which demonstrate that subjects involved in litigation are less likely to perform consistently on retesting, indicate that an approach based on the consistency of retest scores is highly promising. Retest mean scores of the litigation group were always lower than the initial mean scores, and some of these changes were statistically significant. Considering the fact that the nonlitigants had better means on every test on the second testing (although not always significantly better), it is apparent that a scale reflecting direction of change would differentiate strikingly between the two groups.

Study 2: Consistency of Responses to Test Items

In Study 1 (Reitan & Wolfson, 1997) our approach to identifying malingerers was based on a comparison of a subject's test scores on two examinations (retest

TABLE 4. Standard Deviations and *t* Ratios Based on Scaled Scores Transformed from Difference Scores

Group		Comp	PA	Digit Symbol	Category	Trails B	TPT-Loc	Total
Nonlitigation	M	2.55	2.40	1.55	2.25	2.20	2.15	13.10
	SD	1.23	1.23	0.51	1.12	1.01	1.42	2.67
Litigation	M	3.55	3.85	4.00	3.70	3.75	3.65	22.50
	SD	1.39	1.18	0.92	1.38	1.37	1.27	4.12
	t	2.40	3.80	10.43	3.65	4.08	3.52	8.55
	p<	.025	.001	.001	.001	.001	.005	.001
								16/17 cutoff

consistency). Study 2 (Reitan & Wolfson, 1995b) compared subjects' responses on individual test items on two examinations (response consistency). Again, our basic hypothesis was that a subject who is malingering or not putting forth the best possible effort (as might occur among persons involved in litigation) will respond less consistently than a subject who is not adversely influenced (as might be presumed of subjects not involved in litigation). In the present investigation of this hypothesis, however, the evaluation was based on responses to individual items, presuming that a subject who was not putting forth his or her best effort would not remember specific responses originally given and thus demonstrate inconsistency of responses on two testings.

The Retest Consistency Index (Reitan & Wolfson, 1995b) showed the most striking intergroup differences on tests that were particularly sensitive to cerebral damage, such as Digit Symbol, the Category Test, and Part B of the Trail Making Test. However, a measure that evaluates the consistency of responses on individual items on two testings would have to use tests that require much more specific responses (such as the Verbal subtests of the Wechsler Scale).

Procedure

In Study 2 we analyzed performances on Information, Comprehension, Arithmetic, Similarities, and Vocabulary from either was WAIS or WAIS-R (whichever version had been administered). For each subject, the same version of the Wechsler Scale (WAIS or WAIS-R) was used for both testings.

A raw consistency score for each subtest was obtained by comparing scores for every item on the two testings. If the subject earned a better score on an item on the second testing, 1 point was assigned to that item. If the subject earned a poorer score on an item on the second testing, 2 points were assigned. If an unequal number of items had been administered on the two testings (as a result of reaching the criterion for discontinuation at different points), failure to qualify for an item yielded a score of 0 for that item. This system yielded a raw consistency score for each subtest for each subject.

The raw consistency scores were then tabulated for the combined groups on each subtest, and a five-point scale was developed for each subtest. A score of 5 was assigned to the 20% of the combined groups (eight subjects) who demonstrated the least consistency, a score of 4 was assigned to the next 20%, and so on, to a score of 1 for the eight subjects who had the greatest consistency on the two testings. Scaled scores on the five subtests were then summed for each subject to produce the Response Consistency Index.

Data Analysis

In each group, means and standard deviations were computed and statistical comparisons of Testing I versus Testing II were performed. Intergroup comparisons of level-of-performance scores were not calculated because of the significant differences noted above between the two groups.

Next, difference score distributions between Testing I and Testing II in each of the two groups were compared, and the consistency scores generated by comparing the responses on individual items on the two testings were evaluated. The procedure described above was used to generate raw consistency scores. Each response that earned a higher score on the second testing was assigned 1 point, and each response that earned a lower score was assigned 2 points.

The raw consistency scores for each subtest were converted to scaled scores using the five-point scale shown in Table 7. This procedure assigned a score of 5 to the least consistent 20% of the combined distributions, ranging to a score of 1 for the 20% of the total sample that was most consistent on the two testings. (Some tied scores made it impossible to adhere perfectly to this procedure, but this categorization was followed as closely as possible.) These conversions allowed the scaled scores for the five subtests to be summed to obtain a Response Consistency Index for each subject. Means and standard deviations were calculated for the scaled scores for each of the five subtests as well as for their sum (Response Consistency Index), and intergroup comparisons were made by computing *t* ratios. Finally, a cutoff point that best discriminated the groups was determined by comparing the distributions of the Response Consistency Index for the two groups.

Results

Table 5 presents means and standard deviations, *t* ratios, and probability levels comparing Testing I versus Testing II in each group, and comparisons of difference score distributions for the two groups based on the two testings. (Table 5 essentially recapitulates the data presented in Tables 1 and 2.)

Although mean values were generally within the normal range for each group on both testings, the direction of change from Testing I to Testing II indicates that the nonlitigation group had higher means than the litigation group on each subtest, whereas the litigation group had lower means than the nonlitigation group in each instance. However, most of these intragroup differences were not statistically significant. A comparison of the difference score distributions of the two groups showed significant differences only on Comprehension ($p < .025$) and Vocabulary ($p < .05$), despite the fact that the direction of change was different in each instance. It is apparent that a level-of-performance approach (comparisons based on how well the subjects performed) reveals little significant information about differences between the two groups.

A rather different picture emerged, however, when response consistency scores were analyzed. Table 6 presents means, standard deviations, and a comparison of the two groups for scores generated by comparing responses to individual items on the two testings.

TABLE 5. Scaled Score Means and Standard Deviations for Testing I and Testing II for Head-Injured Groups Either Involved or Not Involved in Litigation, Together with Comparisons of Difference Score Distributions between Testings for the Two Groups

Group			Inf	Comp	Arith	Simil	Vocab
Nonlitigation	Testing I	M	10.20	10.45	9.10	11.60	10.10
		SD	3.27	3.65	4.91	4.22	3.57
	Testing II	M	10.45	11.30	9.95	11.70	10.20
		SD	3.27	3.80	4.48	4.66	3.93
		t	1.05	1.93	1.47	0.27	0.37
		$p <$	.40	.10	.20	.90	.80
Litigation	Testing I	M	9.75	9.65	8.10	9.25	10.20
		SD	2.07	2.70	2.77	2.84	2.42
	Testing II	M	8.85	8.70	7.65	8.35	9.20
		SD	2.50	2.39	3.30	2.62	2.14
		t	1.69	1.58	0.68	2.20	2.21
		$p <$	.20	.20	.50	.05	.05
Mean difference score comparisons							
	Mean intergroup difference		1.15	1.80	1.30	1.00	1.10
		t	1.98	2.40	1.51	1.89	2.12
		$p <$	.10	.025	.20	.10	.05

For every subtest except Information, the raw consistency mean score for the litigation group was more than twice as large as the score for the nonlitigation group. For each subtest individually considered, the litigation group was less consistent than the nonlitigation group at highly significant levels.

The next step was to use a five-point scale to convert the raw consistency

TABLE 6. Means and Standard Deviations Representing Consistency Raw Scores[a] on Testing II as Compared with Testing I for Head-Injured Groups Involved and Not Involved in Litigation

Group		Inf	Comp	Arith	Simil	Vocab
Nonlitigation	M	4.50	4.55	2.00	4.05	8.00
	SD	1.85	2.13	1.49	3.07	3.80
Litigation	M	8.80	10.15	5.45	8.35	18.20
	SD	5.45	4.48	3.89	2.37	5.98
	t	3.33	5.00	3.71	6.09	6.46
	$p <$	.005	.001	.001	.001	.001

[a]0 for the same score, 1 for a higher score, and 2 for a lower score.

TABLE 7. Conversion of Raw Consistency Scores to Scaled Scores Based on a 5-Point Scale[a]

Scaled score	Inf	Comp	Arith	Simil	Vocab
1	3 or less	4 or less	0–1	2 or less	6 or less
2	4–5	5	2	3–5	7–10
3	6	6–7	3	6–7	11–14
4	7–8	8–10	4–5	8–9	15–19
5	9 or more	11 or more	6 or more	10 or more	20 or more

[a]A score of 1 equals the most consistent performance and a score of 5 equals the least consistent performance.

scores for each subtest to scaled scores. This conversion scale is presented in Table.7.

Table 8 presents means and standard deviations based on the five-point scaled score distributions for each subtest and for the Response Consistency Index (which represents the sum of the scaled scores for each subject) together with intergroup comparisons.

Each intergroup comparison yielded highly significant differences, with the litigation group demonstrating less consistency in responses between Testing I and Testing II in every instance. As would be expected considering the greater degree of stability that tends to characterize summary measures, comparisons based on the Response Consistency Index yielded the largest t ratio.

The Response Consistency Index scores for individual subjects ranged from 6 (most consistent) to 25 (least consistent). The best cutoff score for differentiating

TABLE 8. Means, Standard Deviations, and Probability Levels Based on a 5-Point Scale for Individual Tests and the Response Consistency Index (Total Score) for Head-Injured Groups Involved and Not Involved in Litigation

Group		Inf	Comp	Arith	Simil	Vocab	Response Consistency Index
Nonlitigation	M	2.15	2.05	2.10	2.15	1.95	10.40
	SD	0.93	0.94	1.17	1.23	0.89	2.62
Litigation	M	3.55	4.10	4.05	3.75	4.10	19.55
	SD	1.23	0.91	1.23	0.85	1.02	2.82
	t	4.05	6.97	4.88	4.80	7.12	10.64
	$p <$	.001	.001	.001	.001	.001	.001

the two groups was 15/16, with 100% of the nonlitigation group having scores of 15 or less and 90% of the litigation group earning scores of 16 or more.

Conclusions

The results of this study indicated that subjects involved in litigation were much less consistent between two testings in their responses to individual items on the Information, Comprehension, Arithmetic, Similarities, and Vocabulary subtests than were subjects not involved in litigation. A summary score that represented the sum of scaled scores for the individual subtests (the Response Consistency Index) correctly classified 100% of the nonlitigants and 90% of the litigants. There seems to be little doubt that the groups differ strikingly.

The differences between the litigation group and the nonlitigation group were derived from comparisons of performances on two testings (intraindividual comparisons that in effect used each subject as his or her own control) rather than from intergroup comparisons. The results suggested that level of performance, as evaluated with relation to normative distributions, would have been far less productive of differences between the groups than the evaluation of intragroup changes (the procedure used in this study).

Study 3: The Dissimulation Index

Although Studies 1 and 2 used the same groups of subjects, completely separate data were used in each study. Both studies utilized intraindividual differences based on the scores of the same tests administered at different times. Study 1 was based on scores for six tests and Study 2 was based on consistency of responses to individual test items using five tests. Except for the Comprehension subtest, the tests used in Studies 1 and 2 did not overlap. It appears that the Retest Consistency Index (Study 1) and the Response Consistency Index (Study 2) were essentially independent measures in terms of their procedural considerations. Nevertheless, both measures were remarkably effective in differentiating litigants from nonlitigants.

Under these circumstances, it seemed advisable to combine these two indexes and exploit their possible complementary effect. This combination was done in Study 3 and produced the Dissimulation Index (Reitan & Wolfson, 1996).

Procedure

The Dissimulation Index, obtained by adding the scores for the Retest Consistency Index and the Response Consistency Index, represented the sum of 11 scores, with the range for each score extending from 1 to 5. Therefore, a subject who was inconsistent on each test of the two testings could receive a maximal score

TABLE 9. Distributions of Dissimulation Index for Two Head-Injured Groups, One Involved in Litigation and the Other Not Involved in Litigation

	Dissimulation Index							
	16–20	21–25	26–30	31–35	36–40	41–45	46–50	51–55
Nonlitigation	4	11	5	0	0	0	0	0
Litigation	0	0	0	3	4	8	4	1

of 55. A subject who performed consistently could obtain a score of 11 (the most consistent score possible).

The Dissimulation Index was computed for each of the 40 subjects. Means and standard deviations were determined for each group, and t ratios were computed to compare the distributions. The degree of overlap of the distributions was used to determine the best cutoff scores.

Results

The mean Dissimulation Index was 42.05 (SD = 6.14) for the litigation group and 23.50 (SD = 3.00) for the nonlitigation group, yielding a t ratio of 12.13 ($p <$ .001). These results indicate that inconsistencies between the first and second testings were far more likely to be demonstrated by litigants than by nonlitigants.

The distributions of the two groups showed that the scores ranged from 33 to 55 for the litigation group and from 18 to 29 for the nonlitigation group. The frequency distributions are presented in Table 9.

Scores for the two groups did not overlap; in fact, none of the 40 subjects received scores of 30, 31, or 32, thus revealing a gap between the two distributions. On the basis of these samples, we judged that the best cutoff point would be 31/32.

Conclusions

The results of this study demonstrated that retest performances were far less consistent in litigants than in nonlitigants. As noted, there was a gap in the scores between the two distributions of Dissimulation Indexes. A cutoff point that separated the groups perfectly was identified, although this study, as with any first report, requires cross-validation. It should also be noted that different characteristics of litigants associated with consistency of test–retest performances may eventually be identified. In addition, the method of test–retest consistency should be studied among other groups in which the possibility of malingering may be likely. In any case, the results of this study strongly suggest that using the subject as his or her own control has significant advantages over interpreting the subject's score with relation to the rest of the population.

The approach used to develop the Dissimulation Index has the advantage of bearing no direct relation to the subject's level of performance. Of course, if a subject scored 0 on every item, there would be no evidence of inconsistency. Consistently poor performances might also lower the Dissimulation Index. However, subjects in litigation appear generally to earn fairly adequate scores, with means that are not consistently significantly lower than the means earned by subjects not in litigation (Reitan & Wolfson, 1997), even though in this study the Dissimulation Index perfectly differentiated the litigants from the nonlitigants.

It should be noted that this study was not directly concerned with malingering; it compared persons involved in litigation with persons not involved in litigation. We knew of no reason why the nonlitigation subjects would not put forth their best effort when taking the tests. It is possible, though, that litigants might deliberately, or because of the stress and pressure of the existing circumstances, fail to do their best on a second examination. In any case, the results of this study suggest that these two groups represent quite different samples in terms of the Dissimulation Index, and raise the probability of eventually identifying test results that are not completely valid.

Inspection of test results of the individual litigants in our series suggests that many tests, over and beyond those that contribute to the Dissimulation Index, often show very inconsistent results. Some of these subjects perform very poorly and inconsistently on the Tactual Performance Test as well as other measures. Further research might reveal that additional tests could profitably be added to the Dissimulation Index.

Finally, the limitations of these studies must be noted. The number of subjects was small, and cross-validation of the results necessary. Even if the sensitivity of these indices is confirmed, many additional details, concerned with specificity, will need to be explored. Do different results occur among litigants of different age ranges, male or female gender, with different socioeconomic or education statuses, with different prelitigation histories and neuropsychological or psychiatric status, and so on? Every practical question concerned with human behavior is complex in terms of determinants of the answer, and detection of malingering, dissimulation, or invalid test scores is no exception.

APPLICATION OF THE RETEST CONSISTENCY INDEX, THE RESPONSE CONSISTENCY INDEX, AND THE DISSIMULATION INDEX TO INDIVIDUAL SUBJECTS

We can illustrate the clinical application of the Retest Consistency Index, the Response Consistency Index, and the Dissimulation Index by computing each Index for the cases described earlier in this chapter.

The Case of John Sterling

John Sterling was the truck driver and horse trainer who claimed to be totally disabled as a result of a work-related accident. On the basis of a single examination, an eminent neuropsychologist declared that John would never again be able to work.

The subject earned the following scores on Testings I and II: Comprehension, 7 and 5; Picture Arrangement, 9 and 7; Digit Symbol, 10 and 7; Category, 61 and 81 errors; Trails B, 153 and 280 sec; and TPT–Localization, 1 and 1.

These results reveal that on Testing II John produced poorer performances on every test except TPT–Localization. The difference scores, converted to scaled scores, yielded a Retest Consistency Index of 27. On this Index, a score of 5 is the most consistent score possible and a score of 30 is the least consistent score possible. The Index Summary Sheet shows John's Retest Consistency Index plotted with relation to means for the litigation and nonlitigation groups and the cutoff score for separating the group. John's Retest Consistency Index score of 27 fell far above the cutoff score and well into the range characterizing litigants. (See Figure 3.)

The Index Summary Sheet also plots John's Response Consistency Index, which was derived from comparisons of responses to individual items on all of the Wechsler Verbal subtests except Digit Span. As noted above, the raw response consistency score was generated for each test by assigning 2 points for each item on which a poorer score was earned on the second testing, 1 point for each item on which a better score was earned on the second testing, and 0 points if the response on the two testings earned the same score. Raw consistency scores were converted to scaled scores for each test, with a score of 1 representing the most consistent score and a score of 5 representing the least consistent score.

John earned scores of 4 on Arithmetic and Vocabulary and scores of 5 on all of the other tests, yielding a Response Consistency Index of 23. This is to be compared with the mean of 19.55 for the litigation group, the mean of 10.40 for the nonlitigation group, and the cutoff score of 15/16.

John's Retest Consistency Index of 27 and Response Consistency of 23 combined to produce a Dissimulation Index of 50. The latter was far above the cutoff score of 31/32, and exceeded the mean of 42.05 earned by the litigation group and the mean of 23.50 earned by the nonlitigation group.

The Case of Katherine Gilmore

Katherine Gilmore was the 38-year-old woman who claimed to have sustained memory loss, toxic encephalopathy, urinary infections, acquired immune dysfunction with chemical hypersensitivity, headaches, and pulmonary infection, and had been rendered sick, sore, nervous, neurotic, hysterical, and distressed as a

Name: **John Sterling** Age: **54** Education: **10**

Date of Testing I: ________ Date of Testing II: ________

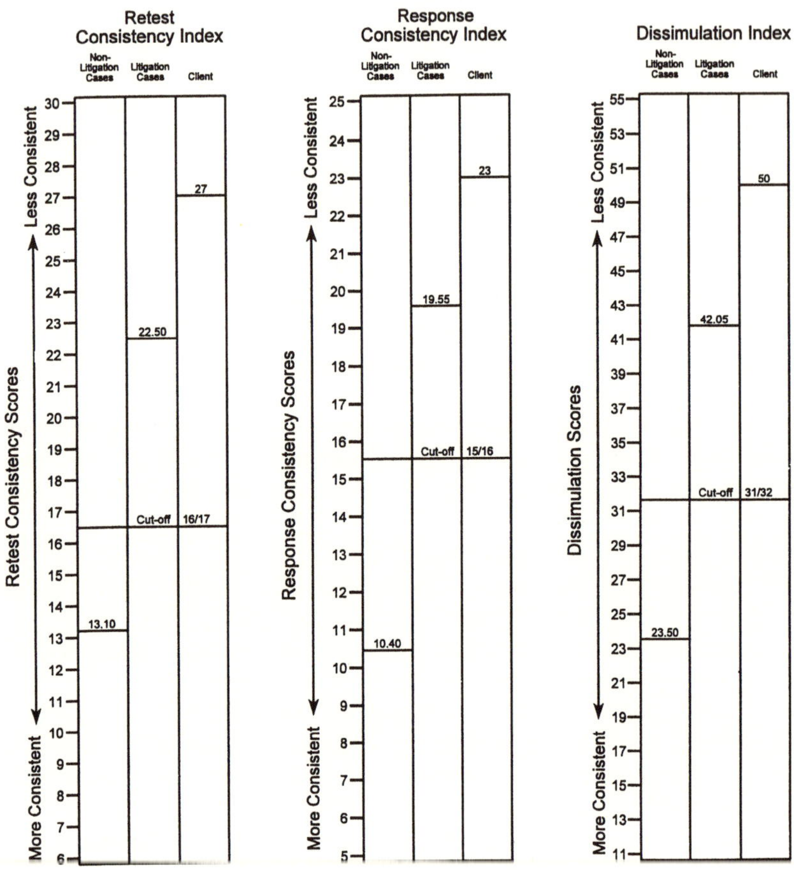

Summary of Client's Scores	
Retest Consistency Index	**27**
Response Consistency Index	**23**
Dissimulation Index	**50**

FIGURE 3. Index summary sheet for John Sterling.

Name: **Katherine Gilmore** Age: **38** Education: **17**

Date of Testing I: ______ Date of Testing II: ______

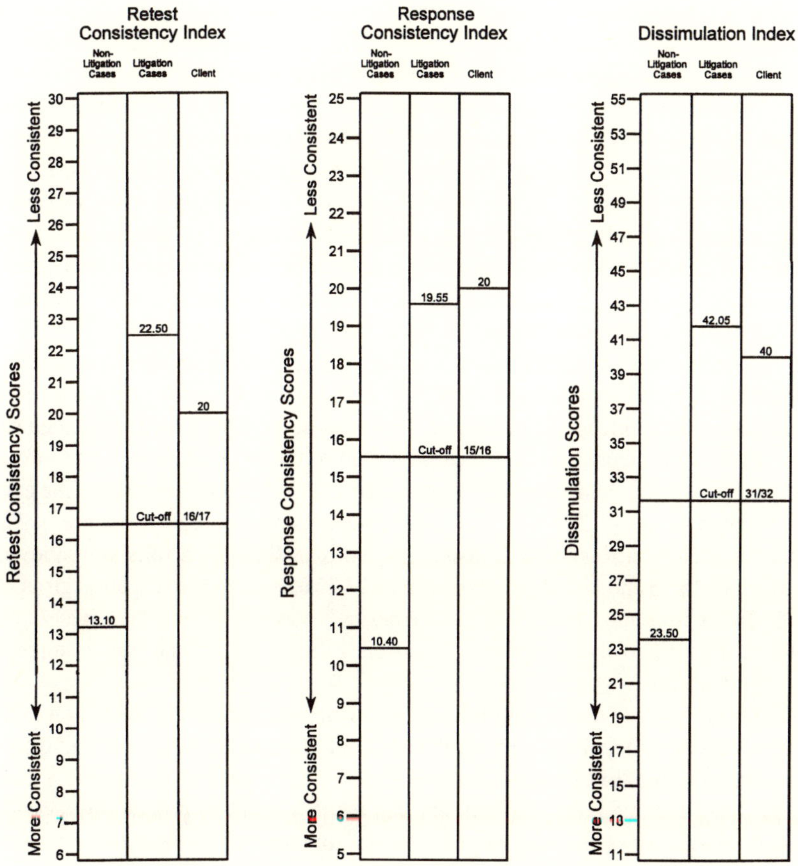

Summary of Client's Scores	
Retest Consistency Index	20
Response Consistency Index	20
Dissimulation Index	40

FIGURE 4. Index summary sheet for Katherine Gilmore.

result of a 3-month exposure to carbon monoxide gas and sulfide gas fumes in her home.

Although this woman had an extensive history of emotional distress and mental instability, we had no reason to believe that she was malingering. Information obtained after this case was completed suggested that the plaintiff genuinely believed that she had been impaired by exposure to the toxic fumes. Nevertheless, as pointed out above, the inconsistency of her responses on serial examinations created serious doubt about the validity of her test results.

Katherine earned the following scores on Testings I and II: Comprehension, 8 and 11; Picture Arrangement, 6 and 11; Digit Symbol, 9 and 4; Category, 53 and 77 errors; Trails B, 110 and 110 sec; and TPT–Localization, 4 and 2. These results reveal striking changes in her performances on five of the six tests. Her performances yielded a Retest Consistency Index of 20, a score somewhat less than the mean of 22.50 for the litigation group, but well above the cutoff of 16/17 and the mean of 13.10 for the nonlitigation group. These comparisons are graphically illustrated on the Index Summary Sheet (see Figure 4).

An evaluation of Katherine's scores on individual items of the Wechsler Information, Comprehension, Arithmetic, Similarities, and Vocabulary subtests also revealed evidence of inconsistent responses. Katherine earned a scaled score of 5 (the most inconsistent score possible) on Arithmetic, a score of 4 on Information, Similarities, and Vocabulary, and a score of 3 on Comprehension. She earned no scaled scores of 2 or 1 (scores that represent consistent performances). These values yielded a Response Consistency Index of 20, which falls well above the cutoff of 15/16 and just above the mean of 19.55 earned by the litigation group (see the Index Summary Sheet). Thus, Katherine's scores on both the Retest Consistency Index and the Response Consistency Index fell in the range suggesting invalid results.

Katherine's Dissimulation Index of 40 was just below the mean of 42.05 for the litigation group, but far above the cutoff of 31/32 and the mean of 23.50 earned by the nonlitigation group.

There seemed to be little doubt that using a standard procedure to compare Katherine's test results on two different examinations demonstrated inconsistencies in performances that sharply undercut a presumption of their validity.

REFERENCES

American Psychiatric Association. (1994). *Diagnostic and statistical manual of mental disorders* (4th ed.). Washington, DC: Author.

Babcock, H. (1930). An experiment in the measurement of mental deterioration. *Archives of Psychology, 18*, 5–105.

Binder, L. M. (1990). Malingering following minor head trauma. *The Clinical Neuropsychologist, 4*, 25–36.

Binder, L. M. (1993). Assessment of malingering after mild head trauma with the Portland Digit Recognition Test. *Journal of Clinical and Experimental Neuropsychology*, *15*, 104–107.

Cullum, C., Heaton, R. K., & Grant, I. (1991). Psychogenic factors influencing neuropsychological performance: Somatoform disorders, factitious disorders, and malingering. In H. O. Doerr & A. S. Carlin (Eds.), *Forensic neuropsychology: Legal and scientific bases* (pp. 141–171). New York: Guilford Press.

Faust, D., Ziskin, J., & Hiers, J. B. (1991). *Brain damage claims: Coping with neuropsychological evidence. Vol. I. The scientific and professional literature*. Los Angeles: Law and Psychology Press.

Franzen, M. D., Iverson, G. I., & McCracken, L. M. (1990). The detection of malingering in neuropsychological assessment. *Neuropsychology Review*, *1*, 247–279.

Goebel, R. A. (1983). Detection of faking on the Halstead–Reitan Neuropsychological Test Battery. *Journal of Clinical Psychology*, *39*, 731–742.

Heaton, R. K., Smith, H. H., Jr., Lehman, R. A. W., & Vogt, A. T. (1978). Prospects for faking believable deficits on neuropsychological testing. *Journal of Consulting and Clinical Psychology*, *46*, 892–900.

Hom, J., & Reitan, R. M. (1982). Effect of lateralized cerebral damage upon contralateral and ipsilateral sensorimotor performances. *Journal of Clinical Neuropsychology*, *4*, 249–268.

Hom, J., & Reitan, R. M. (1984). Neuropsychological correlates of rapidly vs. slowly growing intrinsic neoplasms. *Journal of Clinical Neuropsychology*, *6*, 309–324.

Hunt, H. F. (1943). A practical clinical test for organic brain damage. *Journal of Applied Psychology*, *27*, 375–386.

Mittenberg, W., Rotholc, A., Russell, E., & Heilbronner, R. (1996). Identification of malingered head injury on the Halstead–Reitan Battery. *Archives of Clinical Neuropsychology*, *11*, 271–281.

Nies, K. J., & Sweet, J. J. (1994). Neuropsychological assessment and malingering: A critical review of past and present strategies. *Archives of Clinical Neuropsychology*, *9*, 501–552.

Reitan, R. M. (1955). Affective disturbances in brain-damaged patients: Measurements with the Minnesota Multiphasic Personality Inventory. *AMA Archives of Neurology and Psychiatry*, *73*, 530–532.

Reitan, R. M. (1964). Psychological deficits resulting from cerebral lesions in man. In J. M. Warren & K. A. Akert (Eds.), *The frontal granular cortex and behavior* (pp. 295–312). New York: McGraw–Hill.

Reitan, R. M. (1967). Psychological assessment of deficits associated with brain lesions in subjects with normal and subnormal intelligence. In J. L. Khanna (Ed.), *Brain damage and mental retardation: A psychological evaluation* (pp. 137–159). Springfield, IL: Thomas.

Reitan, R. M., & Fitzhugh, K. B. (1971). Behavioral deficits in groups with cerebral vascular lesions. *Journal of Consulting and Clinical Psychology*, *37*, 215–223.

Reitan, R. M., & Wolfson, D. (1988). *Traumatic brain injury: Vol. II. Recovery and rehabilitation*. Tucson, AZ: Neuropsychology Press.

Reitan, R. M., & Wolfson, D. (1989). The Seashore Rhythm Test and brain functions. *The Clinical Neuropsychologist*, *3*, 70–77.

Reitan, R. M., & Wolfson, D. (1993). *The Halstead–Reitan Neuropsychological Test Battery: Theory and clinical interpretation* (2nd ed.). Tucson, AZ: Neuropsychology Press.

Reitan, R. M., & Wolfson, D. (1995a). The Category Test and the Trail Making Test as measures of frontal lobe functions. *The Clinical Neuropsychologist*, *9*, 50–56.

Reitan, R. M., & Wolfson, D. (1995b). Consistency of responses on retesting among head-injured subjects in litigation versus head-injured subjects not in litigation. *Applied Neuropsychology*, *2*, 67–71.

Reitan, R. M., & Wolfson, D. (1996). The question of validity of neuropsychological test scores among head-injured litigants: Development of a Dissimulation Index. *Archives of Clinical Neuropsychology*, *11*, 573–580.

Reitan, R. M., & Wolfson, D. (1997). Consistency of neuropsychological test scores of head-injured subjects involved in litigation compared with head-injured subjects not involved in litigation: Development of the Retest Consistency Index. *The Clinical Psychologist, 11*, 69–76.

Trueblood, W., & Schmidt, M. (1993). Malingering and other validity considerations in the neuropsychological evaluation of mild head injury. *Journal of Clinical and Experimental Neuropsychology, 15*, 578–590.

Wechsler, D. (1955). *Manual for the Wechsler Adult Intelligence Scale*. New York: The Psychological Corporation.

7

Detection of Feigning of Head Injury Symptoms on the MMPI-2

DAVID T. R. BERRY AND JAMES N. BUTCHER

Current epidemiological data indicate that head injury is the most common acute neurological disorder in the United States (Kraus & Sorenson, 1994). These data also indicate that head injuries vary considerably in severity. Although a number of alternative indices are available, the most well-accepted indicator of initial head injury severity is the Glasgow Coma Scale (GCS), which quantifies disturbance of consciousness on a scale ranging from 3 to 15 (Eisenberg & Weiner, 1987). Head injuries producing GCS scores in the moderate (9–12) to severe (3–8) range often involve significant morbidity or mortality (Adams & Victor, 1993). Head injuries resulting in GCS scores of 13–15 are classified as mild, and approximately 80% of all head injuries fall in this category (Kraus & Sorenseon, 1994). In contrast to the outcome literature on moderate to severe head injury, the largest and best-controlled studies to date suggest that by 1 year postinjury, neuropsychological and psychosocial outcome for patients suffering an uncomplicated mild head injury (disturbance of consciousness lasting no more than 1 hour and no other indicators of neurological disturbance) is comparable to that experienced by patients suffering general trauma not involving brain injury (Dikmen, Machamer, Winn, & Temkin, 1995; Dikmen, Ross, Machamer, & Temkin, 1995). Of course, the general trends observed in group studies, however methodologically sound, do not preclude the possibility of poor outcome in selected individual cases. Nonetheless, the scarcity of such cases in large well-controlled outcome studies should sound a

---

DAVID T. R. BERRY • Department of Psychology, University of Kentucky, Lexington, Kentucky 40506. JAMES N. BUTCHER • Department of Psychology, University of Minnesota, Minneapolis, Minnesota 55415.

Detection of Malingering during Head Injury Litigation, edited by Reynolds. Plenum Press, New York, 1998.

cautionary note in a situation where a patient with a history of mild head injury without neurological complications complains of severe disabilities.

An enduring enigma in the area of head injury outcome has been the fact that some patients who experience mild head injury without demonstrable objective indicators of neurological dysfunction may subsequently complain of prominent cognitive, behavioral, emotional, or somatic difficulties for months or even years following the event. This condition is often referred to as *postconcussive syndrome* (PCS) (Binder, 1986). In most of these cases, subjective complaints are the only sign of dysfunction. Despite the scarcity of objective evidence for neurological dysfunction in mild uncomplicated head injury, these cases have become a growing source of personal injury litigation, and publications serving attorneys often carry articles describing the common features of PCS. For example, in a recent issue of *Trial*, Galski (1995) reviewed the clinical presentation of mild head injury and recommended neuropsychological evaluation involving cognitive and psychological testing as a method of objectively identifying deficits and determining the validity of symptom complaints.

Although neuropsychological and psychological testing may potentially provide objective indicators of head injury sequelae, critics have pointed out that valid results from these procedures require the cooperation and honesty of the patient undergoing assessment. Faust, Ziskin, and Hiers (1991) quoted Rogers (1984): "the extent to which the results of a psychological evaluation impact upon individual's lives will directly and negatively impact their honesty. A litigant's motive to falsify or exaggerate disorder to gain some advantage is obvious" (p. 409). Thus, a prudent neuropsychologist or psychologist evaluating a mild head injury patient in the context of litigation should assess the cooperation and veracity of the patient. Potential indicators of compliance and motivation during neuropsychological testing are explored in other chapters in this volume. The present chapter will address the evaluation of possible feigning of psychological symptoms by head injury patients. The discussion will focus on the MMPI/MMPI-2, a test of personality and psychopathology that is widely used in general psychological assessment (Lubin, Larsen, & Matarazzo, 1984).

In addition to its widespread acceptance in psychological evaluations, the MMPI/MMPI-2 is currently the most commonly used test of personality and psychopathology in general forensic evaluations (Lees-Haley, 1992a), as well as in forensic neuropsychological assessments (Lees-Haley, Smith, Williams, & Dunn, 1995). The popularity of the MMPI/MMPI-2 in forensic contexts is probably related, at least in part, to the presence of well-developed validity scales for assessing the possibility of response sets in answering test questions (Pope, Butcher, & Seelen, 1993). In fact, the MMPI-2 includes seven standard scales for assessment of possible invalid approaches to the test. A literature spanning nearly half a century provides impressive documentation and guidance for use of many of these validity scales. Following discussion of more general issues in assessment of dissimulation and review of data on clinical scale patterns in head injury patients, the application of research on MMPI/MMPI-2 validity scales to forensic head injury cases will be explored and a systematic clinical strategy will be presented along with example cases.

CONCEPTUAL ISSUES IN THE ASSESSMENT OF MALINGERING

Conceptual Models of Malingering

Theoretical conceptualizations of clinical phenomena can be useful guides for research and practice. Rogers (1988) edited an entire volume on conceptualization and detection of malingering. At present, there appear to be three leading models of malingering as applied to head injury. DSM-IV (APA, 1994) defined malingering as the intentional production of false or grossly exaggerated physical or psychological symptoms, motivated by external incentives such as avoiding military duty, avoiding work, obtaining financial compensation, evading criminal prosecution, or obtaining drugs. In the DSM system, malingering must be distinguished from factitious disorder, which involves voluntary production of symptoms apparently to fulfill the sick role and thus receive medical attention. Additionally, malingering must be distinguished from somatoform syndromes such as conversion disorder, in which it is thought that intrapsychic needs fuel the unconscious production of symptoms that are typically neurological in nature. Patients with mild, uncomplicated head injuries who subsequently become involved in litigation could potentially be evaluated within this DSM framework.

Rogers (1990) reviewed empirical and theoretical issues in the assessment of malingering and criticized the DSM model as unduly moralistic and unsupported by research. Rogers suggested that this conceptualization is unified only by a theme of "badness." Thus, the DSM model is said to involve "a bad person (sociopath) in a bad situation (forensic assessment), who is a bad participant (lack of cooperation)." Additional concerns that arise in application of the DSM model are the inherent difficulty in objectively determining the extent to which a symptom is under "conscious" control as well as the fact that the same behavior (exaggerating or fabricating symptoms) may be classified as malingering in one context (seeking compensation) but as a factitious disorder in another context (seeking medical attention).

In place of the DSM model, Rogers offered a tripartite "adaptational model." The adaptational model assumes that the evaluee perceives the assessment as adversarial, that he or she has something to gain or lose from the evaluation, and that no alternative means of achieving the desired outcome is perceived to be available. Although aspects of this model may also be criticized as also involving ultimately "unknowable" information (such as the extent to which the subject perceives a lack of alternative means to achieve desired goals), the emphasis on dissimulation as a reinforcement-driven behavior is potentially helpful. In the present context, head injury patients who have been involved in an accident and experienced transient physical or emotional sequelae may feel justified in pursuing compensation for their suffering and perhaps even for "revenge" on persons or organizations that are perceived to have mistreated them. From the perspective of the adaptational model, continuing postconcussional complaints may be maintained by the reinforcers made contingent on them. In the case of protracted litigation following a mild head injury, the possibility of financial gain might constitute a powerful reinforcer for symptom complaints.

Recently, another model has been proposed that emphasizes the role of psychosocial factors in the development and maintenance of chronic complaints following head injury. Putnam and Millis (1994) noted that somatic complaints are common following head injury, and that the underlying etiology of these symptoms may involve a combination of neurological, social, and psychological factors. Putnam and Millis noted that the majority of head injury patients report such problems only transiently, but that a small minority continue to complain of them for months or years following injury. Interestingly, these persisting postconcussional complaints may be more common in mildly injured patients. Further examination of the base rates of similar complaints in the general population reveals that substantial levels of somatic complaints similar to those reported in PCS are voiced by individuals without neurological illness (Kellner & Sheffield, 1973, cited in Putnam & Millis, 1994), and by litigating personal injury patients who did not have a neurological injury as a basis for their claim (Lees-Haley & Brown, 1993). The authors suggested that PCS patients may misattribute somatic symptoms experienced by many individuals without neurological disease as secondary to their head injury. "Symptom reporting may develop into a self-perpetuating and self-validating cognitive scheme that becomes increasingly refractory to intervention while producing a disabled lifestyle in which the patient can avoid performance demands in a socially acceptable manner" (p. 9). The authors drew a parallel to chronic pain syndromes in which psychological factors are thought to play an important role. They suggested that persisting PCS may be a type of somatoform disorder in which there is no conscious volitional component but which includes an important psychological etiology. Clearly, such a somatoform disorder, falling within the DSM scheme, must be distinguished from malingering by the nonvoluntary nature of symptom production. Unfortunately, determining the relative conscious versus unconscious determinants of postconcussional complaints is likely to be a significant challenge for clinicians working with such patients.

Potential Sources of False Symptom Reports

Identification of false or grossly exaggerated psychological complaints following head injury presumes that feigning patients are producing complaints based on sources other than accurate self-reports. Thus, it may be useful to review possible etiologies of such false reports. One possible source of overreporting might involve exaggeration of actual experiences (dysphoria presented as a clinically significant level of depression). Alternatively, symptom reports may reflect difficulties experienced immediately following injury but which have since remitted. Another potential source of false symptom reports might involve complaints "borrowed" from role models such as fellow patients or other acquaintances who have experienced considerable head injuries. False symptom reports may be gleaned from popular media outlets such as books or movies featuring characters experiencing a head injury or other neurological disorder. Finally, health care workers who ask detailed questions regarding the presence of commonly experienced head injury sequelae may inadvertently provide information on symptoms the patient "should be" experiencing. Thus, the dissimulator has many potential sources on which to base inaccurate symptom reports. To date, relatively little work has been published on detection strategies based on rationally derived potential sources of false symptom reports in postconcussional patients. Future research might explore the possibility of differential strategies intended to identify specific types of false symptom reports.

HEAD INJURY AND MMPI/MMPI-2 CLINICAL SCALES

Psychopathology following Head Injury

Psychopathology potentially seen following head injury has been reviewed by Prigatano (1992). Disturbances sometimes seen after a head injury include irritability, agitation, belligerence, anger, violence, impulsiveness, impatience, restlessness, social inappropriateness, lability, anxiety, sensitivity to noise, suspiciousness, delusions, paranoia, mania, spontaneity, sluggishness, loss of interest, loss of drive, fatigue, and depression. Obviously, any single personality/psychopathology inventory would be hard-pressed to capture this entire range of disturbance, and the MMPI/MMPI-2 is not likely to be sensitive to every problem noted by Prigatano. Thus, to capture the diversity of disturbance following head injury, the MMPI/MMPI-2 should be supplemented as needed by other procedures such as clinical interview, collateral interviews, behavioral observations, and quantified ratings such as the Neurobehavioral Rating Scale (Levin et al., 1987) or the Neuropsychology Behavior and Affect Profile (Nelson et al., 1989). However, the MMPI/MMPI-2 does provide a means for evaluating more classic aspects of psychopathology, and thus, as noted above, has often been used in assessment of head injury patients.

Psychopathology following Head Injury and the MMPI

Gass and Ansley (1995) provided a useful overview of personality assessment in neurologically impaired patients. They note that, in general, these patients tend to show elevated scores on scales 1, 2, 3, 7, and 8. Review of published studies in this area generally confirms the view that these scales are among the most frequently elevated in head injury patients (Alfano, Neilson, Paniak, & Finlayson, 1992; Alfano, Paniak, & Finlayson, 1993; Bornstein, Miller, & van Schoor, 1988, 1989; Diamond, Barth, & Zillmer, 1988; Dikmen & Reitan, 1977; Fordyce, Roueche, & Prigatano, 1983; Gass, 1991; Gass & Russell, 1991; MacNiven & Finlayson, 1993; Novack, Daniel, & Long, 1984). However, perusal of individual studies reveals that significant elevations may occur on virtually any clinical scale for various subgroups of head injury patients (Bornstein et al., 1988). Further, a wide variety of two-point codetypes encompassing virtually all clinical scales has been reported for head injury patients (Alfano et al., 1992). This heterogeneity may be secondary to any of a number of factors present in head injury that could possibly impact on MMPI/MMPI-2 results, such as severity of injury, location and extent of brain damage, premorbid personality characteristics, possible compensation-related factors, chronicity of the injury, extent of neuropsychological impairment, gender composition of the sample, and age of the patients. Thus, it appears that there is no consistent "head injury" profile on the MMPI/MMPI-2. With no pathognomonic profile available, it follows that a clinician suspecting feigning of symptoms on the test cannot rely solely on clinical profile inspection to provide incontrovertible evidence of malingering on the basis of an "impossible" MMPI-2 profile.

Neurological Content and the MMPI

A further potential complication in evaluating clinical profiles of MMPI/MMPI-2 results from head injury patients involves the issue of neurologically related content. MMPI items were originally developed through a strict empirical criterion keying method, whereby items were added to a scale if response patterns to that item differentiated a target psychiatric patient group from normals. When applying such an item pool to neurological patients, it is possible that individuals accurately reporting problems might endorse certain items for nonpsychiatric reasons. Thus, accurate responses by neurological patients might make their MMPI/MMPI-2 profiles appear more psychopathological than is actually the case. Several papers have explored this issue. Gass and Russell (1991) asked three board-certified neurologists to review the MMPI item pool for questions that, in their opinion, could represent actual physical effects commonly produced by head injury. A total of 42 items were identified by at least two of the three judges as tapping physical problems present in 25% or more of head injury patients and termed NRI (neurologically related items). Scales 1, 2, 3, 7, and 8 had the highest number of NRI items from the rationally identified group. Gass and Russell suggested that simply deleting these 42 items from the protocol was likely to underestimate psychopathology, and thus calculated the percentage of non-NRI items endorsed by each of 58 head injury patients. This percentage was multiplied by the number of NRI items on each clinical scale, with the resulting number added to the raw score of non-NRI items on each scale. This allowed the contribution of NRI items that might have been endorsed as a result of nonphysical (psychopathological) sources to be factored in to the appropriate MMPI clinical scales. Comparison of original and "corrected" profiles indicated significant differences on scales 1, 2, 3, 7, and 8, suggesting that genuine neurological causes might significantly impact on these scales. Codetype frequencies were also significantly different for original versus corrected profiles. Gass (1991) compared item responses from 75 closed head injury patients to the MMPI-2 normative sample and found 23 items with statistically and clinically significant differences in endorsement rates. A principal components analysis revealed two factors. Factor 1 accounted for approximately 25% of the variance, and included 14 items with loadings exceeding .30. Inspection of item content led this factor to be labeled Neurologic Complaints. The second factor accounted for approximately 4% of the variance, with 5 items exceeding a .30 loading. Item content inspection led this factor to be named Psychiatric Complaints. As in the previous study, these items came most commonly from scales, 1, 2, 3, 7, and 8. Gass recommended that MMPI-2 profiles be scored twice, the first time using standard procedures and the second after deleting the 14 NRI items from each scale they loaded on. Alfano et al. (1993) followed a methodology similar to that of Gass and Russell (1991) in that 14 medical specialists from clinical neuroscience areas reviewed the MMPI item pool and identified items that they believed reflected the construct of neurological dysfunction. A total of 44 items were so rated by at least two-thirds of the judges. The responses of 102 moderate to severe closed head injury patients were inspected for each of these items. For 24 of the 44 items, a minimum of at least 30% of the head injury patients answered in the "pathological" direction. A principal components analysis indicated a two-factor solution. The first factor accounted for 25% of the variance and included 13 items. Inspection of item content resulted in this factor being labeled a Neurobehavioral Factor. The second factor accounted for approximately 8% of the variance and had 10 items loading at .41 or above. This factor was labeled an Emotional/Somatic factor. Rescoring of MMPI protocols following deletion of the 13 Neurobehavioral Factor items resulted in significant differences relative to original protocols on several scales, particularly 2 and 8. Significant codetype differences were found between original and neurocorrected profiles as well. Alfano et al. recommended scoring the MMPI twice for head injury patients, once using original procedures and a second time deleting the 13 neurobehavioral items. Dunn and Lees-Haley (1995) compared endorsement rates for neurologically related items in forensic head injury patients versus non-head injury patients and found that responses to only 5 items differentiated the two groups. Rescoring of the protocols after deletion of the 5 items did not result in significant differences on clinical scales. These authors recommended against using the neurocorrection in forensic head injury cases.

Currently available studies raise the possibility that certain MMPI/MMPI-2 items may have higher endorsement rates in head injury patients secondary to accurate report of neurological symptoms, and thus may, to some extent, be inaccurate in their reflection of psychopathology. Although the available evidence is important, several conceptual and practical issues remain to be resolved. First, deletion of neurologically related items from a protocol precludes these items being endorsed and scored as a reflection of psychopathology. For some subset of neurological patients, "neurological" items may be endorsed for "psychopathological" reasons. Gass and Russell (1991) addressed this possibility by adding raw score points from neurological items based on the percentage of nonneurological items endorsed on each scale. This procedure may minimize deflation of the protocol by deletion of all neurological items. A second issue involves the codetype changes resulting from deletion of neurological items. As suggested by Alfano et al. (1993), the relative accuracy of original versus corrected codetypes as behavioral descriptors in head injury patients is an empirical question. Further research is clearly needed to address the relative accuracy of behavioral inferences drawn from standard versus neurocorrected MMPI/MMPI-2 profiles of head injury patients. A final issue from the perspective of clinicians evaluating PCS patients involves the possible contribution of psychological factors to symptom complaints. Although it is possible that in some cases, continuing symptoms may be secondary to occult neurological dysfunction, it is also possible that a psychological etiology may be a factor in other cases. If this is true, then deletion of neurological items from a protocol reduces the probability of accurately identifying psychopathology in such a case because of deflation of scale scores. Thus, correction for neurological content may obscure, to some extent, possible psychological issues in a patient group for whom such factors could be making an important contribution to the overall picture. At present, research does not provide unambiguous answers to these complex questions. As suggested by both research groups, scoring of MMPI/MMPI-2 protocols using both original and corrected methods may be the most conservative approach to the problem, along with an interpretive caveat that neurological complaints might be impacting on the findings.

RESPONSE SETS AND THE MMPI/MMPI-2

As noted above, one of the major attractions of the MMPI/MMPI-2 for forensic psychologists has been the availability of well-developed validity scales for detection of response sets. Response sets are present when a testee produces answers that are not meaningfully related to questions or are distorted in some important way. Nichols, Greene and Schmolck (1989) divided response sets on the MMPI into two major categories: content nonresponsiveness (CNR) and content-responsive faking (CRF). CNR is present when answers bear no meaningful relationship to questions. Omitted or double-marked answers as well as random responding fall into this category. This may occur when a testee is unable for some reason to respond to an item or when answers are marked randomly. Uncooperativeness, poor reading comprehension, or psychosis may result in CNR responding. The defining feature is that answers cannot be interpreted because they are not meaningfully related to questions. CRF occurs when a testee distorts responses based on the content of the questions. There are two major categories of CRF: underreporting psychopathology and overreporting psychopathology. In the former case, the testee answers question in such a way that psychological problems are denied or minimized. Because this is rarely a controversial issue in litigation involving mild head injury patients, it will not be addressed further here, although interested readers may review a series of papers addressing detection of underreporting of symptoms on the MMPI/MMPI-2 (Baer, Wetter, & Berry, 1992, 1995; Baer, Wetter, Nichols, Greene, & Berry, 1995). In the case of overreporting of psychopathology, the testee responds with the goal of exaggerating or fabricating psychological problems, and this response set may be an important issue in mild head injury cases evaluated for forensic purposes.

Response Sets and the MMPI: CNR

On the MMPI, CNR was originally detected using the F scale, which consisted of 64 items selected for their low endorsement rate in the normative sample. Thus, less than 10% of the normative sample answered an F scale item in the scored direction. Additionally, F items were selected to represent a wide variety of problems and content areas so that individuals reporting genuine psychological disturbances were thought to be unlikely to endorse more than a few of these items (Dahlstrom, Welsh, & Dahlstrom, 1972). Given 64 items on the F scale, a totally random protocol would result in F raw scores in the range of 28–36. Later research revealed that F scale elevations could occur for reasons other than random responding. Severe psychopathology could elevate the F scale (Gynther, 1961) as could overreporting of symptoms (Gough, 1947). To address these issues, Buechley and Ball (1952) introduced the TR index, composed of 16 repeated items that occurred on the machine-scorable form of the MMPI. The assumption was that individuals who elevated F secondary to random responding would have a number of discordant responses to repeated TR items, as they were not responding to item content. Greene (1978) described the CLS scale consisting of 12 pairs of items with similar or opposite content. Again, discordant responses suggested the presence of random responding. Nichols et al. (1989) found hit rates of 85–92% for discriminating totally random protocols from valid protocols using a combination of the TR and CLS indices. Additionally, Gallucci (1985) studied MMPI protocols from VA patients involved in disability determinations. The patients were classified into four groups based on their presumed motivation to overreport symptoms inferred from their status in the disability determination system. The groups differed significantly in predicted ways on overreporting scales but showed no significant differences on the TR and CLS scales. These results suggested that the two CNR scales were insensitive to CRF. Thus, the interpretation of an elevated F scale can be clarified by reference to the TR and CLS indices. An elevated F in combination with elevated TR and CLS indices strongly implies random responding, whereas an elevated F in combination with average TR and CLS scores suggests that random responding is not the cause of the F scale rise.

Response Sets and the MMPI: CRF

Turning to detection of overreporting on the MMPI, a number of scales have been employed for this purpose. The F scale, described above, has been used to detect overreporting. Additionally, the F − K index, which involves subtraction of the raw K score from the raw F score, was suggested by Gough (1950). The F − K index contrasts the tendency to overreport problems as indexed by the F scale with the tendency to underreport problems as indicated by the K scale (an indicator of subtle denial of problems). A relative tendency to overreport problems will result in a higher F scale score, and thus in a more positive F − K scale value. Gough (1954) described another overreporting index termed the Dissimulation scale (Ds). The Ds scale was developed by contrasting responses from normal individuals asked to fake a neurotic disturbance on the MMPI with the responses of psychiatric patients diagnosed with neurotic disorders. Seventy-four items endorsed at higher rates by normals faking disorder relative to patients actually diagnosed with the disorder formed the Ds scale. Another popular index of feigning psychological disorders on the MMPI was based on the Subtle and Obvious subscales described by Wiener (1948). Wiener reviewed MMPI items and classified them as obvious or subtle in terms of their face valid relationship to psychopathology. Thus, an obvious item had a clearly pathological response direction, whereas a subtle item did not. The assumption was that individuals faking psychopathology would tend to endorse many obvious items in the scored direction as they attempted to overreport problems on the MMPI, whereas they would be unsure of the pathological direction for subtle questions and hence endorse far fewer of these items. Weiner identified 146 obvious and 110 subtle items on the MMPI. Only five MMPI clinical scales included sufficient numbers of both obvious and subtle items to allow contrast of the two types: 2, 3, 4, 6, and 9. Responses to obvious subscales may be contrasted with responses to subtle subscales, with a large difference in favor of obvious subscales suggesting dissimulation. Thus, there are a number of MMPI validity scales of potential use for detection of overreporting of problems, including the F, F − K, Ds, and Obvious/Subtle subscales, and the question arises as to which are the most effective.

Berry, Baer, and Harris (1991) meta-analytically reviewed available publications on detection of overreporting using MMPI validity scales. They used effect sizes as a metric for overall effectiveness of these scales in differentiating groups of individuals answering honestly from groups of individuals known or presumed to be overreporting problems. The *d* statistic indicates the mean difference between the two groups standardized in terms of the pooled standard deviation of scores on the scale for the two groups. Berry et al. found that the mean overall effect size collapsing across all reports was 2.1, indicating that, on average, groups answering with an overreporting response set were 2.1 pooled standard deviation units higher on overreporting scales than those known or presumed to be answering accurately. This finding supported the overall validity of these scales. Inspection of the mean *d* scale scores for individual overreporting scales indicated that the highest overall *d* score was for the F scale (2.3) followed by the Ds scale (2.2) and F − K scale (1.9). Other overreporting scales such as the shortened Ds scale (Dsr) and the Subtle/Obvious subscales had much lower *d* scores and caution was recommended in their use.

Although these results provided encouragement regarding the effectiveness of these scales at a group level, clinicians must make decisions about individuals. Berry et al. reviewed cutting scores published in each study for the identification of overreporting on the MMPI. Although it was possible to identify clusters of optimal cutting scores, they were unable to find specific cutting scores that were consistently supported in the literature. Thus, although increasing elevations of overreporting scales should lead to growing concern about the possibility of overreporting, there are no clear cutting scores that conclusively indicate presence of the response set in all populations. Thus, a clinician encountering an elevated F scale on a head injury patient's MMPI should be concerned about the possibility of an overreporting response set, but should not automatically conclude that feigning is present.

Response Sets and the MMPI-2

In the late 1980s, the revised MMPI was released as the MMPI-2 (Butcher, Dahlstrom, Graham, Tellegen, & Kaemmer, 1989). The MMPI-2 consists of 567 items and has been revised to eliminate objectionable items, clarify ambiguous or previously outdated content, include a large and nationally representative normative sample, employ uniform *T*-score scaling which results in equivalent percentile rankings across clinical scales, and, most important for present purposes, include additional validity scales to assist in identification of response sets. The seven MMPI-2 validity scales include several standard scales retained from the MMPI: Cannot Say (omitted or double-marked items), L (15 items involving denial of common flaws), F (60 items rarely endorsed in normative sample, 4 items deleted from original scale), and K (30 items tapping subtle defensiveness). Three additional standard validity scales have been introduced on the MMPI-2. Back F (Fb), which consists of 40 items appearing toward the second half of the test, was developed in a fashion similar to that used for the F scale. The Variable Response Inconsistency scale (VRIN) consists of 67 pairs of responses that are scored when inconsistent answers are noted to question pairs with either similar or opposite content. High VRIN scores thus reflect inconsistent or random responding that is occurring independent of item content. Finally, the True Response Inconsistency scale (TRIN) includes 23 item response pairs from questions with exclusively opposite content. TRIN reflects the tendency to respond either true or false independent of item content (yeasaying or naysaying), and thus is another type of inconsistent responding potentially invalidating an MMPI-2 protocol.

Response Sets and the MMPI-2: CNR

The majority of the standard MMPI-2 validity scales are sensitive to CNR. The Cannot Say scale, as was true for the MMPI, involves simply adding the number of omitted or double-marked answers. One change in the instructions given to subjects taking the MMPI-2 has probably contributed to a drop in the number of omitted items. The instructions now state "Remember, try to respond to every statement." The examiner may also attempt to minimize cannot say answers by scanning the answer sheet as soon as the subject has turned it in and requesting clarification of any double-marked answers and encouraging a second attempt to respond to any omitted items. Although little empirical work has been published to date on the impact of various levels of omitted or double-marked answers on the MMPI-2, Graham (1993) noted that "the MMPI-2 manual suggests that protocols with thirty or more omitted items must be considered highly suspect, if not completely invalid." He went on to note that his practice is to interpret with great caution any protocol with more than 10 omitted items and not to interpret protocols with 30 or more omitted items. Pending publication of empirical work on the question using the MMPI-2, this seems a reasonable strategy.

A number of publications have examined the detection of random responding on the MMPI-2. Berry, Wetter, et al., (1991) found that F, Fb, and VRIN scales were all quite sensitive to the presence of random responding in an analog study investigating the detection of various levels of partially random responding. Paolo and Ryan (1992) confirmed these findings in clinical samples. Berry et al. (1992) found that these same validity scales were significantly correlated with self-estimates of number of random responses given during MMPI-2 administrations under standard instructions, supporting the ecological validity of CNR scales. Wetter, Baer, Berry, Smith, and Larsen (1992) found that although F, Fb, and VRIN were all sensitive to random responding, VRIN was insensitive to overreporting of symptoms, suggesting that VRIN functioned on the MMPI-2 as TR and CLS did on the MMPI. Gallen and Berry (1996) examined positive and negative predictive powers for F, Fb, and VRIN at various base rates of random responding. They concluded that, at a 5% base rate of random responding, a raw VRIN cutting score of ≥ 13 had the highest overall hit rate in detecting random responding as well as a 100% positive predictive power. Given the sensitivity of F and Fb to overreporting of symptoms, as well as the differential sensitivity of VRIN to random responding, the use of VRIN to clarify the source of an elevated F score is recommended for routine and forensic clinical practice.

The last CNR index from the MMPI-2 to be discussed is TRIN. As noted earlier, TRIN is calculated from responses to pairs of items with opposite content and is intended to be sensitive to "yeasaying" or "naysaying." Little research has been published on the characteristics of TRIN. However, Wetter and Tharpe (under review) investigated the impact of various levels of random true or random false answers on MMPI-2 clinical and validity scales. They found good support for the sensitivity of TRIN to this analog model of yeasaying and naysaying, and recommended use of the cutting scores published in the manual for rejection of invalid protocols with significant levels of this type of response set. Based on this research as well as recommendations made in the MMPI-2 manual, protocols with TRIN raw scores ≤ 5 or ≥ 13 should be rejected as invalid.

Response Sets and the MMPI-2: CRF

Detection of overreporting of symptoms has received a great deal of attention since the publication of the MMPI-2. As noted earlier, a number of scales are available for this purpose. The F scale, which received the strongest support in the meta-analysis by Berry, Baer, and Harris (1991) described earlier, has remained relatively intact on the MMPI-2, with deletion of 4 items bringing the total down to 60 items. The F − K index is also retained on the MMPI-2, and should have similar properties as on the MMPI, although cutting scores may need to be adjusted in response to different underlying distributions of F and K (Rothke et al., 1994). The 40-item Fb scale, constructed to emulate the F scale in the latter part of the test, should have similar properties. The Ds scale suffered the loss of 16 items, bringing its total down to 58 items. The Obvious/Subtle scales had a number of items edited for the revision, but should function in a comparable fashion on the MMPI-2. Finally, a new validity scale, Fp, has been described by Arbisi and Ben-Porath (1995). The Fp scale consists of 27 items that were rarely endorsed by psychiatric inpatients as well as the normative sample. Thus, elevations of the Fp scale should not occur secondary to severe psychopathology and/or distress. Fp may therefore function as an additional scale for clarifying the source of an elevated F, although this scale should probably be used cautiously until further documentation of its characteristics becomes available.

Rogers, Sewell, and Salekin (1994) reported a meta-analysis of 15 studies investigating detection of malingering on the MMPI-2. Their analyses paralleled those of Berry, Baer, and Harris (1991). Results indicated strong effect sizes overall as well as continuing support for the F ($d = 3.0$) and F − K scales ($d = 2.5$). The Fb scale was also supported by a mean effect size of 2.3. In the largest departure from the findings of the earlier meta-analysis, the Obvious/Subtle scales had a strong effect size of 3.1 in this report, comparable to that found for the F scale. The Fp scale was not examined because of an insufficient number of studies published in the short time since its initial appearance. Overall, these results provide continuing support for the detection of malingering on the MMPI-2 using the traditional scales, as well as promising support for the Fb scale. The strong results reported for the Obvious/Subtle scales must be tempered by the severe criticism of these scales by Timbrook, Graham, Keiller, and Watts (1993), who found that they provided no increment in classification accuracy over that of the F and L scales, whereas these two standard scales did provide a significant increment in classification accuracy relative to the Obvious/Subtle scales.

Rogers et al. (1994) also examined the issue of cutting scores for identification of malingering in individual cases. As in the earlier meta-analysis, optimal cutting scores varied widely. The authors' suggested use of a mean cutting score collapsed across all reports. Obviously, neither the clustering approach nor the averaging approach is an ideal solution to this problem. Instead, further research is necessary to identify moderating factors such as gender (Graham, Watts, & Timbrook, 1991) or setting (Berry, 1995) which could be contributing to the heterogeneity of scores from various populations. Hopefully, such research will allow identification of cutting scores for particular populations that will consistently and accurately identify feigning. Until such research is available and supported by independent work, the MMPI-2 overreporting scales may best be viewed as sensitive warnings of the possibility of this response set, with increasing scores raising progressively stronger concerns.

MMPI-2 VALIDITY SCALES AND FEIGNING OF HEAD INJURY SYMPTOMS

Most studies of the utility of MMPI-2 validity scales for the detection of overreporting of head injury symptoms have methodological roots in a seminal report by Heaton, Smith, Lehman, and Vogt (1978). Heaton et al. asked 20 normal individuals to feign head injury during an evaluation that included neuropsychological testing as well as the MMPI. These analog malingerers were given a plausible historical scenario, instructed to fake a severe deficit, asked to imagine they were in litigation to compensate them for their impaired work abilities, and offered $25 for their efforts in the study as well as the possibility of winning a $5 bonus for successful faking. Of the 20 subjects initially included in the analog malingering group, 4 were dropped from analyses because no sign of impairment was noted on their neuropsychological tests, leaving 16 subjects. Seven of these 16 were noted by technicians to have given questionable levels of effort during testing. Results from the analog malingerers were compared with data from 16 demographically matched head injury patients drawn from file reviews. All of these patients had sustained a significant head injury as indicated by a minimum of at least 12 hours of unconsciousness and all had been rated as putting forth adequate effort by technicians. None of these patients was involved in seeking compensation at the time of evaluation. The two groups were comparable on summary indices from the Halstead–Reitan Neuropsychological Battery (Average Impairment Rating and Halstead Impairment Index). Malingering subjects scored significantly lower than actual head injury patients on tests tapping motor and sensory abilities. Additionally, analog malingering subjects had significantly higher scores on the MMPI F, 1, 3, 6, 7, 8, and 0 scales. Review of the 32 protocols by 10 neuropsychologists asked to identify malingered versus genuine results yielded accuracy rates that ranged from chance to 20% better than chance. However, discriminant function analyses resulted in equations based on neuropsychological tests that correctly classified all subjects. A discriminant function based solely on MMPI results correctly classified all but 2 subjects (1 from each group).

The Heaton et al. study had a number of important implications for feigning of head injury symptoms. One significant finding was that relatively untrained individuals were able to fake a level of impairment that was quite comparable to that of actual head injury patients. A startling finding was that neuropsychologists were unable, on the basis of test results alone, to discriminate feigned from actual head injury protocols with any impressive degree of accuracy. Heaton et al. did find patterns of findings differentiating the two groups using neuropsychological or MMPI results. Although it was not possible to cross-validate these equations, the accuracy of discrimination of "real" versus feigned protocols was only slightly lower using the MMPI than using neuropsychological test results, suggesting that the MMPI might have some utility for detecting feigning during a neuropsychological evaluation.

With the advent of the MMPI-2, a number of research groups began exploring the detection of feigning of head injury symptoms on the test. Villanueva and Binder (1993) studied 15 patients with known traumatic brain injury (TBI) who were not seeking compensation. Additionally, a group of 36 mild, uncomplicated head injury patients who were seeking compensation were divided into two groups based on their scores on the Portland Digit Recognition Test (PDRT), which is sensitive to inadequate effort on cognitive testing (Binder, 1993). Twenty-one of the mild head injury patients were classified as poorly motivated based on PDRT results, and 15 were classified as well motivated. All patients had received an MMPI-2. Mean F scale scores were 56 for the TBI patients, 53 for the well-motivated mild head injury patients, and 63 for the poorly motivated mild head injury patients. A statistically significant difference was found between the two groups of mild head injury patients. Additionally, performance on the PDRT "hard items" was negatively correlated with F scale scores ($r = -.38$, $p < .01$)

across all subjects. Although modest in magnitude, the significant correlation between F and PDRT results suggests some relationship between feigning on cognitive and psychological testing.

Millis, Putnam, and Adams (1995) studied 20 uncomplicated mild head injury patients who were seeking compensation and had scored significantly below chance on a forced-choice test of recognition memory. Millis et al. contrasted their MMPI-2 results with those from 20 patients who had moderate to severe head injuries. After correction for multiple comparisons, the mild head injury group with strong evidence for faking on neuropsychological procedures had significantly higher scores on the F and F − K scales. Additionally, significantly higher scores were observed for this group on the Fake Bad Scale (FBS; Lees-Haley, English, & Glenn, 1991) and two of the Harris–Lingoes subscales (Hy4 and Sc6). A trend was noted for similar differences on the Fp scale, although this was not significant after the correction for multiple comparisons. Cutting scores for prediction of group membership were also investigated. Setting specificity at 90%, an F cutting score of >75 had a sensitivity of 60%, and an F − K cutting score of >0 had a sensitivity of 65%. The highest overall hit rate was achieved with a cutting score of >22 on the FBS (sensitivity 95%, specificity 90%). The authors recommended caution in the use of FBS for this purpose until further validation work had been published. Additionally, they noted that the concordance between unequivocal evidence of neuropsychological feigning and MMPI-2 overreporting scales was modest, and suggested that different patterns of feigning might be present in different individuals. Thus, some feigning individuals might dissimulate on cognitive measures but not psychological tests, some might distort both types of tests, and some might malinger only on psychological tests.

Greiffenstein, Gola, and Baker (1995) compared 68 factitious brain injury patients with 56 severe brain injury patients and 53 patients with persistent PCS who were seeking compensation for medical bills only. Factitious brain injury patients were all involved in compensation seeking for mild head injuries and had either improbable histories or unlikely symptom patterns as defined by the authors. These authors administered a comprehensive battery that included neuropsychological tests, motivational procedures, and the MMPI-2. Overall, motivational tests provided the maximum power to detect patients who were inferred to be feigning deficits. The MMPI-2 Obvious scale and scale 8 were also reliably different between severe brain injury patients and presumed feigners. The F scale achieved only borderline significance ($p < .05$, one-tailed test) in the contrast between severe brain injury patients and presumed feigners, using a conservative $p < .01$ threshold. A principal components analysis of motivational and MMPI-2 scales produced a two-factor solution, with MMPI-2 scales loading on the first factor and motivational tests loading on the second factor. The authors concluded that patients feigning head injury symptoms may selectively dissimulate on neuropsychological tests and regard psychopathology as not a plausible component of their dissimulated deficits. They did note, however, that a subset of feigners might malinger psychopathology and thus possibly elevate MMPI-2 overreporting scales.

Berry et al. (1995) studied MMPI-2 patterns in several groups of subjects: normals answering under standard instructions, normals feigning head injury, head injury patients seeking compensation, and head injury patients not seeking compensation. The analog head injury malingerers were given information about head injury symptoms, took a quiz to ensure mastery of the material, were offered prizes for successful simulation, and were screened for compliance with instructions. The head injury patients were divided into two groups based on whether or not they were seeking any kind of compensation for their injury at the time of evaluation with the presumption that, as a group, those seeking compensation had a stronger motivation to overreport symptoms. Although the two head injury groups were matched on time since injury, compensation-seeking patients had significantly briefer durations of loss of consciousness, implying less severe injuries than experienced by non-compensation-seeking patients. After correction for multiple comparisons, significant differences were noted across groups for a number of MMPI-2 overreporting scales, including F, Fb, F − K, Ds2, and Fp. The highest mean scores on these scales were obtained by the analog malingering group, followed at a much lower level by compensation-seeking head injury patients. Compensation-seeking head injury patients had significantly higher mean scores than non-compensation-seeking patients on the F, Fb, F − K, and Ds scales. The authors concluded that MMPI-2 overreporting scales were sensitive to fabrication of head injury symptoms, and pending confirmation from additional research, sensitive to exaggeration of head injury symptoms.

Overall, available evidence suggests that MMPI-2 validity scales are sensitive to feigning of psychological symptoms, but not necessarily to feigning of cognitive deficits. Several authors have suggested that head injury dissimulators often may not see psychological symptoms as part of the head injury syndrome pattern they "should be" displaying, and thus they do not necessarily overreport these problems on the MMPI-2. The lack of consistent evidence for concordance between MMPI-2 overreporting scales and motivational tests in known or inferred groups of head injury malingerers is compelling evidence for the need to consider these two types of feigning separately. That is, based on currently available research, dissimulation of psychological symptoms is not necessarily predictive of dissimulation of cognitive deficits. Similarly, feigning of cognitive deficits is not necessarily predictive of feigning of psychological symptoms.

The Impact of Coaching on Malingering of Head Injury Symptoms on the MMPI/MMPI-2

One issue bearing on use of the MMPI-2 in forensic head injury cases that has recently received a good deal of attention involves possible preevaluation exposure to specific information that might increase a person's ability to avoid detection while feigning psychological symptoms of head injury. Hare (1985) raised concern that detailed information on the MMPI was available to prison inmates undergoing psychological evaluation. Ziskin and Faust (1988) as well as Lees-Haley (in press) expressed concern that overt or covert delivery of information on specific psychological disorders might influence a litigant's ability to malinger successfully. Youngjohn (1995) reported that an attorney representing a head injury plaintiff admitted in court that he had "coached" his client regarding motivational testing. Wetter and Corrigan (1995) surveyed practicing attorneys in two states regarding their opinions on provision of information on psychological tests and validity scales to their clients. They found that the majority of the practicing attorneys felt that clients referred for psychological testing should be given specific information about test procedures and that nearly half felt that clients should be informed of the presence of validity scales on psychological tests. Taken together, these sources suggest that the possible coaching of clients undergoing psychological or neuropsychological testing is potentially of concern to forensic clinicians.

Lamb, Berry, Wetter, and Baer (1994) examined the effect of two types of information on feigning of head injury on the MMPI-2. In this analog study, college students were given a plausible scenario, offered prizes for successful simulation, and screened for compliance with procedures. A factor of presence or absence of information on head injury symptoms was crossed with a factor of presence or absence of information on MMPI-2 validity scales. The highest clinical and validity scale scores were obtained by subjects feigning with information on head injury symptoms alone. The next highest validity and clinical scale scores were obtained by subjects feigning with no information at all. The third highest validity and clinical scale scores were obtained by subjects feigning with information on both head injury symptoms and validity scale characteristics. The lowest scores overall were obtained by subjects feigning with information on validity scales alone.

These results suggested that normals fabricating psychological symptoms of head injury can be aided by provision of information on the MMPI-2 validity scales, but are not greatly aided by information on specific symptoms experienced by head injury patients. These results are consistent with reports by Rogers, Bagby, and Chakraborty (1993) and Wetter, Baer, Berry, Robison and Sumpter (1993) who found that information on symptoms of posttraumatic stress disorder and schizophrenia did not assist analog malingerers in faking the target disorder successfully on the MMPI-2. Additionally, Rogers et al. (1993) also found that information on validity scales greatly improved the success of analog malingerers in escaping detection by the validity scales.

Researchers investigating the impact of different types of coaching on the success of analog malingerers face a dilemma pointed out by Ben-Porath (1994), who noted that provision of data on specific faking strategies ran the risk of compromising the integrity of the psychological test involved, which violates APA guidelines on protection of test content. Berry, Lamb, Wetter, Baer, and Widiger (1994) agreed with this concern and discussed several possible solutions to the problem. The needs of clinicians working with populations at risk for coached malingering must be balanced with the ethical imperative to protect the content of the test being studied. One proposed solution is for authors publishing in this area to take care not to reveal detail on successful coaching strategies in their publications. These details could be provided on request to other researchers agreeing to be bound by the APA ethical guidelines to protect test content.

Summary of Empirical Literature on Feigning of Head Injury Symptoms on the MMPI/MMPI-2

The currently available literature on detection of feigning of head injury symptoms on the MMPI/MMPI-2 suggests the following conclusions:

1. The MMPI/MMPI-2 contains a number of scales with demonstrated sensitivity to overreporting of psychological symptoms. Overall, the scale with the most consistent support for success in this task is the F scale. The F − K, Ds/Ds2, and Fb also have moderate support from the literature. Promising additional scales that currently have less available support are Fp and FBS. Caution is recommended for these last two scales until additional empirical support appears.

2. Analog studies suggest that individuals fabricating and possibly exaggerating psychological symptoms of head injury tend to show elevated MMPI-2 overreporting scales. Although several MMPI/MMPI-2 scales have good support for sensitivity to overreporting of symptoms, consistently supported cutting scores are not available. Therefore, these scales cannot be used alone to conclusively identify malingering of psychological symptoms. However, increasingly elevated scores on these scales should raise increasingly strong concerns regarding overreporting of symptoms. As a rule of thumb, after ruling out inconsistent responding with the VRIN and TRIN scales, F scale T scores in the 80s should begin to raise concern about the possibility of an overreporting approach to the MMPI-2. T scores in the 90s and beyond clearly signal the need for special attention to the possibility of dissimulated symptoms. However, given the lack of firm cutting scores, the diagnosis of feigning of psychological symptoms requires converging evidence from other domains such as historical data, behavioral observations, and specialized procedures (e.g., the Structured Interview of Reported Symptoms) (Rogers, Bagby, and Dickens, 1992).

3. Studies of mild head injury patients with strong evidence for malingering of cognitive deficits suggest that only a subset also overreport psychological symptoms. Feigning of cognitive deficits and fabrication of psychological symptoms may be independent dimensions in individuals malingering head injury. Thus, dissimulation of cognitive deficits cannot be inferred from feigning of psychological symptoms. Similarly, fabrication of psychological symptoms can-

not be inferred from malingering of cognitive deficits. Thus, both types of malingering should be independently evaluated in head injury patients with important results hinging on the outcome of their neuropsychological evaluations.

4. There is evidence that some head injury patients may arrive for their neuropsychological evaluations forewarned regarding specific procedures for evaluating the integrity of their presentation. Unfortunately, empirical methods for detecting this type of tampering with patient presentation are not yet available. However, forensic examiners must consider this possibility as they interpret obtained results.

CLINICAL STRATEGIES FOR ASSESSMENT OF POSSIBLE FEIGNING OF HEAD INJURY SYMPTOMS ON THE MMPI/MMPI-2

As noted earlier, feigning of cognitive and psychological deficits may be separable dimensions in dissimulating head injury patients. Therefore, administration of procedures assessing the possibility of both types of malingering is recommended for forensic head injury cases.

Assessment of possible feigning of psychological symptoms of head injury begins with review of MMPI/MMPI-2 validity scales. First, the possibility of CNR is evaluated through review of the Cannot Say, VRIN, and TRIN scales. Cutting scores reviewed above may be considered for use in the identification of CNR, although clinicians should consider the impact of varying base rates on their utility and adjust cutting scores accordingly (Berry, 1995). If CNR is ruled out, the possibility of CRF is evaluated through reference to the L, K, and F scales. Because generally accepted cutting scores are not available for detection of overreporting using these scales in isolation, they should be regarded as sensitive warnings of the possibility of this response set. Converging evidence should be sought from other domains, such as historical data (e.g., reports of other clinicians, videotapes), or behavioral observations. Finally, administration of the Structured Interview for Reported Symptoms (Rogers et al., 1992) may be considered for additional data bearing on possible malingering of psychological symptoms.

FEIGNING OF PSYCHOLOGICAL SYMPTOMS OF HEAD INJURY ON THE MMPI-2: CASE EXAMPLES

Four case examples involving the question of possible feigning of psychological and/or cognitive symptoms of head injury will be reviewed next.

Case 1 involves R., a 37-year-old white, right-handed male who had graduated from high school and worked for 20 years as an equipment operator in underground coal mines. Mr. R. was seen for an independent neuropsychological evaluation as part of his lawsuit following an accident in the mines. He had been trapped against the roof of a tunnel when his "scoop" hit an obstruction. Mr. R. stated that he had hit his head against the roof of the tunnel and been briefly dazed. When he regained his senses, he experienced a panic attack that lasted for approximately 20 minutes until he was able to wriggle free of the machine. He complained of pain, memory problems, confusion, depression, and anxiety symptoms following the accident. Neurological examination as well as neuroimaging procedures were negative. However, he was unable to return to work and filed a workers' compensation claim as well as a lawsuit. His premorbid history was unremarkable and he denied substance abuse, previous neurological disorder, and premorbid psychiatric disorder. Mr. R.'s neuropsychological results were remarkable for memory deficits, motor slowing, defective visuomotor integration, and impairment of frontal/self-regulatory abilities. However, on the Digit Memory Test (Hiscock & Hiscock, 1989) his overall percent correct was 68, with performance on the three blocks at 79, 69, and 57%. As these scores were far below those reported for well-motivated severe head injury patients (Guilmette, Hart, & Giuliano, 1993) and showed a declining performance across trials characteristic of individuals dissimulating memory disorder (Prigatano & Amin, 1993) a motivational impairment was felt to be present and neuropsychological results were not interpreted. Mr. R.'s MMPI-2 profile appears in Figure 1. Supplementary validity scale scores were as follows: VRIN (57), TRIN (50), Fb (120), and Ds2 (80). Because the validity scales suggested the possible presence of an overreporting response set, Mr. R. was administered the Structured Interview of Reported Symptoms (SIRS). SIRS results indicated three scales elevated into the probable feigning range (Subtle Symptoms, Selective Symptoms, and Severity of Symptoms). According to the SIRS manual, the presence of elevation of three scales into the probable feigning range has a positive predictive power of 98% for identification of malingering. As suggested in the manual, these results were interpreted as follows: "This combination of elevated scores is characteristic of individuals who are feigning a mental disorder, and is rarely seen in clients responding truthfully." The report noted that these results did not rule out the presence of either cognitive deficits or psychopathology, but rather precluded interpretation of the data because of the apparent presence of inadequate motivation as well as an overreporting response set.

This case illustrates the occurrence of possible feigning of cognitive deficits as well as probable feigning of psychopathology. The Digit Memory Test results were strongly suggestive of poor effort and possible deliberate manipulation of performance on memory testing. The elevated MMPI-2 F scale combined with the normal range inconsistency indicators (VRIN and TRIN) signaled the high likelihood of the presence of overreporting. Follow-up testing with the SIRS was strongly suggestive of feigning of psychopathology, confirming the suggestion of the MMPI-2 F Scale.

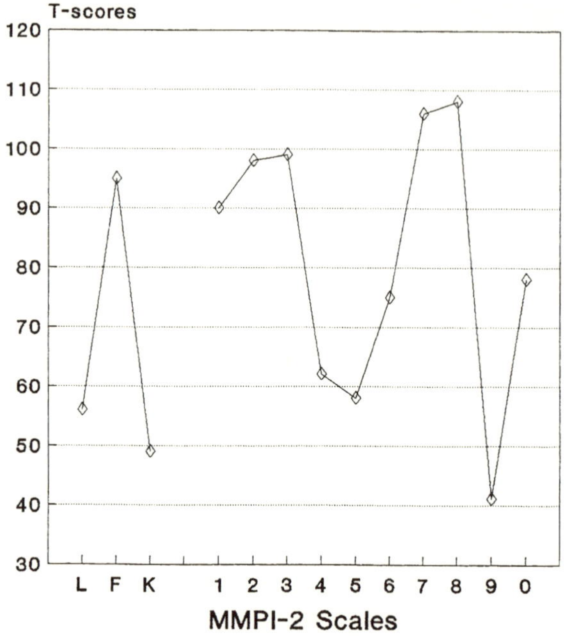

FIGURE 1. MMPI-2 profile of Mr. R., a 37-year-old equipment operator being assessed following a mining accident.

The second case is of a 37-year-old white, right-handed male who graduated from high school and was a qualified electrician employed as a foreman and supervisor in underground coal mines. S. had been involved in an automobile accident in which he suffered a dislocated jaw and a possible brief loss of consciousness. Neuroimaging had not been carried out, although neurological examination was negative. Premorbid history was reported to be unremarkable. Despite the fact that S. had driven several hours by himself to the test site, his neuropsychological examination suggested significant impairments that included disorientation to season of the year, severe impairment of memory, and motor slowing. However, observed effort was noted to be poor and Digit Memory Test overall percent correct at 26% was significantly below chance. Thus, his cognitive test results were not interpreted. His MMPI-2 profile is given in Figure 2. His supplementary validity scores were as follows: VRIN (57), TRIN (65), Fb (67), and Ds2 (58). Although the TRIN score is technically in the significant range, his raw score of 11 fell below the recommended cutting score of ≥13. Mr. S. was also given a Beck Depression Inventory, and his score of 16 falls in the moderate

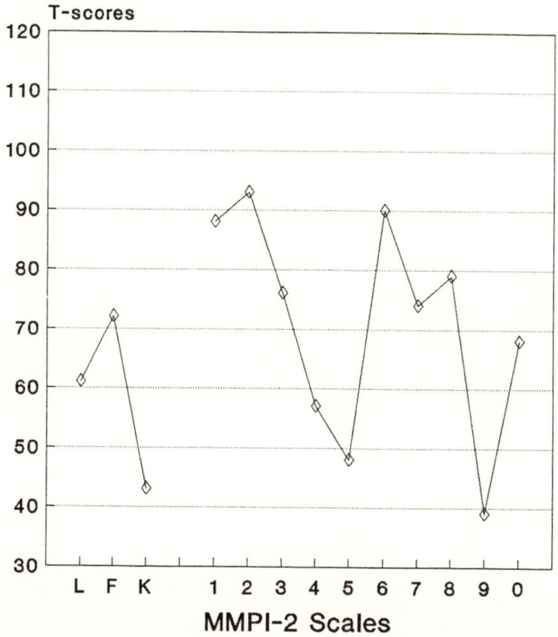

FIGURE 2. MMPI-2 profile of Mr. S., a 37-year-old electrician being assessed following an automobile accident.

depression range. Mr. S. was referred for psychiatric evaluation to address the possibility of affective disorder.

This case illustrates the presence of apparent deliberate feigning of cognitive deficits without accompanying overreporting of psychopathology.

Case 3 involves N., a 41-year-old white, right-handed male who had graduated from high school and worked as a mechanic for a large transportation company. Mr. N. experienced a mild head injury with a reported brief loss of consciousness in an automobile accident. He was involved in a lawsuit for compensation for his deficits secondary to the accident. His premorbid history was unremarkable as were neurological examination and neuroimaging procedures. Neuropsychological results revealed mild deficits involving defective perception of speech sounds, motor slowing, and inability to inhibit a dominant response on a Stroop task. His Digit Memory Test results were excellent at 96% overall, and thus not suggestive of motivational impairment. His MMPI-2 profile is shown in Figure 3. In addition to his elevated F scale, his supplementary scale scores were as follows: VRIN (46), TRIN (57), Fb (120), and Ds2 (90). In light of the elevated

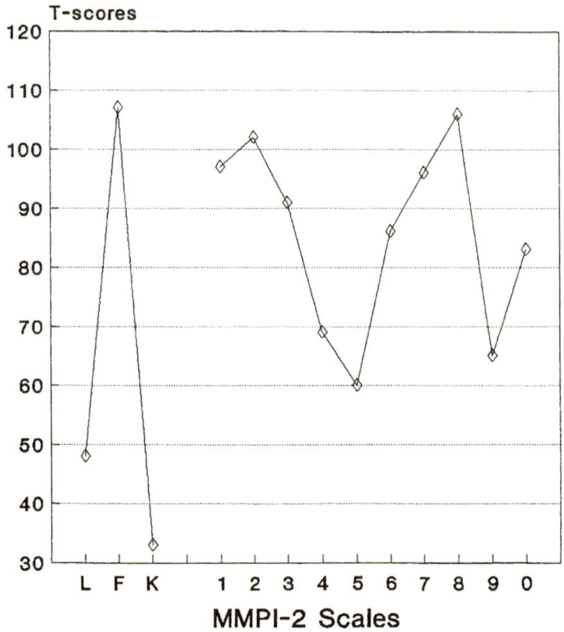

FIGURE 3. MMPI-2 profile of Mr. N., a 41-year-old mechanic being assessed following an accident in which he claimed to have suffered a head injury.

MMPI-2 overreporting scales, Mr. N. was given the SIRS. He elevated two scales into the definite feigning range and three additional scales into the probable feigning range. These findings were interpreted as consistent with dissimulation of psychological complaints.

This case illustrates the presence of overreporting of psychopathology without evidence for feigning of cognitive deficits. Apparently, Mr. N. was fabricating or grossly exaggerating psychopathology but did not manipulate his level of effort on motivational testing.

These first three cases illustrate the potential independence of feigning of cognitive and psychological problems. Taken together with the research reviewed earlier, these cases suggest that forensic neuropsychologists should remain alert to the possibility of both types of malingering when evaluating litigating head injury patients.

Case 4, although not involving a head injury, involves another type of neurological insult that posed an interesting validity scale question. Mr. Z. was a 35-year-old white computer engineer with 16 years of education who suffered carbon monoxide poisoning that killed four family members. Mr. Z. was comatose

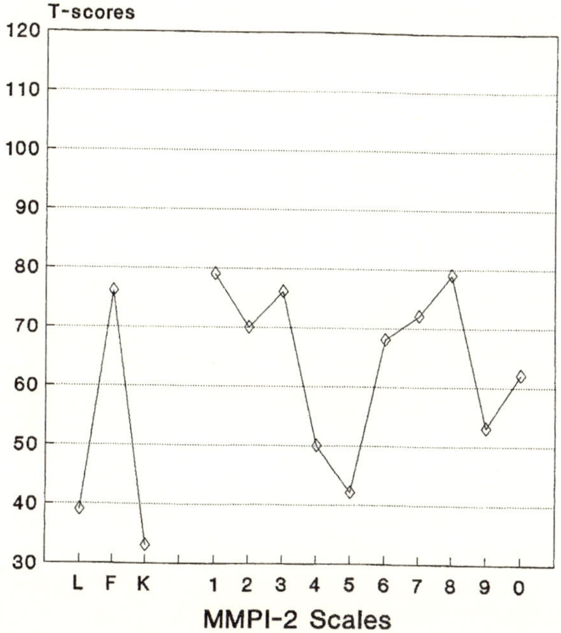

FIGURE 4. MMPI-2 profile of Mr. Z., a 35-year-old computer engineer with 16 years of education being assessed following a situation in which he suffered severe brain damage as a result of carbon monoxide poisoning.

for 3 weeks following the accident and has significant residual impairment that includes a gait disorder. He filed a lawsuit over the defective stove that leaked the carbon monoxide and was given an MMPI-2 as part of his evaluation. His clinical profile is shown in Figure 4. Additional validity scales were as follows: VRIN (65), TRIN (72), and Fb (108). The discrepancy between his F and Fb scores was remarkable with a 30-point difference in favor of Fb. Because Fb is sensitive to malingering as well as random responding (Wetter et al., 1992), and because Fb items may tap somewhat different content areas from F, it was possible that this difference reflected a selected overreporting of problems. To address this problem, Mr. Z.'s responses to VRIN item pairs that both occurred in the first 370 items were contrasted with his responses to VRIN item pairs that both occurred after item 370. Mr. Z. inconsistently endorsed 5 out of 31 VRIN item pairs from the first part of the test. For the second part of the test, 5 of 15 VRIN item pairs were endorsed inconsistently. The ratio of inconsistent responding was thus .161 for the first part of the test versus .333 for the second part of the test. These results suggested that a higher level of inconsistent responding was present for the last part of the test. It seems probable, on this basis, that the elevated Fb came about because of increased random responding toward the end of the test, rather than because of selective overreporting. The length of the MMPI-2 may mean that neurological patients with decreased stamina secondary to their injury tire after a period of time and produce increased random responding toward the rear of the test (H. Klove, personal communication, 1994). This possibility can potentially be examined through scoring of VRIN subscales as outlined above (Gallen & Berry, 1997).

CAVEAT

This chapter has reviewed currently available data on feigning of psychopathology in head injury cases. Although failure to detect malingering has potentially significant costs to society and the individuals involved, it should be emphasized that diagnosing malingering usually has drastic consequences for the person being evaluated. Thus, this conclusion should never be reached without careful consideration of available data, the presence of converging evidence from two or more sources, and thorough evaluation of possible alternative explanations. Additionally, even in the presence of strong indicators of malingering, the clinician should bear in mind that feigning of psychological deficits does not preclude the presence of genuine psychopathology.

REFERENCES

Adams, R., & Victor, M. (1993). *Principles of neurology* (5th ed.). New York: McGraw–Hill.

Alfano, D., Neilson, P., Paniak, C., & Finlayson, M. (1992). The MMPI and closed-head injury. *The Clinical Neuropsychologist*, *6*, 134–142.

Alfano, D., Paniak, C., & Finlayson, M. (1993). The MMPI and closed head injury: A neurocorrective approach. *Neuropsychiatry, Neuropsychology and Behavioral Neurology*, *6*, 111–116.

American Psychiatric Association. (1994). *Diagnostic and statistical manual of mental disorders* (4th ed.). Washington, DC: Author.

Arbisi, P., & Ben-Porath, Y. (1995). An MMPI-2 infrequent response scale for use with psychopathological populations: The F(p) scale. *Psychological Assessment*, *7*, 424–431.

Baer, R., Wetter, M., & Berry, D. (1992). Detection of underreporting of psychopathology on the MMPI: A meta-analysis. *Clinical Psychology Review*, *12*, 509–525.

Baer, R., Wetter, M., & Berry, D. (1995). Effects of information about validity scales on underreporting of symptoms on the MMPI-2: An analog investigation. *Assessment*, *2*, 189–200.

Baer, R., Wetter, M., Nichols, D., Greene, R., & Berry, D. (1995). Sensitivity of MMPI-2 validity scales to underreporting of symptoms. *Psychological Assessment*, *7*, 419–423.

Ben-Porath, Y. (1994). The ethical dilemma of coached malingering research. *Psychological Assessment*, *6*, 14–15.

Berry, D. (1995). Detecting distortion in forensic evaluations with the MMPI-2. In Y. S. Ben-Porath, J. Graham, G. Hall, R. Hirschman, & M. Zaragoza (Eds.), *Forensic evaluations with the MMPI-2* (pp. 82–102). Newbury Park, CA: Sage.

Berry, D., Baer, R., & Harris, M. (1991). Detection of malingering on the MMPI: A meta-analysis. *Clinical Psychology Review*, *11*, 585–598.

Berry, D., Lamb, D., Wetter, M., Baer, R., & Widiger, T. (1994). Ethical considerations in research on coached malingering. *Psychological Assessment*, *6*, 16–17.

Berry, D., Wetter, M., Baer, R., Larsen, L., Clark, C., & Monroe, K. (1992). MMPI-2 random responding indices: Validation using a self-report methodology. *Psychological Assessment*, *4*, 340–345.

Berry, D., Wetter, M., Baer, R., Widiger, T., Sumpter, J., Reynolds, S., & Hallam, R. (1991). Detection of random responding on the MMPI-2: Utility of F, back F, and VRIN scales. *Psychological Assessment*, *3*, 418–423.

Berry, D., Wetter, M., Baer, R., Youngjohn, J., Gass, C., Lamb, D., Franzen, M., MacInnes, W., & Buchholz, D. (1995). Overreporting of closed head injury symptoms on the MMPI-2. *Psychological Assessment*, *7*, 517–523.

Binder, L. (1986). Persisting symptoms after mild head injury: A review of the postconcussive syndrome. *Journal of Clinical and Experimental Neuropsychology*, *8* 323–346.

Binder, L. (1993). Assessment of malingering with the Portland Digit Recognition Test after mild head injury. *Journal of Clinical and Experimental Neuropsychology*, *15*, 170–182.

Bornstein, R., Miller, H., & van Schoor, J. (1988). Emotional adjustment in compensated head injury patients. *Neurosurgery*, *23*, 622–627.

Bornstein, R., Miller, H., & van Schoor, J. (1989). Neuropsychological deficit and emotional disturbance in head-injured patients. *Journal of Neurosurgery*, *70*, 509–513.

Buechley, R., & Ball, H. (1952). A new test of validity for the group MMPI. *Journal of Consulting Psychology*, *16*, 299–301.

Butcher, J., Dahlstrom, W., Graham, J., Tellegen, A., & Kaemmer, B. (1989). *MMPI-2: Manual for administration and scoring*. Minneapolis: University of Minnesota Press.

Dahlstrom, W., Welsh, G., & Dahlstrom, L. (1972). *An MMPI handbook: Vol. I. Clinical interpretation.* Minneapolis: University of Minnesota Press.

Diamond, R., Barth, J., & Zillmer, E. (1988). Emotional correlates of mild closed head injury: The role of the MMPI. *International Journal of Clinical Neuropsychology*, *10*, 35–40.

Dikmen, S., Machamer, J., Winn, H., & Temkin, N. (1995). Neuropsychological outcome at 1-year post head injury. *Neuropsychology*, *9*, 80–90.

Dikmen, S., & Reitan, R. (1977). Emotional sequelae of head injury. *Annals of Neurology*, *2*, 492–494.

Dikmen, S., Ross, B., Machamer, J., & Temkin, N. (1995). One year psychosocial outcome in head injury. *Journal of the International Neuropsychological Society*, *1*, 67–77.

Dunn, J., & Lees-Haley, P. (1995). The MMPI-2 correction factor for closed-head injury: A caveat for forensic cases. *Assessment*, *2*, 47–51.

Eisenberg, H., & Weiner, R. (1987). Input variables: How information from the acute injury can be used to characterize groups of patients for studies of outcome. In H. Levin, J. Grafman, & H. Eisenberg (Eds.), *Neurobehavioral recovery from head injury* (pp. 13–29). London: Oxford University Press.

Faust, D., Ziskin, J., & Hiers, J. (1991). *Brain damage claims: Coping with neuropsychological evidence*. Marina del Rey, CA: Law and Psychology Press.

Fordyce, D., Roueche, J., & Prigatano, G. (1983). Enhanced emotional reactions in chronic head trauma patients. *Journal of Neurology, Neurosurgery, and Psychiatry*, *46*, 620–624.

Gallen, R., & Berry, D. (1996). Detection of random responding in MMPI-2 protocols. *Assessment*, *3*, 171–178.

Gallen, R., & Berry, D. (1997). Partially random MMPI-2 protocols: When are they interpretable? *Assessment*, *4*, 61–68.

Gallucci, N. (1985). Influence of dissimulation on indexes of response consistency for the MMPI. *Psychological Reports*, *57*, 1013–1014.

Galski, T. (1995, March). Mild traumatic brain injury: When symptoms linger. *Trial*, pp. 76–79.

Gass, C. (1991). MMPI-2 interpretation and closed head injury: A correction factor. *Psychological Assessment, 3*, 27–31.

Gass, C., & Ansley, J. (1995). Personality assessment of neurologically impaired patients. In J. Butcher (Ed.), *Clinical personality assessment: Practical approaches* (pp. 192–210). London: Oxford University Press.

Gass, C., & Russell, E. (1991). MMPI profiles of closed head trauma patients: Impact of neurological complaints. *Journal of Clinical psychology, 47*, 253–260.

Gough, H. (1947). Simulated patterns on the MMPI. *Journal of Abnormal and Social Psychology, 42*, 215–225.

Gough, H. (1950). The F minus K dissimulation index for the MMPI. *Journal of Consulting Psychology, 14*, 408–413.

Gough, H. (1954). Some common misconceptions about neuroticism. *Journal of Consulting Psychology, 18*, 287–292.

Gouvier, W., Uddo-Crane, M., & Brown, L. (1988). Base rates of postconcussional symptoms. *Archives of Clinical Neuropsychology, 3*, 273–278.

Graham, J. (1993). *MMPI-2: Assessing personality and psychopathology* (2nd ed.). London: Oxford University Press.

Graham, J., Watts, D., & Timbrook, R. (1991). Detecting fake good and fake bad MMPI-2 profiles. *Journal of Personality Assessment, 57*, 264–277.

Greene, R. (1978). An empirically derived MMPI consistency scale. *Journal of Clinical Psychology, 34*, 407–410.

Greiffenstein, M., Baker, W., & Gola, T. (1994). Validation of malingered amnesia measures with a large clinical sample. *Psychological Assessment, 6*, 218– 224.

Greiffenstein, M., Gola, T., & Baker, W. (1995). MMPI-2 validity scales versus domain specific measures in the detection of factitious traumatic brain injury. *The Clinical Neuropsychologist, 9*, 230–240.

Guilmette, T., Hart, K., & Giuliano, A. (1993). Malingering detection: The use of a forced-choice method in identifying organic versus simulated memory impairment. *The Clinical Neuropsychologist, 7*, 59–69.

Gynther, M. (1961). The clinical utility of invalid MMPI F scores. *Journal of Consulting Psychology, 25*, 540–542.

Hare, R. (1985). Comparison of procedures for the assessment of psychopathy. *Journal of Consulting and Clinical Psychology, 53*, 7–16.

Heaton, R., Smith, H., Lehman, R., & Vogt, A. (1978). Prospects for faking believable deficits on neuropsychological testing. *Journal of Consulting and Clinical Psychology, 46*, 892–900.

Hiscock, M., & Hiscock, C. (1989). Refining the forced-choice method for the detection of malingering. *Journal of Clinical and Experimental Neuropsychology, 11*, 967–974.

Kellner, R., & Sheffield, B. (1973). The one-week prevalence of symptoms in neurotic patients and normals. *American Journal of Psychiatry, 130*, 102–105.

Kraus, J., & Sorenson, S. (1994). Epidemiology. In J. Silver, S. Yudofsky, & R. Hales (Eds.), *Neuropsychiatry of traumatic brain injury* (pp. 3–42). Washington, DC: American Psychiatric Press.

Lamb, D., Berry, D., Wetter, M., & Baer, R. (1994). Effects of two types of information on malingering of closed-head injury on the MMPI-2: An analog investigation. *Psychological Assessment, 6*, 8–13.

Lees-Haley, P. (1992a). Psychodiagnostic test usage by forensic psychologists. *American Journal of Forensic Psychology, 10*, 25–30.

Lees-Haley, P. (1992b). Efficacy of MMPI-2 validity scales and MCMI-II modifier scales for detecting spurious PTSD claims: F, F − K, Fake Bad Scale,Ego Strength, Subtle–Obvious subscales, DIS, and DEB. *Journal of Clinical Psychology, 48*, 681–689.

Lees-Haley, P. (in press). Attorneys influence expert evidence in forensic psychological and neuropsychological cases. *Assessment.*

Lees-Haley, P., & Brown, R. (1993). Neuropsychological complaint base rates in 170 personal injury claimants. *Archives of Clinical Neuropsychology, 8*, 203–209.

Lees-Haley, P., English, L., & Glenn, W. (1991). A fake bad scale on the MMPI-2 for personal injury claimants. *Psychological Reports, 68*, 203–210.

Lees-Haley, P., Smith, H., Williams, C., & Dunn, J. (1995). Forensic neuropsychological test usage: An empirical survey. *Archives of Clinical Neuropsychology, 11*, 45–52.

Levin, H., High, W., Goethe, K., Sisson, R., Overall, J., Rhoades, H., Eisenberg, H., Kalisky, Z., & Gray, H. (1987). The Neurobehavioral Rating Scale: Assessment of the behavioral sequelae of head injury by the clinician. *Journal of Neurology, Neurosurgery, and Psychiatry, 50*, 183–193.

Lubin, B., Larsen, R., & Matarazzo, J. (1984). Patterns of psychological test usage in the United States: 1935–1982. *American Psychologist, 39*, 451–454.

MacNiven, E., & Finlayson, M. (1993). The interplay between emotional and cognitive recovery after closed head injury. *Brain Injury, 7*, 241–246.

Millis, S., Putnam, S., & Adams, K. (1995). *Neuropsychological malingering and the MMPI-2: Old and new indicators*. Presented at the 30th Annual Symposium on Recent Developments in the Use of the MMPI, MMPI-2 and MMPI-A, St. Petersburg Beach, FL.

Nelson, L., Satz, P., Mitrushina, M., Van Gorp, W., Cicchetti, D., Lewis, R., & Van Lancker, D. (1989). Development and validation of the Neuropsychology Behavior and Affect Profile. *Psychological Assessment, 1*, 266–272.

Nichols, D., Greene, R., & Schmolck, P. (1989). Criteria for assessing inconsistent patterns of item endorsement on the MMPI: Rationale, development, and empirical trials. *Journal of Clinical Psychology, 45*, 239–250.

Novack, T., Daniel, M., & Long, C. (1984). Factors related to emotional adjustment following head injury. *International Journal of Clinical Neuropsychology, 6*, 139–142.

Paolo, A., & Ryan, J. (1992). Detection of random response sets on the MMPI-2. *Psychotherapy in Private Practice, 11*, 1–8.

Pope, K., Butcher, J., & Seelen, J. (1993). *The MMPI, MMPI-2 & MMPI-A in court*. Washington, DC: American Psychological Association.

Prigatano, G. (1992). Personality disturbances associated with traumatic brain injury. *Journal of Consulting and Clinical Psychology, 60*, 360–368.

Prigatano, G., & Amin, K. (1993). Digit Memory Test: Unequivocal cerebral dysfunction and suspected malingering. *Journal of Clinical and Experimental Neuropsychology, 15*, 537–546.

Putnam, S., & Millis, S. (1994). Psychosocial factors in the development and maintenance of chronic somatic and functional symptoms following mild traumatic brain injury. *Advances in Medical Psychotherapy, 7*, 1–22.

Rogers, R. (1984). Towards an empirical model of malingering and deception. *Behavioral Sciences and the Law, 2*, 93–111.

Rogers, R. (1988). Researching dissimulation. In R. Rogers (Ed.), *Clinical assessment of malingering and deception* (pp. 309–327). New York: Guilford Press.

Rogers, R. (1990). Models of feigned illness. *Professional Psychology: Research and Practice, 21*, 182–188.

Rogers, R., Bagby, R., & Chakraborty, D. (1993). Feigning schizophrenic disorders on the MMPI-2: Detection of coached simulators. *Journal of Personality Assessment, 60*, 215–226.

Rogers, R., Bagby, R., & Dickens, S. (1992). *Structured Interview of Reported Symptoms: Professional manual*. Odessa, FL: Psychological Assessment Resources.

Rogers, R., Sewell, K., & Salekin, R. (1994). A meta-analysis of malingering on the MMPI-2. *Assessment, 1*, 227–239.

Rothke, S., Friedman, A., Dahlstrom, W., Greene, R., Arredondo, R., & Mann, A. (1994). MMPI-2 normative data for the F−K index: Implications for clinical, neuropsychological, and forensic practice. *Assessment, 1*, 1–15.

Timbrook, R., Graham, J., Keiller, S., & Watts, D. (1993). Comparison of Wiener–Harmon Subtle–

Obvious scales and the standard validity scales in detecting valid and invalid MMPI-2 profiles. *Psychological Assessment, 5*, 53–61.

Villanueva, M., & Binder, L. (1993). *Association between MMPI-2 validity indices and the Portland Digit Recognition Test.* Presented at the 21st Annual International Neuropsychological Society Meeting, Galveston, TX.

Wetter, M., Baer, R., Berry, D., Robison, L., & Sumpter, J. (1993). MMPI-2 profiles of motivated fakers given specific symptom information: A comparison to matched patients. *Psychological Assessment, 5*, 317–323.

Wetter, M., Baer, R., Berry, D., Smith, G., & Larsen, L. (1992). Sensitivity of MMPI-2 validity scales to random responding and malingering. *Psychological Assessment, 4*, 369–374.

Wetter, M., & Corrigan, S. (1995). Providing information to clients about psychological tests: A survey of attorney's and law student's attitudes. *Professional Psychology: Research and Practice, 26*, 474–477.

Wetter, M., & Tharpe, B. (under review). Detection of acquiescence and counteracquiescence on the MMPI-2: The utility of the TRIN scale.

Wiener, D. (1948). Subtle and obvious keys for the MMPI. *Journal of Consulting Psychology, 12*, 164–170.

Youngjohn, J. (1995). Confirmed attorney coaching prior to neuropsychological evaluation. *Assessment, 2*, 279–283.

Ziskin, J., & Faust, D. (1988). *Coping with psychiatric and psychological testimony* (Vol. 2, 4th ed.). Marina del Rey, CA: Law and Psychology Press.

8

Clinical Detection of Malingering

LAWRENCE C. HARTLAGE

There is no question that malingered data must be recognized and dealt with if neuropsychological data are to be accepted as representing valid indices of diagnostic, etiological, and prognostic phenomena. As neuropsychologists are increasingly drawn into the forensic arena, the veridicality and reliability of data generated by neuropsychological examination have increasingly been brought under scrutiny and into question (Satz, 1988). Interestingly, there have been suspicions for many years of secondary gain or malingering motivation following injuries of all types, described in law and psychiatric literature under such names as "accident aftermath, litigation or profit neurosis; compensation hysteria; post-accident syndrome; or unconscious malingering" (Mendelson, 1987), so that at least a modicum of skepticism in evaluating postinjury sequelae under litigation is not only prudent but requisite for accurate interpretation of findings.

The issue of supposed or potential malingering following neurological injury is confounded by the symptoms often presenting as sequelae of such injury. Many problems realistically attributable to sequelae of neurological injury can be cited as evidence of malingering. Ability to recall some historical information with high particularity while having poor recall for other such information, or ability to perform well on some tests of memory (e.g., remote) while performing poorly on other memory (e.g., short-term) tasks are examples likely familiar to most neuropsychologists. Another confounding factor involves variable attentional components of given tasks. Tests of arithmetic ability, for example, may suggest relatively intact residual ability (e.g., on acquired ability measures such as WRAT-III tests with only moderate attentional component) and concurrently showing poor

LAWRENCE C. HARTLAGE • Augusta Neuropsychology Center, Augusta, Georgia 30809.

Detection of Malingering during Head Injury Litigation, edited by Reynolds. Plenum Press, New York, 1998.

residual ability (e.g., on WISC-III tests with higher attentional demands) as a result of differential attentional components of the ability presumably being measured. Similarly, patients with attentional problems may show variable attention to various aspects of given mental tasks, to produce a pattern not grossly dissimilar from what might result from variable effort or haphazard responding. Fortunately, the broad and comprehensive array of data typically available to the neuropsychologist permits opportunity for overview of data sources and types for evaluation—often at leisure and in retrospect of examination—to interpret these possible confounds and contamination of data. However, it is common (and probably desirable) for the clinician to make initial and ongoing appraisal of the veridicality of information being collected, as is done in the course of interview data and clinical observations, preparatory to consideration of actual test data. This is actually the manner in which information relevant to potential malingering is typically elicited, processed, and evaluated in the course of psychiatric interview, without benefit of subsequent test data (Othmer & Othmer, 1994). This is, in fact, the basis of imputations concerning insensitivity to malingering posited by such critics as Ziskin and Faust (1988).

Historical estimates of malingered symptoms following injury have ranged from 1% (Keiser, 1968) to greater than 50% (Miller & Cartlidge, 1972), with more recent estimates clustered toward the lower of these two figures. Whatever the actual incidence, neuropsychologists involved in postinjury assessment of patients need to be aware of and provide safeguards against possible contamination of neuropsychological data by incorporating factitious, fallacious, or fictitious information; or accepting spurious or suboptimal performance on test items into the diagnostic conclusion.

A problem inherent in clinical detection of malingering involves the vagueness of criteria for malingering. Unfortunately, most empirical approaches to the topic consider malingering as a dichotomous phenomenon; i.e., groups are classified as "malingerers" (as in the case of college students told to emulate brain injury symptoms) versus "nonmalingerers," whereas in the world of the forensic neuropsychologist the phenomenon is more likely to represent a continuum (Price, 1995). Popular press reports, such as a recent (1994) *Time* magazine survey, indicate that the "average" person averages two and a half "lies" per day; by Faust and Zitkin criteria everyone could thus be classified as a malingerer. Although nonforensic situations readily tolerate slightly less than total veridicality (e.g., "I enjoyed your snail casserole," "What a lovely dress," or even "The check is in the mail"), deviations from total truth in a forensic neuropsychological context may be used to impeach truthfulness and support implications of malingering (e.g., Berry, Baer, & Harris, 1991; Brandt, 1992; Green, Astner, Kiss, & Allen, 1993; Hall & Pritchard, 1995; Nies & Sweet, 1994; Roberts & Resnick, 1989; Rogers, 1988).

Before addressing the issue of clinical approaches to detection of malingering, it is relevant to define the terms as they will be pursued. *Clinical approaches* as discussed in this chapter refer to nonactuarial, nonstatistical approaches that rely on (1) clinical observations; (2) consideration of congruence (or lack of same) among cognate abilities and relationship (or lack) among diverse tests or measures related to function of given cortical areas or functional systems; and (3) contextual phenomena such as patient expectancies and examiner instructions or comments. The exclusion of actuarial and statistical approaches reflects no disdain for their utility, but rather a recognition that the complex factors in those approaches properly belong in the purview of those neuroscientist practitioners specializing in such matters.

Unlike examinations for personality, aptitude, or achievement, which are addressed to "typical" or "representative" performance, neuropsychological examination, like intellectual assessment, is addressed to "optimal" performance, and thus the issue of malingering or suboptimal performance is central and crucial to valid assessment. As a result, neuropsychologists are, by necessity, sensitive and attuned to any clinical cues that might suggest or even raise questions of suboptimal performance, and such issues have been recommended as considerations to be taken into account in the content, process, and sequence of neuropsychological examination (Hartlage, 1990; Klebe & Davis, 1995; Millis, Putnam, & Adams, 1995; Ruchinskas, Barth, & Diamond, 1995). Whereas experienced neuropsychologists have incorporated procedures for eliciting valid data into their clinical practice, it is interesting that clinical studies of malingering in neuropsychology have tended to be much scarcer than artificial scenarios comparing absolute test performance of individuals (e.g., college students) told to "fake head injury" with those of real patients with documented head injury. Review of abstracts of papers dealing with malingering that were presented at recent National Academy of Neuropsychology meetings in the 1994 and 1995 *Archives of Clinical Neuropsychology*, for example, reveals the overwhelming majority involved either artificial or simulated patients, or individuals assessed actuarially rather than clinically; with only one clearly clinically diagnosed case (Ribbler, 1995). Interestingly, the clinical neuropsychological examination's validity was demonstrated in a clinical context rife with potential for misdiagnosis because of malingering in this one case.

CLINICAL OBSERVATIONS

Neurological abnormalities, dysfunctions, and impairments provide the observant clinician a wealth of relevant diagnostic information. Indeed, many neurological syndromes have such unique presentation that diagnostic impressions can be formulated mainly by looking at the patient (e.g., *Atlas of Mental Retardation Syndromes*).

Other neurological conditions present with obvious clues to status of the central nervous system in such symptoms as plegias, tremors, or spasticity, whereas many patients with more subtle neurological impairments reveal symptoms in their gait, speech, or purposive movements. Interaction, even on a superficial basis, may reveal symptoms involving decreased verbal fluency, bradyphrenia, attentional and memory problems, and phrenasthenia.

Much of early clinical neurology was based on observation of such anomalies, and early incursions by psychology into parameters of neuropsychology involved fairly straightforward observations of patients' ability to articulate, copy, imitate, repeat, or execute fairly simple commands, with the dimension of systematic examination procedure and recording added to the sorts of clinical assessments historically used by neurologists (Bernat, 1994; Corey-Brown, 1996; Schiffer, 1996).

Interestingly, as neuropsychology began to flourish as an emerging independent science, the focus was shifted from clinical observation to systematic, standardized data collection procedures incorporated into a comprehensive battery assessment procedure, whose data could be collected by technicians (Reitan, 1955). For purposes of scientific validation, the interpretation of battery data was done by blind analysis to preclude the neuropsychologist from utilizing clinical clues in formulating a diagnosis, in effect putting the burden of proof on the battery and the objective data it contained (Reitan & Wolfson, 1985). As with so many innovative procedures, even after the comprehensive neuropsychological battery had repeatedly demonstrated its diagnostic accuracy and robustness in a variety of settings and with a wide range of patients and thus obviated the need for blind interpretation, many practitioners new to the field adopted the (unspoken and typically unrecognized) motto "If it's good enough for the 1950s, it's good enough for now."

The influx of clinically trained psychologists into neuropsychological training programs, internships, fellowships, and practice helped resurrect an interest in clinical observation in neuropsychological assessment. Perhaps of even greater importance, as neuropsychologists increasingly became drawn into the forensic arena, there was increased interest in utilizing all available relevant data, so as to enhance prediction to ecological validity criterion measures and to ensure that their test data were relevant to real-world questions at issue. The following pages list some selective factors relevant to this aspect of clinical observation.

Occasionally a patient's *demeanor* presents a powerful clue concerning validity of his or her performance. Obviously a haphazard or at least submaximal effort may be anticipated from the patient who makes comments disparaging the test, the test situation, the examiner, or the setting in which the examination is being conducted. Potentially relevant clues may be found in comments disparaging the legal profession, or given attorney, or the insurance industry, in that such comments may reflect an unwillingness to cooperate with the object of disparagement, or may merely reflect an anger that would not necessarily preclude valid performance on the tests. In either case, such verbal clues toward patient attitude can alert the examiner to be especially attuned to possible instances of suboptimal effort. More importantly, they indicate to the examiner a need to clarify to the patient the importance of attempting best performance on all measures. If any questions concerning validity of data resultant from questionable patient compliance remain, noting the specific verbalizations made by the patient, and at what stage of the examination, can be of help if subsequent question arises.

Nonverbal communication by patients, although more difficult for less well trained or experienced examiners to detect, can similarly provide clues to the attitude of patients concerning their performance on specific (or even all) aspects of tests involved in the examination. Obvious signals include overt activities such as surreptitious breaking of pencil lead or dropping or knocking over test manipulanda or other items. Yawning, requiring encouragement to keep on task, looking around the room for distractions, or frequently looking at a watch or clock are other obvious clues. More subtle nonverbal clues can be noted in facial expressions, body kinesics and position; spontaneous activity level; and psychomotor speed for on- versus off-task activities. Claimed inability to respond to simple items presumably within the repertoire of even severely impaired patients is another obvious clue, and has been fairly extensively reported (e.g., Bectar & Williams, 1995; Bernard & Fowler, 1990; Wiggins & Brandt, 1988).

More subtle nonverbal clues can come from observations of regularity of pace maintained over timed test sequences; consistency over repeated trials of tasks like rate of finger oscillation; and on no signs of fatigue over trials like grip strength wherein expenditure of maximum levels of effort might reasonably produce accumulative decrement in performance levels.

Although often overlooked, behaviors involved in getting into or out of cars, managing stairs, or negotiating crowded hallways can provide clues concerning balance and motor coordination. Behaviors in waiting room (e.g., reading the *Wall Street Journal*) can be compared with comments concerning reading difficulty/concentration problems, or with subsequent data from reading tests to assess congruence. Attitudes of family members toward the patient (e.g., protective, supportive, apprehensive) may provide clues to the patient's typical out-of-examination-room behavior, and serve as a basis for formulation of questions. As a general rule, a typical neuropsychological examination provides an entire day's opportunity to observe a patient's nonverbal behavior in the context of both social interaction and test performance, and thus provides the neuropsychologist with sustained access to behaviors that can potentially be masked, avoided, or suppressed during the course of a 50-minute psychiatric interview, or neurological examination, and full advantage should be made of the opportunity (Landau, 1996; Weintraub, 1996).

Verbal comments, such as inquiry concerning how many more tests there are or how much time remains, disparaging comments about the test or test context, or threats to terminate are obvious indicators of less than optimum motivation, and although they do not necessarily invalidate the data are clear caveats that considerable care must be exercised in evaluating data at least temporally related to such utterances, and quite possibly all data. Similarly, it is not uncommon for patients involved in litigation to have developed a tendentious approach to their problems. Perhaps conditioned by their interaction with attorneys, patients may well give an "all or nothing" history, wherein they were supranormal and exquisitely happy before their injury but have become disabled and depressed since suffering the injury. When such a pattern is noted in verbal reports or reconstructions, it may be necessary to obtain data concerning preinjury status from uninvolved external sources (e.g., employers, ministers) to a somewhat greater extent than usual. Conversely, statements expressing concern, doubt, or frustration may, in content, suggest positive achievement orientation or motivation and, if perceived as credible by the examiner, can support impressions concerning validity of data. Occasional comments like "I was always good at figures," "My brother and I used to play games to see who could recall more digits," or "I never was good at art or drawing" can help place apparently incongruent or uneven test performances in context.

Direct observation of implausible "floor effect" phenomena represents an approach for identification of individuals at risk for producing invalid data. Tests that reveal deficits of unlikely severity, such as the Wiggins and Brandt (1988) interviews or the Rey 15-Item Visual Memory Test, are examples of approaches to such floor effect indicators of malingering (Bernard & Fowler, 1990; Goldberg & Miller, 1986; Hays, Emmons, & Lawson, 1993; Lee, Loring, & Martin, 1992; Schretlen, Brandt, Krafft, & Van Gorp, 1991). The Wiggins and Brandt inventory uses a dozen questions that can reasonably be expected to be answered correctly by anyone, including individuals with brain injury, with incorrect or implausible answers to questions such as:

What is your name?
What is your age?
What is your birthdate?
What is your telephone number?
What is your address?
What is your mother's first name?
What is your mother's maiden name?
What is your father's first name?
What is your brother's and/or sister's name?

being highly associated with malingering. The National Academy of Neuropsychology Research Consortium has developed a 17-item Personal History/Orientation Questionnaire covering some of the same items as the Wiggins and Brandt inventory, with addition of questions involving colors in the U.S. flag, our first president, our current president, and the current month and year, i.e., representing facts likely known by most individuals. The consortium is also studying a 21-item test (Iverson, Franzen, & McCracken, 1991) that consists of two lists of nouns, one read to the patient and a second used as a distractor or foil on the recognition task. Both free recall and forced-choice recognition trials are given.

Perhaps one of the more commonly used "floor" tests for clinical detection of malingering involves the 15-item test (Rey, 1941, 1964), which presents the patient with 15 items in five rows of three characters per line, e.g.,

A	B	C
1	2	3
a	b	c
○	△	□
I	II	III

with 10-second exposure followed by request to reproduce. Interestingly, review suggests that this test is likely to detect only a minority of unsuspected malingerers (Rogers, Harrell, & Liff, 1993). Somewhat better research support has been presented for the use of a 16-item format (Iverson & Franzen, 1991) with items presented in the following format:

A	B	C	D
1	2	3	4
a	b	c	d
I	II	III	IV

After a 10-second memorization/study period, the patient is asked to copy as much as can be remembered. Obviously the patient need recall only three or four ideas to reintegrate most of the items, and use of a cutting score of 6 correctly classified 100% of normal and 100% of memory-impaired patients, but only 40% of malingerers. Other "floor" types of tests used for clinical detection of factors relating to validity of neuropsychological test results include the Porch Index of Communicative Ability (PICA), Dot Counting or Word Recognition (Rey, 1941).

Another screening approach involves a forced-choice format, such as the Portland Digit Recognition Test (Binder, 1993a,b) or the forced-choice components of the 21-Item Test (Iverson, Franzen, & McCracken, 1991, 1994), whereby patients performing at worse than chance levels may be suspected of making intentionally wrong responses (Hiscock & Hiscock, 1989; Iverson, Nailler, & Franzen, 1993; Millis, 1992; Millis & Putnam, 1994). Alternatives or variants to this forced-choice format have been reported (e.g., Ruchinskas et al., 1995) for use in cases where a standardized test for malingering may not be feasible. In cases where recall on Story Recall Testing appears to be depressed beyond what might be expected from clinical observations, for example, I add a 10-question forced-choice questionnaire of story content after delayed recall testing: More than chance recall errors or discordance with delayed recall performance may document malingering.

Observations of level of performance on given tests from the Halstead–Reitan Neuropsychological Battery have also been used under this general (forced-choice) paradigm. The Rhythm Sense test represents an obvious forced-choice format, and has been used for determination of validity (Millis et al., 1995; Trueblood & Schmidt, 1993) and malingering (Gfeller, Craddock, & Falkenhain, 1994). Less direct observations (i.e., multichoice) of Category Test and Speech Perception Test performance by means of cutoff scores have been shown to have some utility in the detection of malingering (e.g., Iverson, Myers, & Adams, 1994; Millis et al., 1995; Tenhula & Sweet, 1994) and Charter (1994) has identified procedures for detection of random responding for Category, Speech Perception, and Rhythm Tests.

Yet another approach to observation of test performance as a clue to possible malingering involves automaticity of responses, whereby an automatic implicit memory task is presented, with suppressed performance on a primary task suggestive of malingering. Klebe and Davis (1995), for example, demonstrated that on tasks like mirror image reading malingerers are not able to decrease performance when instructed to do so. Although such examination procedures are not typically included in most neuropsychological examinations, they offer further evidence that clinical observations of test performance can offer an effective and parsimonious approach to detection of malingering in the examination setting.

Impressionistic notations, although perhaps lacking in demonstrated validity, can be very helpful in reconstructing possible instances wherein suboptimal functional level may have spuriously lowered performance on given tasks. For example, examiner notes concerning word finding difficulties, paraphasias, or apparent frustration concerning inability to find a word on vocabulary or information types of tests may relate to subsequent apparent inconsistencies wherein the patient misses easier items but successfully responds to more difficult ones. Similarly, a note reflecting apparent impulsive responding on picture completion types of items, absent such notation for other types of items, could help indicate those subtests of questionable validity compared with other tests for which there was no such question. This can be especially helpful for dealing with cross-examination wherein the attorney cites references showing typical congruence between a test on which the patient did poorly and one reflecting intact ability. Indeed, many neuropsychologists include in their behavioral observations such conclusive statements as "Very good levels of cooperation were maintained over extended examination," "Levels of performance on Tests X and Y, given late in examination, may have reflected accumulative fatigue," "There appeared to be special subjective difficulty with test items involving . . . ," or "Fluctuations in attention, apparently nonvolitional, were noted on . . . ."

Obviously, such interpretive and conclusive statements depend to a considerable extent on the skill, experience, and sophistication of the clinician. For purposes of litigation, such conclusions are typically best supported when the examination has been personally conducted by the neuropsychologist, although exceptionally skillful technicians can in some instances provide appropriate impressionistic data.

CONGRUENCE AMONG AND ACROSS NEUROPSYCHOLOGICAL TESTS

Congruence (or lack of same) among and across tests provides neuropsychologists with a compelling and powerful opportunity for clinical detection of possible malingering, an opportunity not typically available to psychiatrists or clinical psychologists dependent on observation and inferences based on level of performance. In but one of many papers documenting this fact, Anderson and Bigler (1994), using CT, MR, and neuropsychological data, demonstrated that a within-subjects design can be more sensitive to differences than a between-subjects design, for both cognitive outcome and morphological criterion measures. Similarly, among populations such as healthy older adults, although occasional single test performance may fall within a range suggestive of impairment, overview of all data in configured context can identify likelihood of misclassification related to malingering or other sources of Type I error (Palmer, Boone, Lesser, & Wohl, 1995).

Because neuropsychological assessment measures functions that are anatomically based and verifiable, as opposed to the sorts of hypothetical constructs commonly measured by tests of intelligence or personality, the data resulting from neuropsychological assessment lend themselves to validation and verification by analysis of their degree of adherence to (deviation from) their neuroanatomic substrates. Basic motor functions, for example, can be conceptualized as dependent on integrity of contralateral cerebral cortex area just anterior to the Rolandic fissure, with damage to that anatomic area supported by corresponding data from relevant motor system testing. Similarly, because certain neurocognitive functions tend to show correlation with cerebral hemisphere on a lateralized basis, such as typical specialization of some language functions to the dominant cerebral hemisphere, there is the opportunity to relate observed test findings to neuroanatomical functional units.

Specific examples from common neuropsychological instruments may help make such concepts obvious.

Sensory data such as the ability to recognize which finger was touched; recognize basic geometric shapes; and identify numbers written on fingertips can, by themselves, provide excellent first-line clues to malingering. First, in the anterior portions of the parietal lobe just posterior to the Rolandic fissure, such (sensory) information is communicated from fingers and hand along cervical nerves with discrete representation. Cervical nerves six, seven, and eight, for example, convey information from the thumb side of the hand to the small finger side of the hand in a known pattern (e.g., Netter, 1958, p. 55). Consistency in sensory misperceptions (e.g., missing numbers written on C6 distribution and correctly identifying those on C7 and C8) not only can segregate peripheral from central etiology underlying graphaesthesia, but can also yield potent clues relevant to effort versus malingering. Perhaps even more obviously, presence of sensory impairments such as glove anesthesia offers evidence of nonanatomic distribution of complaints, not referable to functional neuroanatomic systems.

Using sensory data in combination affords a second level of clinical detection of malingering, by comparing data obtained through different methods for evaluating similar anatomic substrates. An individual who can correctly identify numbers written on all fingertips, for example, but who cannot correctly identify which fingertip has been touched is likely not demonstrating signs of central nervous system injury, and in fact may be evidencing signs potentially referable to malingering. Similarly, an individual who performs within good time limits on the tactual performance test with a given hand, but is found unable to identify simple shapes or recognize stimulation to the corresponding hand may be malingering or at least producing uneven levels of effort. Conversely, good congruence on ipsilateral performance involving measures of graphaesthesia and astereognosis (e.g., fingertip number writing and tactual performance test or finger recognition measures) provides some support for inferences suggestive of commensurate and compatible levels of effort across referent tasks.

Motor measures, in similar manner, provide clinical data regarding congruence of findings. With most individuals, motor performance involving grip strength and finger oscillation rate tends to show clear ipsilateral performance superiority/inferiority, with performance of the dominant hand usually in the range of 5–10% greater than for the nondominant hand (Hartlage & Telzrow, 1986). Occasional variations, such as might result from quite recent injury impairing finger oscillation rate but before reflecting disuse or other muscle atrophy, are obvious exceptions. Other expectations might involve specific use patterns, such as exhibited by some string musicians. Absent anamnestic data supporting possible basis for unexpected motor findings, however, lack of optimal effort must remain a viable consideration to be confirmed or excluded by subsequent examination.

Grip strength can be a simple yet solid indicator of consistency of maximal effort, insofar as with maximal effort some degree of fatigue over trials is likely. An individual who can, with encouragement, exceed prior grip strength, obviously did not perform at maximum level on the previous trial. Yet such obvious truisms can be overlooked by psychologists who slavishly refer to normative data (e.g., Heaton, Grant, & Matthews, 1991) and ignore the wealth of clinically relevant information available by simple observation. Typically, there will be a slight but gradual decrement in kilogram/grip strength with closely successive efforts, providing that absolute optimum efforts were expended on each trial. Differential configuration—even with widely diverse findings discarded before averaging—

obviously must be evaluated with respect to their implications for malingering or at least evidence of less than optimum effort on at least some trials.

Finally, constructional praxis tasks, whether involving copying from stimuli or from memory, can be sensitive to malingered efforts. On Bender Gestalt reproductions, for example, it was possible to identify attempted simulation by attending to the specific sorts of errors typically unique to organically impaired patients (e.g., simplification, parallel distortion, variability and intersection/rotation) (Bruhn & Reed, 1975). Similarly, types of errors discriminated simulators from brain injury patients on the Benton Visual Retention Test, in that patients made more errors of omission (especially small peripheral figures) whereas simulators made more distortions (Benton & Spreen, 1961).

Clinical comparison of combined motor and sensory data represents another sound basis for inferences concerning malingering. For most neurologically intact individuals, it is reasonable to expect some degree of congruence between ipsilateral sensory and motor functions, typically involving somewhat stronger levels of performance of upper extremity functions contralateral to the dominant cerebral hemisphere. Certain neurological impairments such as may occur from coup-contrecoup blows to the head or focal neurological insults can obviously interrupt this pattern of expected symmetry, as can an occasional neurodevelopmental anomaly. Absent anamnestic data compatible with such etiology, especially when such mixed performance or sensory and motor functions are incongruent with other neuropsychological test data, it is reasonable to regard malingering as a possible contributory factor.

Multitest patterns of test data represent the strongest and most compelling basis for clinical detection of malingering, in that such patterns provide for overviews and syntheses of all relevant data for which clinical observations have already been made and assembled. The possible permutations of such multitest pattern analyses are quite numerous, and thus provide multiple opportunities for multiple cross-validations of within-subject data configurations.

A brief review of some research findings in this area may help put such approaches into perspective regarding the relevance of such approaches to clinical detection of malingering.

In a discriminant analysis of neuropsychological test results for brain-damaged, postconcussive, and malingering subjects, Baker, Gola, and Greiffenstein (1995) found that analysis including only five scales (RAVLT recognition; short delay; dominant hand fingertapping; dominant hand grooved pegboard; WMS-R Visual Recognition I) provided a correct classification rate of 86% overall, with highest discrimination for the malingerers (89.3%). These findings are compatible with and update the findings of Heaton, Smith, Lehman, and Vogt (1978) that the pattern of results produced by malingerers can be differentiated from brain-damaged patients. Similar conclusions were reported by Mittenberg, Rotholc, Russell, and Heilbronner (1994) using the Halstead–Reitan Battery, replicating the Heaton et al. (1978) methodology on a larger sample. Reitan and Wolfson (1985) presented workshops on malingering and age/education norms in which they demonstrated sensitivity of the Halstead–Reitan Neuropsychological Test Battery configurations to malingering. In their chapter in this volume, they report data showing the development of a "Retest Consistency Index" and a "Response Consistency Index," which are both combined into a "Dissimulation Index." The Retest Consistency Index showed classification rates of 90% for litigants and 95% for nonlitigants, and the Response Consistency Index correctly classified 100% of nonlitigants and 90% of litigants, suggesting that careful attention to configurations of data from the Halstead–Reitan Neuropsychological Battery without attention to collateral data can provide potent clues for the identification of potential malingering.

Other, more specialized configural analyses have similarly shown sensitivity to simulation of neuropsychological symptoms. Using rate of decay across Raven's Standard Progressive Matrices, Gudjonsson and Shackleton (1986) found a sensitivity of 82.8% with a specificity of 95.1% for 81 military simulators, controls, and neuropsychological patients.

With common measures such as Wechsler IQ and memory scales, configural analysis has shown fair sensitivity to detection of malingering. Using 67 head injury patients matched with 67 simulators on FSIQ and age, Mittenberg, Zielinski, Fichera, Heilbronner, and Youngjohn (1993) compared Vocabulary–Digit Span subtest difference scores, and found that whereas head trauma patients showed similar levels of performance on both scales, simulators showed exaggerated decrement on Digit Span performance. Comparable findings were reported by Mittenberg, Theroux-Fichera, Zielinski, and Heilbronner (1995). Similarly, Mittenberg, Azrin, Millsaps, and Heilbronner (1993) found that malingerers could be detected by comparing measures of attention relative to their own memory scores. Comparing 39 head injury patients with 39 age-matched subjects instructed to simulate head injury, they found 83.3% correct classification by using the difference between WMS-R memory and attention/concentration scores, according to the following weighting:

Difference between general memory and attention/concentration scores	Malingering probability
35	.99
32	.95
30	.92
25	.85
19	.75
09	.60
02	.50

Other investigators (Bectar & Williams, 1995) have found Memory Assessment Scales to identify malingerers on virtually all scales, through simulator response style characterized by either intentional wrong or random response pattern; and Larrabee (in press) has reported on the efficacy of using modified configurations of standard memory tests (e.g., Continuous Recognition Memory Test; Continuous Visual Memory Test; Verbal Selective Reminding Test; Rey Auditory Verbal Learning Test; California Verbal Learning Test; Recognition Memory Test) for producing cutting scores indicative of malingering.

Because it is impractical to describe all of the possible permutations of test data, a sample of one small and one intermediate-size data set should suffice to provide sufficient basis for exposition of the value of such analysis.

A not unreasonable nor uncommon configuration of test data might include performance IQ some 10 points lower than verbal; left hand perhaps 15% poorer than right on motor function; reaction time to left visual stimuli slower than to right; more neglect or distortion errors on left than right peripheral figures on Benton Visual Retention Test; tactual performance time on left (nondominant) hand approximately equal to that of time for the dominant hand; astereognosis and graphaesthesia on nondominant upper extremity; greater difficulty with visual than verbal memory; and history of insult to central nervous system mainly involving the nondominant cerebral hemisphere. Comparison of current mental functional status is grossly compatible with prior educational and work history. Further, there are confirmatory findings by electrophysiological, radiographic, and magnetic resonance imaging all compatible with damage to right cerebral hemisphere. No litigation is pending or anticipated. Given such a configuration, with no clinical observation of intentional malingering and no data suggestive of malingering, and further given all MMPI-2 validity scales within normal limits and no F − K ratios suggestive of faking bad, it is possible that even the more skeptical and suspicious neuropsychologist may not immediately suspect fraud, malingering, or prevarication. Obviously, the data appear to "make sense," to "hang together," i.e., they demonstrate apparent congruence. It is the lack of congruence of neuropsychological test data (absent EEG, CT, MRI, data, and litigation status considerations), on the other hand, that offers possible suggestion or likelihood of malingered data, and can provide more than adequate sensitivity to its detection.

A look at deviations from the just-described test data may help put into perspective both false-positive and false-negative opportunities for suspecting malingering. By exclusion, review of peripheral (i.e., nonneuropsychological) data may be an appropriate place to start.

Assume the same configuration of neuropsychological test and anamnestic data, but assume that EEG, CT, and MRI data do not document neurological damage. Although some might assume that the absence of "confirmatory" neuroradiological or electrophysiological findings indicates malingering, the venerable axiom "absence of evidence is not evidence of absence" deserves consideration.

For a number of years, dating at least since findings of lack of congruence between EEG and neurocognitive functions (Hartlage & Green, 1973), there have been numerous studies documenting lack of neuroradiological findings among patients with documented brain injury (e.g., Bigler & Snyder, 1995; Tsushima & Wedding, 1979). Thus, mere lack of support or confirmation from procedures that measure quite different phenomena from those assessed by neuropsychological examination cannot necessarily be considered prima facie evidence of malingering so much as possible supersedence of the sensitivity and accuracy of neuropsychological measures compared with such criterion measures. Assume next that the validity scale of the MMPI-2 shows an elevated F scale, with all other (neuropsychological and anamnestic) data remaining constant. Lack of congruence with other test data is not necessarily lost, for although the F scale indeed detects admission of unusual symptoms, it is oriented toward psychiatric rather than neurological anomalous symptomatology. Indeed, some symptoms included as detectors in the F scale may be reasonable sequelae of brain injury, and so such indices may not necessarily document any intentional malingering of neurological symptoms.

Alterations of the internal configuration of neuropsychological test data in this hypothetical case, however, can point quite directly to malingering, as has been mentioned under sensory, motor, and combined approaches to the detection of malingering. Thus, the internal consistency (or lack of same) of the depth and breadth of typical neuropsychological measures is sufficient, in and of itself, independent of any external criterion variables, to detect attempts to malinger the data. Especially in the case of the Halstead–Reitan Neuropsychological Battery and complementary additional measures, there is a wealth of cross-check, redundancy, and measurement of overlapping and adjacent functions to provide a superlatively sensitive set of successive sieves through which data can be processed to detect malingering.

CONTEXT

The context in which the neuropsychological examination takes place needs to be considered as an important component of the clinical picture. Two aspects are especially relevant to the context in which the neuropsychological examination is done, one aspect involving the patient milieu and the other involving the unique characteristics of a litigation setting (Johnson & Hartlage, 1994).

As Cullum, Heaton, and Grant (1991) lucidly proposed, such intrapersonal factors as somatoform and factitious disorders need to be considered in the context of malingering. In the case of somatoform disorder (Bricquet's syndrome), there is a clear possibility that symptoms may be present in the absence of supportive test data, with symptoms representing unconscious processes not under voluntary control. Although clearly distinct from intentional simulation of symptoms, the clinical presentation may have a number of similarities. Most frequently diagnosed in women, somatization disorder has a prevalence in the range of 20%, and may be suspected as a possibility among patients with a history of repeated visits to numerous physicians, with vague and polysymptomatic complaints (Cloninger, Reich, & Guze, 1975; Perley & Guze, 1962). Differentiation of somatization disorder from neuropsychological abnormalities has been reported with 90% accuracy for neuropsychological patients and 100% of controls (Flor-Henry, Fromm-Auch, Tapper, & Schopflacher, 1981), albeit with a small sample size and a number of methodological limiting factors. Somatization disorder may be distinguished from conversion disorders in that in conversion disorder symptoms tend to be fewer in number and more discrete (Pincus & Tucker, 1985). Prevalence of conversion disorders may be fairly high among patients with prior psychiatric history, with one estimate as high as 24% among psychiatric outpatients (Guze, Woodruff, & Clayton, 1971). Although such patients with "pseudoneurological" symptoms are fairly well detected by comprehensive neuropsychological examination (e.g., only 6% classified as having brain disorder; Matthews, Shaw, & Klove, 1966), patients with such psychiatric disorders can occasionally present difficulty for the neuropsychologist who must defend impressions of test validity. The identification of such "pseudoneurological" patients by comprehensive neuropsychological examination is thus demonstrated to be feasible. However, the neuropsychologist involved in potential litigation is advised to buttress the neuropsychological examination with tests such as the MMPI-2, not only to detect possible somatoform or conversion features but also to identify antisocial or mixed personality disorders, substance abuse, and related character disorders potentially at risk for lying or deliberate distortion of data. Indeed, discriminant analyses involving Halstead–Reitan Neuropsychological Battery and MMPI data support a conclusion that neuropsychological data supplemented with information from the MMPI may help identify suspected malingerers (Heaton et al., 1978). Goebel (1983), extending the findings of Heaton et al., successfully classified 94% differentiation of brain injury versus faking subgroups in blind review, and concluded that it is very difficult for neurologically normal subjects to successfully fake brain damage given combined neuropsychological and MMPI data. Obviously the personal injury litigant attempting to prove damages to dispel skepticism by a claims adjuster or defense attorney is examined in a different context than is an individual who has been recognized as having suffered severe head injury (Youngblood, 1995). In the first instance there may be a realistic tendency to exaggerate weaknesses to "prove" there has been an injury, whereas in the second instance there may be equal compulsion for the patient to "prove" that he or she is going to be okay. Another context might involve a patient in a residential rehabilitation facility who is motivated to perform well to demonstrate progress as a form of appreciation to the therapists who have been providing treatment and support. In both the litigation setting and the rehabilitation setting there may be selective "proving" which can affect results. Personal injury litigants, for example, may be inclined to selectively malinger to prove items specifically scoffed at by adjusters or defense attorneys; rehabilitation facility patients may attempt to put on a good front on test items they see as most resembling the item being emphasized by their therapists.

The neuropsychologist can make initial assessment (and provide opportunity to minimize likelihood) of malingering by asking questions to the effect "Why did your attorney tell you that you were coming here?" If the response involves some apparent notion of need to prove that "I'm really messed up" or that "something is wrong with me," obviously cautionary, corrective comments and subsequent close monitoring for signs of malingering may be needed. Exactly the same precautions should be taken with the patient referred (as for independent medical examination) by defense counsel or insurance company, for in this context the patient may perceive the same need to convince the neuropsychologist or "prove" some type of deficit.

Attention has been directed, and quite properly so, to the base rate phenomenon (Gouvier, Uddo-Crane, & Brown, 1988; Lees-Haley & Brown, 1993) as a contextual factor of considerable relevance to neuropsychological examination interpretation. For example, if 90% of a population suffers from headaches, and a postconccussive injury patient admits to headaches, it may be spurious to attribute the headaches to the injury. Failure by neuropsychologists to consider such factors can create need for insurance companies and defense attorneys to defend against spurious damages (Hartlage, 1995). In this respect, it may be the neuropsychologist's interpretation of preexisting problems as accident-related that in effect turns the patient into a malingerer. At the same time, however, the neuropsychologist must be sensitive to the possibility that symptoms may be suggested to the patient not only by family, friends, or representatives, but also by the questions asked by the neuropsychologist. Especially problematical, for example, can be routinely administered, general-purpose "symptom checklist" or "health history data sheets," which can suggest symptoms to patients by making them aware that such symptoms might be ones they may be expected to have. Neuropsychological batteries given following such symptom lists must be carefully scrutinized to rule out contamination by such suggested symptoms.

The verbal instructions and comments of the examiner need to be fairly standardized so as to provide a context free of unintentional messages concerning expectancy of poor performance. Indeed, examinees without a well-monitored, fairly standardized verbal instruction format may inadvertently cue the patient to suboptimal performance, so that it is pertinent and relevant to monitor instructions to assess whether such cueing may have produced selective poor performance. An examiner, in an attempt to alleviate possible patient anxiety, may make a statement (e.g., after Tests I and II of the Category Test) that "a lot of people have trouble with the next test," which can be interpreted by the patient as a cue to perform less well than on the preceding tests. Although most experienced clinical neuropsychologists are aware of the potential contaminating effect on test data by importune examiner comments to patients, the fairly widespread use of technicians to conduct at least portions of the neuropsychological examination poses considerable risk for contamination of data. Whereas instructions to patients are, hopefully, standardized and consistent; comments, whether extemporaneous, spontaneous, or planned, are rarely standardized, and pose opportunity for influencing test performance which could be classified as malingering. Examples of two such comments gleaned from observations of technician–patient comments, along with their effects on the data, are offered as illustrative of the point. (In both cases, technicians were experienced neuropsychological examiners with more than 3 years' experience, who worked for neuropsychologists in medical school/VA Hospital settings, observed through one-way mirror, for the intended purpose of watching the patients' behavior during testing.)

In the first setting, the patient had been instructed to do as many arithmetic problems (Wide Range Achievement Test-III) as he could, in the time specified. After the patient's glance had lingered over the more difficult portions of the test, and a look of anxiety/frustration flashed across his face, the examiner commented: "I know these are tough, but give it a shot. Don't feel bad if you can't do all that many. I know I couldn't begin to do them all, but take a shot at it." The examiner then left the patient alone for 2–3 minutes to get some coffee. Obviously, to "give it a shot" or "take a shot at it" differs from instructions involving emphasizing doing your best, making your best effort, or similar language used for encouraging maximum performance. Leaving the room may have been interpreted by the patient as indicative of a laissez-faire attitude toward the importance of that test. When reviewing the comprehensive test battery data, the neuropsychological report noted the relatively low score (standard score 83) on the arithmetic portion of the WRAT-III compared with the higher scaled score (10) on the WAIS-R, and concluded from the discrepancy that the patient was malingering, "since he obviously knows the stuff, as evidenced by his intact WAIS-R arithmetic performance." Having observed the face-to-face interactions between patient and examiner during the course of the WAIS-R arithmetic subtest, and witnessed at least two appropriate facilitative comments by the examiner, although I would not categorically rule out "malingering" as a possible contributory factor in the discrepancy between the two measures of mathematical/calculating ability, I would certainly consider alternative explanations involving the context of the testing as being contributory, at least in part, to the discrepancy. Interestingly, as the patient involved was an inpatient, I had opportunity to interview him after reading the neuropsychologist's report. When I raised the issue of how he thought he had done on the tests, he indicated that he thought he had done "OK on the important ones."

In the second setting, the patient was an obviously apprehensive and anxious young woman involved in litigation over an automotive injury in which she sustained a brief loss of consciousness, but radiographic and electroencephalographic studies did not document structural damage. After she had become confused and made two errors on the second scale of the Category Test, the examiner told her "Now this next one is really tough, so I don't want you to feel dumb if you never get it. In fact, I've tested lots and lots of patients who never got the hang of this test. But we've got to do it, so just hang in there and press a button for each picture." After a very poor performance on this scale, similar "support" was given for subsequent Category subscales, with resultant error scores rather in excess of what might have been predicted from other cognate tests. Although the issue of malingering was not raised in this case, it is probably safe to conclude that her performance on these subscales did not represent performance at the highest levels of which she was capable, which in fact is the general operational criterion used to define malingering (Hall & Prichard, 1995; Nies & Sweet, 1994; Price, 1995; Wiggins & Brandt, 1988; Youngblood, 1995).

CONCLUSION

Beginning with simple direct clinical observations of the patient, the neuropsychological examiner can make observations relevant and crucial to possible malingering. Following this clinical observation and combining with it the configurations of test scores, the neuropsychologist has a very powerful repertoire for assessing possible contamination of data by malingering. Neuropsychological data are unique in this respect and much more powerful than psychiatric or clinical psychological sorts of data for detecting malingering. Finally, consideration of the context of the examination can provide a final check on validity of data, to an extent that provides the neuropsychologist with a most formidable armanentarium for detecting and controlling for contamination of conclusions by malingering.

REFERENCES

Anderson, C. V., & Bigler, E. D. (1994). Ventricular dilation as a predictor of cognitive outcome. *Archives of Clinical Neuropsychology*, *9*, 106 (abstract).

Baker, W. J., Gola, T. J., & Greiffenstein, M. F. (1995, November). *Discriminant analysis of neuropsychological tests with brain damaged post concussive and malingering subjects*. Paper presented at the National Academy of Neuropsychology, San Francisco.

Bectar, J., & Williams, J. (1995). Malingering response studies on the memory assessment scales and symptoms validity tests. *Advances of Clinical Neuropsychology*, *10*, 57–72.

Benton, A. L., & Spreen, O. (1961). Visual memory test: The simulation of mental incompetence. *Archives of General Psychiatry*, *4*, 79–83.

Bernard, L., & Fowler, W. (1990). Assessing the validity of memory complaints: Performance of brain damaged and normal individuals on Rey's task to detect malingering. *Journal of Clinical Psychology*, *46*, 432–436.

Bernat, J. L. (1994). *Ethical issues in neurology*. Boston: Butterworths–Heinemann.

Berry, D., Baer, R., & Harris, M. (1991). Detection of malingering on the MMPI: A meta-analysis. *Clinical Psychology Review*, *11*, 585–598.

Bigler, E. D., & Snyder, J. L. (1995). Neuropsychological outcome and quantitative neuroimaging in mild head injury. *Archives of Clinical Neuropsychology*, *10*, 159–174.

Binder, L. M. (1993a). Assessment of malingering after mild head trauma with the Portland Digit Recognition Test. *Journal of Clinical and Experimental Neuropsychology*, *15*, 170–182.

Binder, L. M. (1993b). Assessment of malingering after mild head trauma with the Portland Digit Recognition Test: Erratum. *Journal of Clinical and Experimental Neuropsychology*, *15*, 852.

Brandt, J. (1992). Detecting amnesia's imposters. In L. R. Squire & N. Butters (Eds.), *Neuropsychology of memory* (2nd ed., pp. 156–165). New York: Guilford Press.

Bruhn, A. R., & Reed, M. R. (1975). Simulation of brain damage on the Bender Gestalt by college students. *Journal of Personality Assessments*, *39*, 244–255.

Charter, R. (1994). Determining random responding for the Category, Speech-Sounds Perception, and Seashore Rhythm Tests. *Journal of Clinical and Experimental Neuropsychology*, *16*, 744–748.

Cloninger, C. R., Reich, T., & Guze, S. (1975). The multifactorial model of disease transmission: III Familial relationship between sociopathy and hysteria (Bricquet's syndrome). *British Journal of Psychiatry*, *127*, 23–32.

Corey-Brown, J. (1996, March). *Dementia update: The American Academy of Neurology practice parameters for the evaluation of dementia*. Paper presented at the American Academy of Neurology, San Francisco.

Cullum, C. M., Heaton, R. K., & Grant, I. (1991). Psychogenic factors influencing neuropsychological performance: Somatoform disorders, factitious disorders, and malingering. In H. O. Doerr & A. S. Carlin (Eds.), *Forensic neuropsychology: Legal and scientific bases* (pp. 141–171). New York: Guilford Press.

Flor-Henry, P., Fromm-Auch, D., Tapper, M., & Schopflacher, D. (1981). A neuropsychological study of the stable syndrome of hysteria. *Biological Psychiatry*, *16*, 601–626.

Gellis, S., & Feingold, M. (1968). *Atlas of mental retardation syndromes. Visual diagnoses of facies and physical findings*. Washington, DC: U.S. Department of Health, Education and Welfare.

Gfeller, J. D., Craddock, M. M. & Falkenhain, M. A. (1994, November). *Detecting feigned neuropsychological impairment with the Seashore Rhythm Test*. Paper presented at the National Academy of Neuropsychology, Orlando, FL.

Goebel, R. A. (1983). Detection of faking on the Halstead–Reitan Neuropsychological Test Battery. *Journal of Clinical Psychology*, *39*, 731–742.

Goldberg, J. O., & Miller, H. R. (1986). Performance of psychiatric patients and intellectually deficient individuals on a test that assesses the validity of memory complaints. *Journal of Clinical Psychology*, *42*, 792–795.

Gouvier, W. D., Uddo-Crane, M., & Brown, L. M. (1988). Base rates of post concussional symptoms. *Archives of Clinical Neuropsychology*, *3*, 273–278.

Green, P., Astner, K., Kiss, I., & Allen, I. (1993). *CARB malingering test results in 210 accident/compensation cases with or without head injury*. Paper presented at the National Academy of Neuropsychology, Phoenix, AZ.

Gudjonsson, G., & Shackleton, H. (1986). The pattern of scores on Raven's Matrices during "faking bad" and "non-faking" performance. *British Journal of Clinical Psychology*, *25*, 35–41.

Guze, S. B., Woodruff, R. A., & Clayton, P. A. (1971). A study of conversion symptoms in psychiatric outpatients. *American Journal of Psychiatry*, *128*, 643–646.

Hall, H. A., & Pritchard, D. (1995). *Detecting malingering and deception: Forensic distortion analysis*. Delray Beach, FL: St. Lucie Press.

Hartlage, L. C. (1990). *Neuropsychological assessment of head injury*. Sarasota, FL: Professional Resource Exchange.

Hartlage, L. C. (1995). Neuropsychological complaint base rate in personal injury, revisited. *Archives of Clinical Neuropsychology*, *10*, 279–280.

Hartlage, L. C., & Green, J. B. (1973). The EEG as a predictor of intellective and academic performance. *Journal of Learning Disabilities*, *6*(4), 42–45.

Hartlage, L. C., & Telzrow, C. F. (1986). *Neuropsychological assessment and intervention with children*. Sarasota, FL: Professional Resource Exchange.

Hays, J. R., Emmons, J., & Lawson, K. A. (1993). Psychiatric norms for the Rey 15-Item Visual Memory Test. *Perceptual and Motor Skills, 76*, 1331–1334.

Heaton, R. K., Grant, I., & Matthews, C. G. (1991). *Comprehensive norms for an expanded Halstead–Reitan Battery*. Odessa, FL: Psychological Assessment Resources.

Heaton, R.K., Smith, H. H., Jr., Lehman, R. A., & Vogt, A. T. (1978). Prospects for faking believable deficits on neuropsychological testing. *Journal of Consulting and Clinical Psychology*, *46*, 892–900.

Hiscock, M., & Hiscock, C. K. (1989). Refining the forced-choice method for the detection of malingering. *Journal of Clinical and Experimental Neuropsychology*, *11*, 967–974.

Iverson, G.L., & Franzen, M. D. (1991, November). *Applying several objective measures to the detection of malingered memory deficits*. Paper presented at the National Academy of Neuropsychology, Dallas, TX.

Iverson, G. L., Franzen, M. D., & McCracken, L. M. (1991). Evaluation of an objective assessment technique for the detection of malingered memory deficits. *Law and Human Behavior*, *15*, 667–676.

Iverson, G. L., Franzen, M. D., & McCracken, L. M. (1994). Application of a forced-choice memory procedure designed to detect experimental malingering. *Archives of Clinical Neuropsychology*, *9*, 437–450.

Iverson, G., Myers, B., & Adams, R. (1994, November). *Specificity of the Category Test for detecting malingering*. Paper presented at the National Academy of Neuropsychology, Orlando, FL.

Iverson, G. L., Nailler, T. R., & Franzen, M. D. (1993). Detecting simulated memory deficits with the Recognition Memory Test. *Archives of Clinical Neuropsychology*, *8*, 234–235.

Johnson, D. J., & Hartlage, L. C. (1994, November). *Litigation status and behavior changes reported following TBI*. Paper presented at the National Academy of Neuropsychology, Orlando, FL.

Keiser, L. (1968). *The traumatic neurosis*. Philadelphia: Lippincott.

Klebe, K., & David, H. (1995, November). *Automaticity of memory tasks as determined by the ability to malinger*. Paper presented at the National Academy of Neuropsychology, San Francisco.

Landau, W. (1996, March). *A clinical perspective on somatization and malingering*. Paper presented at the American Academy of Neurology, San Francisco.

Larrabee, G. J. (in press). On modifying recognition tests for detecting of malingering. *Neuropsychology*.

Lee, G. P., Loring, D. W., & Martin, R. C. (1992). Rey's 15-Item Visual memory Test for the detection of malingering: Normative observations on patients with neurological disorders. *Psychological Assessment*, *4*, 43–46.

Lees-Haley, P. R., & Brown, R. S. (1993). Neuropsychological complaint base rates of 170 personal injury claimants. *Archives of Clinical Neuropsychology*, *8*, 203–209.

Matthews, C. G., Shaw, D. J., & Klove, H. (1966). Psychological test performances in neurologic and "pseudoneurologic" subjects. *Cortex*, *2*, 244–253.

Mendelson. (1987). Accident neurosis. *International Journal of Law and Psychiatry*.

Miller, H., & Cartlidge, N. (1972). Simulation and malingering after injuries to the brain and spinal cord. *Lancet*, *1*, 580–585.

Millis, S. R. (1992). The Recognition Memory Test in the detection of malingered and exaggerated memory deficits. *The Clinical Neuropsychologist*, *6*, 406–414.

Millis, S. R., & Putnam, S. (1994). The Recognition Memory Test in the assessment of memory impairment after financially compensable mild head injury: A replication. *Archives of Clinical Neuropsychology*, *9*, 163.

Millis, S., Putnam, S., & Adams, K. (1995, November). *Speech-Sounds Perception Test and Seashore Rhythm Test as validity indicators in the neuropsychological evaluation of mild head injury*. Paper presented at the National Academy of Neuropsychology, San Francisco.

Mittenberg, W., Azrin, R., Millsaps, C., & Heilbronner, R. (1993). Identification of malingered head injury on the Wechsler Memory Scale-Revised. *Psychological Assessment, 5*, 34–40.

Mittenberg, W., Rotholc, A., Russell, E., & Heilbronner, R. (1994, November). *Identification of malingered head injury on the Halstead–Reitan Battery*. Paper presented at the National Academy of Neuropsychology, Orlando, FL.

Mittenberg, W., Theroux-Fichera, S., Zielinski, R., & Heilbronner, R. (1995). Identification of malingered head injury on the Wechsler Adult Intelligence Scale-Revised. *Professional Psychology: Research and Practice, 26*, 491–498.

Mittenberg, W., Zielinski, R. E., Fichera, S. M., Heilbronner, R., & Youngjohn, J. R. (1993, November). *Identification of malingered head injury in the Wechsler Adult Intelligence Scale-Revised*. Paper presented at the National Academy of Neuropsychology, Phoenix, AZ.

Netter, F. H. (1958). *Nervous system* (Vol. 1). The CIBA Collection of Medical Illustrations. Elsevier, Amsterdam.

Nies, K., & Sweet, J. (1994). Neuropsychological assessment and malingering: A critical review of past and present strategies. *Archives of Clinical Neuropsychology, 9*, 501–522.

Othmer, E., & Othmer, S. (1994). *The clinical interview using DMS-IV: Volume 2. The difficult patient*. Washington, DC: American Psychiatric Press.

Palmer, B., Boone, K., Lesser, I., & Wohl, W. (1995, November). *Deficient neuropsychological test performance among healthy older adults*. Paper presented at the National Academy of Neuropsychology, San Francisco.

Perley, M. J., & Guze, S. B. (1962). Hysteria—The stability and usefulness of clinical criteria. A quantitative study based on a follow-up of six to eight years in 39 patients. *New England Journal of Medicine, 266*, 421–426.

Pincus, J. H., & Tucker, G. J. (1985). *Behavioral neurology* (3rd ed.). London: Oxford University Press.

Price, J. R. (1995, November). *Identification of malingering and symptom exaggeration*. Workshop presented at the National Academy of Neuropsychology, San Francisco.

Reitan, R. (1955). An investigation of the validity of Halstead's measures of biological intelligence. *Archives of Neurological Psychiatry, 73*, 28–35.

Reitan, R., & Wolfson, D. (1985). *The Halstead–Reitan Neuropsychological Test Battery: Theory and clinical interpretation*. Tucson: Neuropsychology Press.

Rey, A. (1941). L'examen psychologique dans les cas d'encephalopathie traumatique. *Archives de Psychologie, 28*, 286–340.

Rey, A. (1964). *L'examen clinique en psychologie*. Paris: Presses Universitaires de France.

Ribbler, A. (1995). The use of neuropsychological evaluation in the detection and treatment of a patient with Munchausen's syndrome. *Archives of Clinical Neuropsychology, 10*, 383 (abstract).

Roberts, A. C., & Resnick, P. I. (1989). Malingering closed head injury symptoms. In A. Taylor (Ed.), *Litigating head trauma cases*. Eau Claire, WI: Professional Education Systems.

Rogers, R. (Ed.). (1988). *Clinical assessment of malingering and deception*. New York: Guilford Press.

Rogers, R., Harrell, S.H., & Liff, C. D. (1993). Feigning neuropsychological impairment: A critical review of the methodological and clinical considerations. *Clinical Psychology Review, 13*, 255–274.

Ruchinskas, R. A., Barth, J. T., & Diamond, R. (1995, November). *Forced-choice paradigms and the detection of somatosensory symptom exaggeration*. Paper presented at the National Academy of Neuropsychology, San Francisco.

Satz, P. (1988). Neuropsychological testimony: Some emerging concerns. *The Clinical Neuropsychologist, 2*, 89–100.

Schiffer, R. (1996, March). *A bedside mental status examination*. Paper presented at the American Academy of Neurology, San Francisco.

Schretlen, D., Brandt, J., Krafft, L., & Van Gorp, W. (1991). Some caveats in using the Rey 15-Item Memory Test to detect malingered amnesia. *Psychological Assessment, 3*, 667–672.

Tenhula, W. N., & Sweet, J. J. (1994, February). *Identifying malingering through analyses of multiple components of the Category Test.* Paper presented at the International Neuropsychological Society, Cincinnati, OH.

Trueblood, W., & Schmidt, M. (1993). Malingering and other validity considerations in the neuropsychological evaluation of mild head injury. *Journal of Clinical and Experimental Neuropsychology, 15*, 578–590.

Tsushima, W. T., & Wedding, D. (1979). A comparison of the Halstead–Reitan Neuropsychological Battery and computerized tomography in the identification of brain damage. *Journal of Nervous and Mental Disease, 167*, 704–707.

Weintraub, M. (1996, March). *Fraud, chronic pain, litigation—An emerging problem.* Paper presented at the American Academy of Neurology, San Francisco.

Wiggins, E., & Brandt, J. (1988). The detection of simulated amnesia. *Law and Human Behavior, 12*, 57–78.

Youngblood, J. (1995). Confirmed attorney coaching prior to neuropsychological evaluation. *Assessment, 2*, 279–283.

Ziskin, J., & Faust, D. (1988). *Coping with psychiatric and psychological testimony* (vol. 1,2,3). Venice, CA: Law and Psychology Press.

9

Common Sense, Clinicians, and Actuarialism in the Detection of Malingering during Head Injury Litigation

CECIL R. REYNOLDS

With the explosion of civil litigation related to personal injury over the last 25 or so years, the issue of malingering has grown substantially as well. There is little agreement as to base rates for malingering in the population of patients seen by neuropsychologists or psychologists generally. The base rate in the general patient population seen by neuropsychologists is almost certain to differ substantively from the base rate for malingering among patients seen during litigation related to a claim of brain injury[1] (see Pritchard, 1997). Estimates for base rates of malingering range from 1 to 50% among the population of head injury litigants, according to other authors in this volume.

This disparity in estimates will go unresolved because malingerers will not self-identify with complete accuracy nor are we likely to devise foolproof methods for detection of malingering. That the base almost certainly exceeds the lower-bound 1% estimates is clear from the results of a meta-analysis by Binder and Rohling (1996) and supported in various prior traditional reviews (e.g., Binder,

[1]Brain injury and head injury are used synonomously in this work as has become customary in the field; nevertheless it is recognized clearly that the head can be injured in many different ways while the brain goes unscathed.

CECIL R. REYNOLDS • Department of Educational Psychology, Texas A&M University, College Station, Texas 77843.

Detection of Malingering during Head Injury Litigation, edited by Reynolds. Plenum Press, New York, 1998.

1990) and specific research studies (e.g., Youngjohn, Burrows, & Erdal, 1995). Contributing to the disparate estimates of base rates is the issue of definition. As discussed by Faust and Ackley (this volume), the issue of definition is important and other authors in this volume (e.g., Gouvier, Hayes, & Smiroldo; Williams; and Hartlage) have presented definitions and discussed some of the issues of defining malingering. Not all arrive at the same definition, a problem clearly present in the broader literature. Some (e.g., Binder & Rohling, 1996) avoid the definitional issue and discuss instead "the effects of financial incentives on recovery" (p. 7), which will be, as is malingering, a contextually related issue.

Definitions are important to any scientific inquiry, for scientists must first agree on a phenomenon before studying it en masse. Early in the scientific process, there is commonly debate over defining constructs, although psychology seems to have more than its share of such problems (e.g., try to get psychologists to agree even today on a definition of intelligence). For the less tangible, perhaps more ethereal constructs of psychology, the researchers will devise an operational definition of a construct that allows other researchers to study the same variable, whereas other researchers may study variations of the construct under the same name but with a different operational definition (see Reynolds & Brown, 1984, for a further discussion of how this can impact emotionally laden issues in particular, of which malingering is certainly one). The latter problem is common among researchers and clinicians in the study and assessment of malingering. It is instructive then to examine some definitions of malingering.

DEFINITIONS OF MALINGERING

Dictionaries are often a good place to begin looking for definitions of words that are common to a vocabulary. The *World Book Dictionary* (Barnhart, 1967) defines *malinger* as "to pretend to be sick in order to escape work or duty" (p. 1176). *Webster's New Universal Unabridged Dictionary* (McKechnie, 1983) defines a *malingerer* as a person who "feigns illness in order to avoid duty" (p. 1090). Interestingly, even the unabridged dictionary provides no alternative or secondary definitions. *Roget's International Thesaurus* offers as synonyms *shirker*, *dodger*, and *goldbrick* as colloquial terms (Roget, 1962). The term *malingerer* thus is pointedly defined and using words that clearly carry negative connotations. It is a small move from the person who "feigns illness in order to avoid duty" to the person involved in an accident who feigns symptoms to gain a large monetary settlement thus avoiding work or the duty to support oneself.

The primary diagnostic tool of mental health professionals in the United States is the *Diagnostic and Statistical Manual* series of the American Psychiatric

Association (APA). DSM-IV provides a more detailed instructive definition of malingering in the context of the mental health professions:

> . . . malingering is the intentional production of false or grossly exaggerated physical or psychological symptoms, motivated by external incentives such as avoiding military duty, avoiding work, obtaining financial compensation, evading criminal prosecution, or obtaining drugs. Under some circumstances, malingering may represent adaptive behavior—for example, feigning illness while a captive of the enemy during wartime. . . . Malingering differs from Factitious Disorder in that the motivation for the production in malingering is an external incentive . . . malingering is differentiated from Conversion Disorder and other Somatoform Disorders by the intentional production of symptoms and by the obvious, external incentives associated with it. (APA, 1994, p. 683)

In all of the above definitions, the volitional nature of the false presentation is clear and a requirement for the determination of malingering. Clearly, symptom exaggeration, if volitional and motivated by external incentives, in an injured person is malingering, though almost certainly more difficult to detect than a person malingering all symptoms as opposed to malingering by degree of impairment only.

In all but one instance noted above, the designation *malingerer* carries a negative connotation and is a harsh judgment of another person. As clinicians and health care providers, we are reluctant to make such judgments of our fellow human beings. It is difficult for most in caregiving professions to make harsh diagnoses of a variety of types including malingering and even more traditional and more easily determined diagnoses such as mental retardation that may be perceived as having harsh prognoses or socially/politically negative connotations (see Reynolds, 1987b, for a discussion). Even individuals who have developed methods for detection of malingering report they are reluctant to make the diagnosis and have thus set cutoffs for regarding someone a malingerer very conservatively (e.g., Doty, 1995; also Doty, personal communication, 1996).

DSM-IV (APA, 1994) provides clear, authoritative guidance on the definition of malingering. There is no need for continuing debate over whether the term includes those with legitimate injuries who choose to exaggerate them. It does include the latter under the category of malingerers however harsh this seems. Some differentiate, although vaguely, poor motivation from "outright malingering" (Binder & Rohling, 1996). There is only outright malingering; what differs is the degree of malingering as it may range from complete fabrication to exaggeration. It is not always possible to distinguish the two in clinical practice, just as it is not always possible to detect any degree of malingering. What is most likely to occur, as suggested by experience in forensic settings, is a designation of malingering, but when asked whether the symptoms are fabricated or exaggerated, to respond that because of the lack of complete cooperation in completing the neuropsychological examination (e.g., see Hartlage, this volume) to the best of the patient's ability, the latter question cannot be answered definitively.

Misattribution of Symptoms

Another circumstance, one that has been addressed meagerly in the profession, is the misattribution of symptoms. In this case, the symptoms described by the patient are neither fabricated nor exaggerated but were present premorbidly despite the patient attributing the symptoms to the event subject to current litigation. Consider the case of a woman who slipped and fell on the way to a restroom in a restaurant. Several days later she saw her family physician, an internist, with complaints of headaches, dizziness, and memory problems. Over the next few weeks her self-reported symptoms increased to include rapid mood swings, impulsivity, inability to concentrate, sleep disturbance, and depression. A personal injury suit was filed and a subsequent review of her records indicated that she had eight psychiatric hospitalizations over the prior 10-year period and had diagnoses, premorbidly, of bipolar disorder, major depressive disorder, borderline personality disorder, and alcohol abuse. Each symptom described by her as well as the deficits found on neuropsychological examination had been documented in her voluminous medical records prior to her slip and fall. She had denied the existence of these symptoms prior to the fall in the history given to plaintiff's expert neuropsychologist who was angry and embarrassed to learn of these records on the witness stand before a jury (who ultimately ruled in favor of the defendant). When also considering her pattern of test results, the defense expert argued the symptoms were most likely pre-existing and the patient had engaged in misattribution of symptoms.

Of course, it is possible the patient's symptoms had been in remission prior to the fall or had not been as severe as after the fall. One cannot be 100% certain in any case. Misattribution of the cause of mental or psychological symptoms is very difficult to determine when clear documentation of premorbid states does not exist and remains difficult even in the face of detailed premorbid records. Someone who is impaired premorbidly may also be injured in a new event and made worse. Full patient cooperation is necessary to determine the degree of injury suffered in such circumstances and symptom exaggeration and/or misattribution makes an accurate determination of the degree of injury, if any, extremely difficult.

Causal substitutions, another name for misattribution of symptoms, may be the most difficult form of deception to detect in a litigant or other patient population because of the genuine nature of the pattern and congruence of symptom presentation. In the contentious arena of allegations of child sexual assault, perpetrator substitution is the most difficult of all false allegations to detect and for similar reasons (Hickman & Reynolds, 1994), e.g., the symptom presentation is entirely realistic, and is analogous to the problem of causal substitutions. Under current statutes in all states, however, the burden of proving the causal connection between a specific event and a set of claimed injuries is on the plaintiff. For individuals with premorbid problems with legitimate enhancement of symptoms as a result of the event being litigated, this may well work against them, making their injury more difficult to prove. Conversely, individuals who have been symptomatic in the past have the knowledge and experience to present symptoms in a believable pattern and are potentially more capable of a persuasive misattribution of symptoms or even a very clever fabrication of a symptom complex. A lifelong, detailed history is the clinician's best defense against being misled in such circumstances and histories should be verified when possible.

Should a Litigant Be Penalized for Symptom Exaggeration?

Following a recent evaluation conducted at the request of a defense attorney, I gave what I thought would be the unwelcomed opinion that the plaintiff had in fact suffered an injury that was likely to result in persistent symptoms related to the phenomenon of postconcussion syndrome, but added that although these legitimate injuries were present to neuropsychological examination, the injuries were also being exaggerated to some degree. To my surprise, the attorney (an experienced, senior partner at a respected firm) was delighted, stating, "That's great, because juries don't give money to liars." I do not know if the attorney is accurate in his appraisal of the mood or perhaps even vengeful nature of juries, but this does raise an interesting issue. Should individuals with a legitimate injury be denied compensation altogether or be penalized by way of reduction of a monetary award if they attempt to take advantage of the injury to enhance their compensation by exaggerating the seriousness of the injury or claiming additional symptoms that do not exist or were not the result of the event under litigation?

Whatever answer one gives is a value judgment; this is not a question falling within the expertise of scientists to answer. Perhaps an expert in logic or philosophy could be called to address such a question. One might argue that the penalties of perjury or fraud as criminal acts are enough but realistically these are more difficult to prove for a variety of reasons, but in large part because of the issue of "reasonable doubt" as opposed to "preponderance of the evidence." Symptom exaggeration and symptom fabrication for monetary gain in a jury award are really no different from claiming as "stolen" items on an insurance report following a burglary that were not taken or not even owned by the robbery victim. In such a case, one risks criminal prosecution for fraud or filing a false police report but nonetheless is entitled to recover real losses. Is the attorney correct in his assessment of the predisposition of juries? I know of no data that address this issue. Should the jury behave in this way toward the plaintiff? This is a matter of personal opinion for the scientist and arguably should be deferred to the philosopher for an expert opinion. In actual practice, the answer will lie in the interaction of the individual jury members and the persuasive powers of the attorneys who argue before them.

WHEN SHOULD AN EXPERT EVALUATE FOR MALINGERING?

The answer to this question should not be related to whether the expert is retained by the plaintiff or by the defense. The expert's role is to remain as objective and unbiased *as possible*. However, the expert also has a duty to assist the attorneys, if asked, in unmasking the weaker components of a plaintiff's case including exposing the problems of opposing experts' opinions and the weak spots in these opinions even if in agreement with the opposing experts' views in the case. In head injury litigation, both plaintiff's and defendant's experts should be evaluating malingering if there is cause to suspect it.

When is there cause to suspect malingering? DSM-IV (APA, 1994) argues that malingering should be *strongly* (emphasis in original) suspected when any of four conditions occur in combination:

1. Medicolegal context of presentation (e.g., the person is referred by an attorney to the clinician for examination)
2. Marked discrepancy between the person's claimed stress or disability and the objective findings
3. Lack of cooperation during the diagnostic evaluation and in complying with the prescribed treatment regimen
4. The presence of Antisocial Personality Disorder. (APA, 1994, p. 683)

The APA guidelines above are largely derived from an experiential base and give grounds to "strongly" suspect malingering. Strong suspicions are not necessary to prompt an evaluation of the possibility and probability of malingering. Literature on the effects of financial incentives on symptom development and presentation is instructive in this regard.

With regard to head injury and malingering, the work of Binder, exemplified in Binder and Rohling (1996), is most prominent. Binder and Rohling evaluated, through the methods of meta-analysis, the impact of financial incentives on disability, symptoms, and objective findings after closed-head injury. These scientists searched the literature from 1975 through 1995 for all articles related to closed-head injury and financial incentives using computerized databases and coupled with the old-fashioned search process of reading reference lists of known, relevant papers. Eighteen study groups were evaluated with a total sample size of 2353 subjects for whom effect sizes could be calculated. These were all actual head-injury patients; studies that exclusively employed experimental simulators were excluded by Binder and Rohling. Results of this work revealed that more abnormality and disability were apparent in the neuropsychological performance of patients with financial incentives for poor performance despite less severe levels of initial injury in such patients relative to patients without financial incentives. Binder and Rohling (1996) were particularly impressed (p. 8) that patients with mild injuries and financial incentives to perform poorly, scored below chance levels on very easy, two-choice recognition tests. They also noted that the later the onset of symptoms, the more likely patients were to seek compensation. Late-onset symptoms following a potentially traumatic event are less likely than immediate symptoms to have an organic basis (e.g., Binder & Rohling, 1996; Cartlidge & Shaw, 1981; Fenton, McClelland, Montgomery, MacFlynn, & Rutherford, 1993).

In discussing their results, Binder and Rohling (1996, p. 9) noted that they took a conservatively biased view, consistent with earlier comments that it is emotionally difficult to call a patient a malingerer. Even with such a bias, Binder and Rohling (1996) concluded in part

> . . . patients with less severe injuries, as measured by posttraumatic neurologic data are *more* likely to seek monetary compensation. . . . These data suggest that the effect of monetary incentives is more powerful for patients with mild head injury than for those with moderate or severe injury. (p. 10)

The weighted mean effect size calculated for financial incentives was 0.47 (the unweighted mean effect size was 0.57). In the context of psychological research, an effect size of this magnitude is substantial and is clinically meaningful. Furthermore, the effect is compounded by having a lesser degree of injuries; "financial incentives assume importance in inverse relation to the severity of the brain injury" (Binder & Rohling, 1996, p. 9). Binder and Rohling's meta-analytic results can be interpreted to suggest that 23% of litigants in head injury litigation are malingering even using their conservative approach. Youngjohn et al. (1995) presented empirical data suggesting that 48% of patients in litigation over persistent postconcussion syndrome are malingering.

With regard to the initial question in opening this section, I am thus in agreement with Binder and Rohling (1996). They argue their results suggest the need for clinicians to consider secondary gain as a potentially significant source of variance in *every* case of closed-head injury with special care given to evaluating the effect of financial incentives on symptom presentation in cases of milder injuries where their results were the most profound. Empirical work and experiences in the field are in concert in this instance. The experiential guidelines of DSM-IV (noted above) regarding when to suspect malingering coupled with the findings of Binder and Rohling (1996) and Youngjohn et al. (1995) suggest that malingering should be assessed in all cases with a medicolegal context of presentation wherein reinforcement is a possibility for continued symptom presentation with special emphasis applied when financial incentives may be present.

DETECTING MALINGERING

Throughout this volume, various and at times disparate views of how best to detect malingering have been presented ranging from the more purely empirical approach of Reitan and Wolfson to the more clinically, experientially based approach of Hartlage. All of the approaches nevertheless involve the evaluation of objective findings by a clinician as presented in this work. No one advocates making such decisions on the basis of clinical "intuition" or "gut feelings" about a patient or a patient's presentation. Faust and Ackley, in the opening chapter, emphasize the many conceptual and methodological problems that plague the determination of someone's status as a malingerer. These problems are not at all insignificant and seem nearly insurmountable at times leaving astute clinicians with a sense of hopelessness. However, just as other difficult diagnoses must be made, so must the question of malingering be addressed in forensic consultations, and even more frequently than thought prior to the work of Binder and Rohling (1996).

It is a naive clinician who believes detection of malingering or its absence is an easy or even perfunctory matter involving an interview, a review of records, or a cursory examination of a lot of test scores. The evaluation of malingering requires an astute clinician with good common sense, a broad knowledge base, skilled in one or more actuarial methods of evaluating malingering, and a healthy respect for the possibility that he or she may be wrong in a particular case. At present, the best method of evaluating malingering requires a combination of clinical and actuarial methods coupled with common sense and the ability to combine data from different sources under different methods of collection (i.e., analytical reasoning). The key then to a proper determination consists of three components: congruence, congruence, and congruence! Once data collection and collation are complete, the clinician must evaluate:

1. *Congruence* of the current symptom presentation with the known history and facts surrounding the injury
2. *Congruence* of the symptoms in juxtaposition with one another, i.e., the internal consistency of the symptom presentation
3. *Congruence* of the course of symptom development and history with known (i.e., probabilistic) outcomes or sequelae with like injuries

We now come to the question of method and, as should be obvious by now, multiple methods are typically required, although there is always the exceptional case of the malingerer who is so bad at it, that the lack of congruence in a single area will overwhelm all other needs for data collection and collation. Malingering may be conceptualized as a problem of signal detection, especially in the latter cases, and once the signal has been detected, that detection is sufficient. The appearance of the signal and its background noise will vary considerably, and different methods are important to suppress noise in some cases or enhance the signal in others. Few neuropsychological tests have an adequate signal-to-noise ratio to allow detection of a clever malingerer (e.g., see Reynolds, 1997; Reynolds & James, 1997).

The latter cases belie actuarialism in the traditional sense though it is true that if you hypothesize that all elephants are gray, it takes but one blue elephant to prove definitively that you are wrong. The presenting paraplegic who is later videotaped in the false security of his home, up and dancing with his girlfriend, absent any visible motoric deficiencies, needs no further actuarial investigation. I once evaluated a felony criminal referral in a local county jail who did not recall his name, age, date of birth, mother's name, could not name, when shown, the primary colors, and earned a raw score of zero on the entire WAIS-R. He was "unable" to complete a human figure drawing, never quite figuring out how to hold the pencil without it falling from his hand whenever it came into contact with the paper. At the conclusion of the examination, when told the examiner wanted to contact the inmate's attorney as quickly as possible to have him moved from the jail to a hospital and declared incompetent to stand trial, the inmate's disarticulate speech resolved instantaneously as he recited his attorney's name and telephone number from memory and without error. His school record showed no history of mental retardation or serious emotional disturbance. In such a case there is no substitute for common sense. No lengthy debate or complicated statistical or philosophical analyses are needed. It has been suggested that a form of time series analysis may be of use in the statistical treatment of a case such as described above (L. Harlow personal communication, 1997) and although it may be possible, the circumstances of each such case and the method of discovery of the blue elephant are unique and not always given to quantification. The lack of internal consistency or incongruity of the behaviors observed with the condition claimed is sufficient in such cases to allow the clinician to draw a conclusion with reasonable psychological probability.

Throughout this volume, various methods are touted for evaluating these three moments of congruence in considering a diagnosis of malingering. It is appropriate now to turn to a discussion of how each might be applied. Keep in mind, however, that the nature of psychological testing itself makes the determination of malingering through actuarial testing alone difficult to resolve, especially in the mind of a lay jury.

The Patient History

Several contributors to this volume note, in various ways, the importance of the patient's history in assessing malingering. History is crucial to diagnosis in any case whether malingering is at issue or not; but, in the assessment of malingering, establishing a reasonable view of the individual's premorbid status is necessary to construct a baseline and to consider properly the special case of misattribution of symptoms in particular. Gouvier, Hayes, and Smiroldo, Golden and Grier, and Hartlage in their chapters all note the special importance of a good history.

In the ordinary course of clinical practice, we are not accustomed to verifying most aspects of an oral or written history given by a patient but neither is malingering a high incidence behavior in common clinical practice. In forensic matters, it is best to verify the history given by the patient by obtaining and reviewing records. Every forensic psychologist has had the experience of the patient who, prior to his or her head injury, by self-report had been a high functioning individual, an A or B student in high school, who graduated in the top 10% of his or her class but whose high school transcript shows a GPA below 3.0, a class rank at the 50th percentile, and an SAT below 950.

In a recent case, a woman gave a work history touting herself as the consummate employee, very productive and liked by everyone prior to a fall in a stairwell that caused her to strike the rear of her skull. A significant portion of her damage claim was that since the fall, she could no longer hold a job because of her personality and mood changes. By her own words, she had become "the employee from hell." A review of her employment records revealed that she had been fired from her last two jobs prior to the fall. She was dismissed from one position for her inability to work well with others and from her more recent sales position for a lack of productivity. At a minimum, such a patient is seen to be malingering through symptom exaggeration and misattribution of symptoms.

Base rates of complaints that seem common to mild head injury among the non-head-injured population are also important in evaluating the history and the congruence of history and symptoms. Patients who deny ever having had an episode of forgetfulness, a dysnomic moment, a headache, a mood swing, a relationship problem, or the like are far out of line with the normal problems experienced in day-to-day life. Although these outliers, i.e., individuals who lead charmed lives, probably do exist, such denials are, on an actuarial and on a commonsense basis, more likely to be related to symptom exaggeration or misattribution in the context of litigation to achieve financial gain. It is appropriate to review a patient's medical records for the period prior to the event in litigation to establish presence or absence of particular symptoms premorbidly. Patients do not always provide an accurate history, especially in the context of litigation, so documentation is preferred although certainly it is recognized that all records may not be available and that financial limitations on how much work can be done in a particular case are real.

Table 1 provides a listing of various records the neuropsychologist should consider reviewing in head injury litigation. The relevance of these records varies somewhat from case to case, but it is necessary to establish reasonable estimates of premorbid levels of cognitive, emotional, behavioral, and vocational functioning.

TABLE 1. Records to Consider Reviewing in the Evaluation of Patient's History in the Context of Litigation

Birth and developmental history	Medical records (including premorbid and postmorbid records)
Educational records (including primary, secondary, and postsecondary records; a special request may need to be made for special education and for disciplinary records)	Mental health records (including any prior contact with a mental health professional whether psychiatrist, psychologist, social worker, counselor, etc., including therapy notes, history and intake forms, testing results, reports, and protocols)
Employment records (including job applications completed by the patient, evaluations and disciplinary actions, workers' compensation claims, unemployment claims, and results of any personnel testing done)	Substance abuse treatment (such records are maintained separately because of certain federal privacy laws and may be more difficult to obtain)
Legal records, criminal and civil (including records of any prior personal injury litigation; records of a divorce may also be relevant in some cases)	Military records (including ASVAB, GATB, etc., results)

Insights into interpersonal and related psychosocial skills will also be gleaned from such records. Knowledge of the individual's medical status prior to the event prompting litigation nearly always plays a prominent role in evaluation of premorbid status and in establishing the validity of symptom attribution and damage claims.

Unusual findings sometimes emerge from such reviews. In a case where physical and emotional injuries were being claimed on behalf of a 7-year-old girl with considerable burns to the lower left leg, ankle, and foot, a claim for future vocational limitation was included based on weakness of the musculature and gross motor incoordination of the legs. A careful review of medical records by the neuropsychologist in the case led to records noting the diagnosis of Kugelberg–Weylander disease via deep muscle biopsy at the age of 4 years. This disease begins as a gait disturbance with subsequent weakness in the large muscle masses associated with running, jumping, and climbing. Eventually, placement in a wheelchair is required in adolescence or early adulthood. Although the father knew of this diagnosis, he did not share the information with the mother or the child, and the information was subsequently presented in a confrontational exchange by attorneys in the depositions of the parents. The nature of the disease process in this case made it very difficult to link the burn to the incoordination and gait disturbance with the premorbid diagnosis of Kugelberg–Weylander disease. The premorbid history then provides also an ipsative base rate for certain problems and complaints to supplement the normative base rates provided in other literature.

Symptom Validity Testing

Symptom validity testing (SVT), since its introduction by Pankratz and colleagues (e.g., Pankratz, 1979; Pankratz, Fausti, & Peed, 1975), has been used in a variety of criminal (e.g., Denney, 1996; Moore, 1996) and civil (e.g., Binder, 1993) litigation circumstances. SVT exists in several forms such as the Portland Digit Recognition Test (Binder, 1993), where an easy task designed to look difficult is presented with known rates of nearly 100% correct by mildly to moderately brain-injured patients, to guilty knowledge testing about knowledge and memory of a criminal act using a forced-choice technique with a known random score distribution (e.g., Denney, 1996; Moore, 1996), to direct assessment of the presense of a symptom using a forced-choice paradigm with a known distribution of random scores (e.g., Doty, 1995). In each case, the patient or examinee responds to a test and his or her score is compared with some known distribution or base score of malingerers, simulators, or nonreferred populations.

The SVT approach tends to be very conservative as actually practiced and likely underestimates the presence of malingering. In SVT, the most common format is to provide a multiple-choice format for a set of questions easily answered correctly by a person without an injury or with the claimed symptom. This ends up being a conservative practice as a result of the reliance on traditional significance testing to analyze the results and our previously noted reluctance to make negatively emotionally charged diagnoses such as malingering. As an example of SVT, consider a 40-item, four-choice multiple-choice test wherein none of the correct answers is inherently more attractive than a distractor to someone who does not know the answers to the questions. The most commonly obtained chance or random score on such a test would be 10 correct as can be shown in any basic statistics text that includes a discussion of probability theory (e.g., Hays, 1973; Parzen, 1960). Table 2 shows the probability of chance occurrences of scores of 1–10 on such a test. If the examinee does not know the answer to any of the questions, the probability of getting 10 or more items correct is quite high, being greater than 50%. As scores drop below 10, the probability of the score being a chance or random occurrence drops precipitously with the probability of only 5 or less correct on such a test, as a chance occurrence, being but .043.

As the examinee scores below the chance level, SVT theory argues that the score is not a random or chance occurrence but represents a purposive distortion by the examinee. How does an examinee score substantively below chance on such a test? The examinee must be very, very unlucky in guessing the right answers or know the correct answer and purposely respond with the incorrect answer.

On the University of Pennsylvania Smell Identification Test (UPSIT; Doty, 1995), an examinee is presented with an odor strip, sniffs it, and selects from four possible odors the one just presented. A total of 40 odors are presented. This is of particular interest to neuropsychologists because of the incidence of impaired

TABLE 2. Probability (Frequency) of Occurrence of Scores 0–10 on a 40-Item, Four-Choice Multiple-Choice Test When the Subject Has No Knowledge of the Correct Response and the Keyed Response and the Distractors Are of Equal Affinity

Score, expressed as number correct	Probability as a random occurrence of this or lower score[a,b]
0	.000
1	.000
2	.001
3	.005
4	.016
5	.043
6	.096
7	.182
8	.300
9	.440
10	.584

[a]For specific formulas see Hays (1973) or Parzen (1960, p. 102).
[b]Rounded to three decimals.

smell (known as microsmia) following traumatic brain injury (e.g., Jafek, Eller, Esses, & Moran, 1989; Malloy, Bihrle, Duffy, & Cimino, 1993; Youssem, Geckle, Bilker, McKeown, & Doty, in press). This 40-item four-choice test produces a score distribution for scores of 10 or less by a true anosmic consistent with the distribution in Table 2. Doty (1995) and others (e.g., Denney, 1996) typically apply the traditional inferential level of statistical significance of $p \leq .05$ to determine the presence of malingering. On the UPSIT, this corresponds to a raw score of 5, which has a probability of occurrence of .043. The logic is that to earn a score of 5 or less, the odds are the examinee can smell the odors presented and purposely marks the answers incorrectly (one cannot purposely choose the wrong answer without knowing the right answer). Denney (1996) noted there is nothing magical about $p \leq .05$ and went on to recommend that a score corresponding to $p \leq .01$ "is more remarkable" (p. 598). These are conservative views reflecting our general reluctance to call an examinee a malingerer. Obviously, an examinee may be one of the 5 in 100 true total anosmics who will earn a score of 5 or less on the UPSIT and this is a level of scientific certainty to which we have been conditioned. The legal establishment, however, deals with such concepts as "reasonable psychological probability" and a "preponderance of the evidence." This could be interpreted to mean "more likely than not," meaning lesser p values such as .10, .15, and the like may be quite reasonable.

From a purely actuarial standpoint, any score with a chance probability of occurrence of less than .5 would merit a best judgment or classification of malingering. A strict, rigid interpretation of Meehl (1954) would argue for this position. We are nevertheless reluctant to make such a diagnosis for fear that we may wrongly accuse an honest and injured party of malingering. However, we are seldom limited to a single score on a single test and can combine data in individual cases in unique ways that lead us to valid conclusions (e.g., de Armas, 1996; Kaufman, 1994; Kleinmuntz, 1990; Matarazzo, 1990).

In the above example, the internal consistency of the symptom presentation may be of interest. Suppose that a raw score of 7 is obtained on the UPSIT. The probability of a score of 7 or less in a true anosmic is approximately .182, or about 1 in 5. There is thus a 1 in 5 chance the patient is not malingering, but in making such a judgment on the basis of this score alone we will call a true anosmic a liar (i.e., malingerer) 18% of the time. Being reluctant to make this diagnosis, we are guided in the UPSIT manual to designate this score as reflective of a true microsmia. Suppose, however, the following information is gleaned from the clinical examination and interview.

The patient complained of increased inhibition with some depression on a posttraumatic basis along with decreased interest in sex in particular. His sense of humor seems less evident by his report and that of his spouse. When interviewed about smell and taste, he complains of a complete loss of both. In response to specific questions, the patient denies the ability to taste the hotness of peppers or various chilies and denies the ability to smell or detect ammonia or other household cleaning fluids to which he has been exposed.

These data supplement the SVT, in this case the UPSIT, and lead to a diagnosis of malingering. Although this diagnosis is potentially incorrect, as are all diagnoses, it is supported by the lack of congruence of the patient's symptoms. Anatomically, the most likely cortical area to have concurrent damage with the olfactory bulbs and the olfactory nerves (cranial nerve I) is the orbitomedial and generally inferior surfaces of the frontal lobes. Damage to this region is more likely to result in disinhibition, jocularity, and sexual acting out than it is to present with increased inhibition, depression, decreased sense of humor, and decreased libido. Many individuals relate the loss of smell to taste and the effect is substantial. However, the heat sensation when "tasting" a hot chili is not taste or smell but is a noxious response mediated by the trigeminal nerve (cranial nerve V) as is the detection of ammonia and certain other noxious fumes present in certain household cleaning fluids. When all of this information is coupled with a neurologist's report noting that cranial nerves II–XII are all intact, the results of the examination as a whole make the conclusion of malingering by far the most likely diagnosis. Does this meet the legal requirements of "reasonable psychological probability" and "preponderance of the evidence"? Although the latter is within the province of the finder of fact, the conclusion of malingering in the circumstances described above seems to satisfy this criterion as it is certainly more likely than not. The former criterion is more subjective.

As psychologists practicing in the area of forensics, do we require a $p \leqslant .05$

or $p \leqslant .01$ for a diagnosis or conclusion to be correct? Would $p \leqslant .15$ be sufficient for clinical decision making as has been suggested (e.g., see Kaufman, 1979)? Statistical significance testing has a role to play in such decisions but it is quite variable. In the above example, had the patient earned a raw score of zero on the SVT, the conclusion of malingering would have been difficult to defeat even if other symptoms were internally consistent. The obtained score of 7 with its associated p value of .18 is less conclusive and makes us uncomfortable as clinicians. However, there is no statistical test for the evaluation of the additional clinical data obtained. There is no method then to assess actuarially the combinatorial probability of these events. Nor is it necessary to support the conclusion reached. A significance level of $p \leqslant .05$ has been adopted by convention in the adversarial world of science for a variety of reasons (e.g., Hays, 1973; Reynolds, 1984) but need not apply to a confluence of congruent clinical and empirical data. Common sense cannot be aborted by the inappropriate rigid application of inferential statistics.

SVT can be adapted to individual cases as demonstrated well by Denney (1996) and by Moore (1996). For example, if a patient claims long term memory loss and an accurate history of life events and actions is available, the clinician can devise a series of true–false or other multiple-choice formatted questions about the patient's life. A worse-than-chance performance on such a task would argue in favor of malingering. A similar procedure is used in guilty knowledge testing in criminal proceedings. Facts about a crime that would be obvious to a perpetrator are gathered, formatted into a two-, three-, or four-choice format, and the methods of SVT are then applied to the responses of the examinee. The distribution of random responses in each case is known. However, SVT is a conservative response and will underidentify malingerers. Whether this is desirable or not is discussed later.

Internal Consistency of Symptoms

SVT deals to some degree with the internal consistency or internal congruence of a patient's symptoms, but in a very limited way. A broader, more classic approach to this question is presented in this volume by Hartlage and Berry and Butcher and to a lesser degree by Golden and Grier. The MMPI F scale is a classic approach to evaluation of the internal consistency of a presentation and is commonly used to assess overreporting of symptoms. This approach has been adopted for rating scales and other objective tests as well (e.g., Reynolds & Kamphaus, 1992). Composed of a set of symptoms that are infrequent and that have low interitem correlations, the logic is that the reporting of a large number of such symptoms, occurring when the T score on F is elevated, is actuarially improbable as a representation of a coherent syndrome or even the co-occurrence of several disorders. The collection of items on such a scale is not unidimensional nor internally consistent with regard to a specific illness or condition.

To their credit, Berry and Butcher (this volume) note that head injury patients are the most difficult group of malingerers to detect and this is accurate as regards the use of elevated F on the MMPI/MMPI-2. This is most likely related to the less predictable nature of specific symptoms following a significant traumatic brain injury (TBI) and the heterogeneity of groups of TBI patients in the collective literature and even in individual studies. Even so, the F scale does remarkably well on an actuarial basis. Even in studies where differing ultimate conclusions have been reached, the MMPI-2 F scale has performed well. Greiffenstein, Gola, and Baker (1995) studied a group of severe TBI patients, a group of "probable malingerers" (PM), and a group of persistent postconcussion syndrome patients. The PM group constituted 68 consecutive referrals of individuals with persistent postconcussive complaints more than 1 year after a very mild head injury (defined as 20 minutes or less of amnesia following a deceleration accident; 29% of the sample had no blow to the head and no period of posttraumatic amnesia). Although Greiffenstein et al. (1995) interpreted their results to suggest caution in the use of MMPI-2 validity scales, F included, in neuropsychological contexts, the PM group scored 8.15 *T*-score points above the severe TBI group ($T = 71.35$ versus $T = 63.25$ for the severe TBI group). This is a substantial difference and the severe TBI group's F scale is not considered elevated even by the more lax standards of MMPI-2 versus MMPI; yet, the PM group has an elevated F scale by old and by new standards. Although not reported and an exact percentage being incalculable from data presented in Greiffenstein et al. (1995), under the assumption of a normal distribution, it can be estimated from data presented that 61% of the PM group had an $F > 65$ whereas only 45% of the severe TBI group had an F of this magnitude. The F scale can be seen as not only useful with mild TBI in the detection of malingering but also conservative. In the case of severe TBI, it is less useful but malingering is also a considerably smaller problem in the severe TBI patient population.

The conceptual model of the MMPI F scale can be applied to any set of symptoms presented by a patient, but is less likely to be useful in determining the validity of a patient's presentation with severe injuries. Severe injuries may well produce a pattern of symptoms that is in fact internally inconsistent and clinicians must be on guard against overdiagnosis of malingering in such cases—another reason why the history of the injury and the premorbid status are crucial to accurate diagnosis.

As an example of the latter, consider the patient with a premorbid diagnosis of schizoaffective disorder who suffers a severe TBI that involves a 48-hour deep coma and a spinal cord contusion, the latter leaving a bilateral dysesthesia of the upper extremities. Such a patient may rightfully have an elevated F based on the presence of multiple disorders that are not highly correlated. Although symptom misattribution may become a problem in such a case, a good history should avoid overdiagnosis of malingering and successful misattribution of symptoms by a knowledgeable patient.

The work of Hartlage (this volume) emphasizes internal consistency, within-patient congruence much as is argued by Anderson and Bigler (1994). The latter authors argue that an intrasubject design is more powerful than the typical inter-subject design so common in research on the detection of malingering. Each evaluation of malingering is in fact a study of $N = 1$. The congruence of the symptoms presented by the individual patient is simply crucial to the evaluation process. This evaluation requires a skilled, knowledgeable clinician capable of evaluating a unique set of data for a given patient. In the case of the neuropsychologist, this requires knowledge of the neuroanatomical correlates of behavioral function, the mechanics of TBI, cognitive and behavioral effects of psychiatric disorders and their various psychopharmacotherapies, along with the nature and course of congenital, developmental, and neuropsychiatric disorders. Through this knowledge, the consistency of the patient's presentation can be evaluated.

CONGRUENCE OF CURRENT STATUS WITH KNOWN SEQUELAE OF AN INJURY

The neurosciences, to which neuropsychology and neuropsychiatry belong, are among the most rapidly progressing of the sciences of our age. In the clinical arena, much is known about the cognitive and behavioral sequelae of various neurologically based diseases and traumatic injury to the brain. The predictability of the course of recovery and the sequelae of a brain injury varies substantially as a function of the specific nature of an injury. A small, well-localized stroke or other lesion has the most predictable outcome along with other clearly localized lesions such as produced by a missile wound. Diffuse injuries of various types have known sequelae and outcomes to a significant degree, even such diffuse injuries as an anoxia or prolonged hypoxia, provided certain elements of the injury are estimated in reasonable fashion such as length and degree of loss of consciousness, initial length of the posttraumatic amnesia, and any structural changes in the brain itself. In the case of mild TBI, the sequelae and recovery period are relatively well established, although there will always be exceptional cases at both ends of the spectrum of recovery.

In at least 90% of cases of mild head injury, there is a substantial recovery and a return to work and other significant life pursuits within 6 months of the injury (e.g., see Binder & Rohling, 1996; Greiffenstein, Baker, & Gola, 1996; Greiffenstein et al., 1995; Levinson & Reeves, 1996; McLean, Dikmen, & Temkin, 1993; Prigatano, 1990). Greiffenstein et al. (1995) used the persistence of symptoms past 1 year following minor head injury to classify research subjects as "probable malingerers," a practice also used by other respected researchers (e.g., McLean et al., 1993; Millis, 1992; Prigatano & Amin, 1993). In a study of 650 young adults, Shine, Morse, and Morse (1996) reported the 15% of this group that had a history of prior hospitalization for loss of consciousness did not differ in number of neuropsychological symptoms reported from the remainder of the sample, none of which had received any hospital treatment related to an injury involving loss of consciousness. (Alcohol consumption was, however, related to poorer outcomes.) None of these loss-of-consciousness, previously hospitalized patients were known to be in litigation. Studies of the base rates of certain psychosocial variables following mild head trauma show few chronic residual deficits. McLean et al. (1993) found no difference in the base rate for unemployment between mild TBI patients and social controls at 1-year follow-up. These general classes of findings led to conclusions such as that reached by Greiffenstein et al. (1996), namely, that "a claim of minor head trauma being the proximate cause of joblessness a year later can be termed an improbable outcome" (p. 284). The term used by this group of researchers, *improbable outcome*, is a choice of words speaking directly to the issue at hand. Is the outcome consistent with the known sequelae of an injury? An improbable outcome does not prove beyond all doubt that an individual is malingering—this would require an "impossible outcome." Given what we do know about the predictability of higher cognitive disturbances, impossible outcomes are not seen. Improbable outcomes do support the hypothesis of malingering as the most probable conclusion. Thus, in the case of improbable outcomes, there is a shift in the burden of proof the psychologist or clinician should require in formalizing a diagnosis of true head-injury related symptomatology versus a diagnosis of malingering.

In the case of an improbable outcome (e.g., an incongruity between the presentation of the patient and the known course of recovery or other sequelae of the claimed injury) in a litigation environment, the presumption of malingering is justified, and it is up to the patient and the clinician to disprove the diagnosis of malingering. Although logically consistent, this conclusion receives strong empirical support from the work of Binder and Rohling (1996) and other, perhaps more indirect sources (e.g., Shine et al., 1996). This said, it is notable that severe disability persisting over the long term following mild head injury is possible and will be the correct conclusion in some cases; it is an improbable outcome, not an impossible or even unknown outcome.

Hartlage (this volume) presents a model for clinical evaluation of improbable sequelae. The work of Reitan and Wolfson (this volume) provides a superlative example of an empirical/actuarial approach to this question that, albeit a conservative strategy, has withstood cross-validation. A century of research shows that, following the acute phase of cerebral trauma, people get better[2] and their neuropsychological test performance improves (e.g., see Reitan & Wolfson, this volume,

[2]There are some known exceptions to this general principle but they are typically not associated with external trauma related CNS insult but are related to certain insidious toxins, most prominently carbon monoxide, and diseases that have accompanying iatrogenic neuropsychological complications, e.g., leukemia.

and other works by such authors as Bennett, Dikmen, Diller, Hodes, Levin, Ruff, and others). Based on this knowledge and insights of a pioneer, Reitan and his colleague once again reach out with an empirical solution to an imposing problem. Their approach nevertheless continues to be conservative as their recommended cut scores will minimize the overdiagnosis of malingering at the risk of allowing some malingerers to go undetected. When actuarial methods such as provided by Reitan and Wolfson result in a classification of probable malingering, the probability is extreme that malingering is the correct diagnosis and very powerful evidence would be needed to overcome this diagnosis. This statement applies to any method based on statistical significance testing such as in SVT. The Reitan and Wolfson method of deriving cutoff scores is superior by nature to the SVT approach but continues to be conservative.

In some instances, data are available on the frequency of occurrence of specific outcomes that enables the clinician to make clear actuarial statements. To characterize an outcome as improbable does not require formal statistical significance testing as used by the SVT procedure in its classical form. A simple actuarial count is all that is required.

In some cases, the prudent conclusion will be that of improbable outcome without clear counts. For example, consider a strongly right-handed adult male (see Dean & Reynolds, in press, and Reynolds, in press, for discussions of handedness and lateralization) who suffers a clean missile wound contained within the dorsolateral posterior parietal lobe and adjacent occipital tissue of the right hemisphere. In addition to claims of a visual field defect, decreased sensation on the left side, severe problems with spatial ability and lesser problems with nonverbal reasoning, and a significant visual memory defect, the patient claimed a significant degree of expressive aphasia. During an acute care rehabilitation period and later on an outpatient basis, very little progress was noted in recovery of the aphasia with only small degrees of progress evident in the other areas as well. Approximately 3 years later, the patient is unemployed and his scores on a broad array of language measures show small declines in performance. Is this an impossible outcome in such a case? No. Is it an improbable outcome? Yes. Clearly our knowledge of functional neuroanotomy leads us to the conclusion that the claims of aphasia and declining language scores are unlikely to be related to the injury described despite the lack of an actuarial count of "aphasia" as a sequela of such an injury, particularly an aphasia showing evidence of declining performance in a premorbidly healthy adult with a static injury. In such a scenario, a patient with a legitimate, compensable TBI may be seen reasonably as attempting to take advantage of the injury to claim additional, improbable injuries to bolster a damage claim. The question of whether this constitutes malingering has already been addressed and the answer is yes. Should the patient be penalized by a jury in considering the damage award for this patient/plaintiff? This question has been addressed as well. The answer is that the neuropsychologist has no expert opinion on this matter. This is a matter for the jury to decide, perhaps with expert opinion from a logician or a philosopher being of assistance.

In the case of multiple instances of improbable outcomes, the diagnosis of malingering is bolstered. This is obvious and most defensible when actuarial counts or related statistical data are available, especially in a form where the principles of combinatorial probability can be applied. The principle of combinatorial probability tells us that the probability of two independent events having a contemporaneous occurrence is equal to the product of the probabilities of each event taken singly.[3] This probability value shrinks rapidly with two or more uncommon events. The rate of shrinkage of p is inversely related to the correlation of any two events and there is no shrinkage (i.e., no change) in p (AB) when $r_{AB} = 1.00$. Unfortunately, in the context of neuropsychological assessment and evaluations, when we note improbable outcomes, we do not know the value of r between the two events and our clinical knowledge is left as our guide. Experience, which remains a valid teacher, notes that most practitioners likely underestimate the dramatic change in the probability of an outcome when two or more improbable outcomes are evident in an individual case. This statement is itself without actuarial evidence and deserves investigation beyond the experiential base available. Nevertheless, as more improbable outcomes and unlikely occurrences reveal themselves, the likelihood of malingering as the correct diagnosis improves and at a compelling pace.

WHAT GOOD CLINICIANS DO

When faced with a head injury patient in litigation, clinicians are constantly subject to attempts by attorneys (on both sides) and the patient to view the patient's condition in a particular way. Treating clinicians are apt to be compromised in forensic evaluations as a result of their need to maintain a treatment alliance with the patient and their tendency to be a patient advocate. Clinicians must assess their allegiances carefully in such circumstances and acknowledge the limits of their opinions appropriately. As noted, most individuals in the caregiving professions of psychology are reluctant to make such a negative diagnosis as malingering. What the good forensic scientist practitioner does do is follow the data, looking for the three keys to evaluating the diagnosis of malingering: congruence, congruence, and congruence.

One seemingly frequent error committed in this process is to weigh the consistencies and inconsistencies in a patient's presentation and come down on the side of the most frequent of the two. This is poor logic. A single inconsistency may

[3]For example, if the probability of event A = .01 and the probability of event B = .01 and $r_{AB} = 0$, the probability of A and B occurring for the same individual is $p(A)p(B)$ or 0.0001. Even when $p = .10$ for each event, when $r_{AB} = 0$, the probability of A and B (not A or B) is quite small: when $p(A) = .10$ and $p(B) = .10$, (AB) = 0.01.

be sufficient to warrant a diagnosis of malingering.[4] If a patient claims an inability to speak, one episode of speech is all that one needs document to draw a solid conclusion.

Good clinicians do look for confirming and disconfirming evidence and do not weigh them equally—to do so is logically inconsistent. As clinicians find incongruities in the patient's total presentation (history, presentation, progress in recovery, and so on), the probability of malingering likewise increases. Unfortunately, we do not have actuarial tables that allow us to put a specific probability neatly on all combinations seen but multiple incongruities will fall in the range of more probable than not (which need be defined only as >50%) when considering the diagnosis of malingering. The rigid application of null hypothesis testing as applied to SVT is not salve to our problem although SVT is helpful when it is significant. It does not rule out malingering particularly convincingly when $p > .05$. Formal hypothesis testing is inadequate to the task of the clinician in this regard just as it is inadequate to many needs of the scientist (e.g., see Cohen, 1994)[5] Cumulative science relies on *replication*, not individual tests of statistical significance. Good clinicians rely on replication. Replication is what the analysis of congruence in a patient's total presentation is all about. Evaluation of the congruence of history, internal consistency of symptom presentation, and sequelae of the injury is a search for replication of a true disorder and a failure to replicate points to an improbable outcome. When more than one improbable outcome occurs, the contrarian replication of malingering evidence is confirmed by the clinician who must then step up and make what is an emotionally charged, personally difficult call. This approach to data analysis, which is by far the most appropriate in individual clinical cases (e.g., see Kaufman, 1979, 1994; Wesman, 1968), was championed early by the eminent statistician John Tukey as well. Tukey (1962, 1977) emphasized detective work in the analysis of data as opposed to "sanctification" through significance testing alone. Being a good clinician in the evaluation of malingering in head injury litigation means being a detective who evaluates the congruence of the available data, quantitative and qualitative, seeks replication, and reports, understands, and explains the most probable conclusion but also understands its alternatives and knows he may be wrong.

[4]Some clinicians are so rife with guilt over the diagnosis of malingering, they refer only to "probable malingering." This perhaps more palatable terminology has been avoided because we do not preface other diagnoses with the term probable. We are seldom if ever 100% certain about a diagnosis, be it schizophrenia, bipolar disorder, borderline personality disorder, or post concussion syndrome. Yet, one rarely sees in a neuropsychological report or a patient's chart a final diagnosis that reads: Axis I, probable depression. The use of the phrase probable malingering is a reflection of our continuing optimism about our fellow human beings and our own role as caregivers.

[5]Even Paul Meehl (1967), a name so often associated with statistical proof of group membership and actuarial classification, has voiced his harangue about the overreliance of psychologists on null hypothesis significance testing and how it has retarded progress in the discipline.

WHAT CATEGORY OF ERROR IS PREFERABLE?

It is axiomatic that as long as decisions are made on the basis of data with less than perfect reliability and perfect validity, errors will be made. The diagnostic decisions made in neuropsychology and dependent on neuropsychological assessments, interviews, histories, and the like will thus be imperfect. When a diagnostic decision is made, there are four potential outcomes with regard to accuracy. The clinicians can be: (1) correct about the presence of a disorder, a true-positive condition; (2) incorrect about the presence of a disorder, a false positive condition; (3) correct about the absence of a disorder, a true-negative condition; and (4) incorrect about the absence of a condition, a false-negative condition. These potential decisions are illustrated with respect to malingering in Figure 1.

When determining cutoff scores or deciding on a significance level to determine the presence of a particular diagnosis (e. g., as in the case of malingering and $p \leqslant .05$ in evaluation of malingering), values are often set so as to minimize either false-positive or false-negative errors. Base rates and the relative costs of each type of error in terms of therapeutic outcome, monetary, medical, psychological, and social costs are some of the primary factors considered in deciding which type of error to minimize. As we increase and decrease error rates of different types, the accuracy of true-positive and true-negative diagnostic decision rates will be variably affected as well. In many cases there are clear mathematical and psychosocial reasons to minimize one type of error over another (e.g., see Reynolds, 1984, for a discussion and example).

In the context of the evaluation of malingering during head injury litigation, is it preferable to: (1) overdiagnose malingering in hopes that no true malingerer goes undetected (minimize false negatives) or (2) underdiagnose malingering in hopes that no honest individual is mislabeled a malingerer (minimize false positives)? In a therapeutic setting, the clinician chooses to underdiagnose malingering to provide treatment to the maximum number of patients because the cost of treating a malingerer is small compared with the cost of not providing care to a truly injured

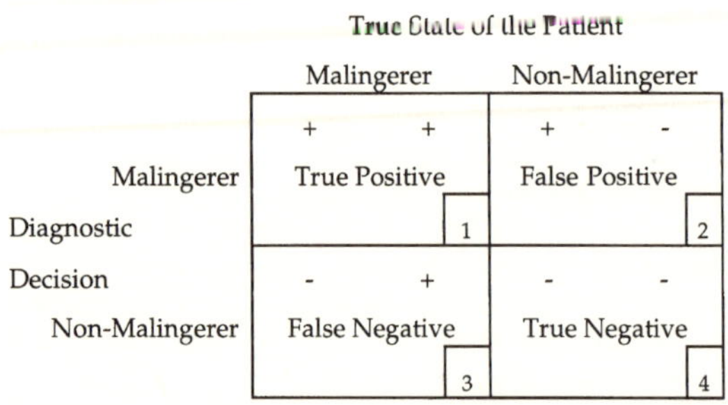

FIGURE 1. Diagnostic outcomes in evaluation of malingering.

patient with legitimate sequelae. In the forensic setting, this balance changes. An innocent party (the defendant) may be greatly penalized financially, psychologically, and socially if a malingerer (the plaintiff) is awarded a large settlement. By the same token, a truly injured party (a legitimately injured plaintiff with long-term sequelae) may be denied compensation and subsequently not be able to receive treatment, support herself or her family, and suffer additional psychological and social damage compounding her injuries if incorrectly diagnosed as a malingerer. Society at large suffers under both circumstances, but in different ways. Obviously, we attempt to minimize all types of errors, but we can seldom establish a perfect balance. SVT interpreted via probability theory will err on the side of underdiagnosis. Using most probable outcome approaches in a rigid application (e. g., remaining jobless 1 year after a mild head injury as a criterion measure for malingering) will overdiagnose malingering. It is incalculable, based on currently available data, how to equate the two diagnostic error rates.

Which is the preferable error? The clinical neuropsychologist has no true scientific basis for answering this question. In the evaluation of malingering in head injury litigation, the decision as to whether it is better to commit a false positive error (Figure 1, box 2) or a false-negative error (Figure 1, box 3) involves moral, social, and perhaps even constitutional values that should be the subject of policy debates. In current forensic settings, it is considered by the finder of fact on a case-by-case basis and a judge or jury may be swayed by the arguments of the attorneys, the facts of the case, and the condition (e.g., financial, social) of the parties. The latter is the primary reason defense attorneys do not allow juries to know of insurance coverage in personal injury litigation. When in doubt, it is easier to take money from a faceless, impersonal insurance company to compensate a questionably injured party than it is to take money or property from another individual facing the jury in the courtroom.

False-positive and false-negative diagnoses of malingering in litigation both have potentially dire consequences. In nonforensic, treatment settings and related arenas where financial incentive or other secondary gain is not at issue, the preference for an error type is clear—false-negative errors are preferred. In the forensic arena, we should present our case for diagnosis, its basis, its philosophy (conservative or liberal), revealing any personal biases and let the litigators do their job. Neither as experts nor as individual clinicians do we need to resolve this question, nor can we on the basis of available data.

INTELLIGENT TESTING AND DIAGNOSIS OF MALINGERING

Faced with decision making when $N = 1$, there is some degree of consensus among otherwise somewhat divergent scholars in the field of testing and assessment. The intelligent testing philosophy of Wesman (1968) and Kaufman (1979,

1994; see also Reynolds, 1987a) seems to capture best the recommended methods of Cohen (1994), Kaufman (1979, 1994), Kleinmuntz (1990), Matarazzo (1990), Tukey (1962, 1977), and Wesman (1968) as they are interpreted here and elsewhere (e.g., Reynolds, 1987a) to apply to individual cases. The intent of the intelligent testing model is to bring together actuarial data, psychometrics, clinical acumen, psychological theories, a solid knowledge base in brain–behavior relationships, and careful reasoning (i.e., good common sense) to build a proper assessment, in context, leading to an accurate diagnosis (broadly conceived) and treatment methods as may be required. This approach to test use and interpretation has been likened to the approach of a psychological detective (Kaufman, 1979) which is precisely our role as scientist-practitioners in a research environment as well (e.g., Cohen, 1994; Tukey, 1962, 1977). Through the elements of clinical skill, psychometric sophistication, and a broad knowledge base, intelligent testing emerges in a synergy of information.

Ever cautious, the forensic neuropsychologist gathers data, clinical, actuarial, and historical, and merges these data, developing competing hypotheses as may be appropriate and pits these hypotheses against one another within the data set available and against the base of knowledge possessed regarding brain–behavior relationships. The knowledge base of the clinical neuropsychologist and the reliability of data provided and collected on examination are crucial to the reliability of the outcome in such cases. In the process of intelligent testing, the search for internal replication is paramount. Congruence of data with conclusions is urgent and requires good common sense. Statistical significance testing, using statistics designed for individual cases, is important but insufficient. There simply is no substitute for common sense and clear reasoning. Cohen (1994) made the point by referring to the researcher who presents a null hypothesis that no cases of a particular type exist with a specific referral population. After gathering data on the population, one case is found. The researcher agonizes over the proper statistical significance test that will allow "scientific" or "statistical" proof for rejection of the null hypothesis. The researcher ignores common sense in the pursuit of such science. We have few such clear-cut cases in forensic neuropsychology and those that are found are not the ones difficult to decipher. The process, however, is the same. The evaluation of malingering in head injury litigation requires intelligent testing; it is a search for congruence across and within assessment domains and demands reasonable interpretation of improbable outcomes.

REFERENCES

American Psychiatric Association. (1994). *Diagnostic and statistical manual of mental disorders*. (4th ed.). Washington, DC: Author.

Anderson, C. V., & Bigler, E. D. (1994). Ventricular dilation as a predictor of cognitive outcome. *Archives of Clinical Neuropsychology*, *9*, 106.

Barnhart, C. L. (Ed.). (1967). *The world book dictionary*. (Vol. 2). Chicago: Field Enterprises Educational Corporation.

Binder, L. M. (1990). Malingering following minor head trauma. *The Clinical Neuropsychologist, 4*, 25–36.

Binder, L.M. (1993). Assessment of malingering after mild head injury with the Portland Digit Recognition Test. *Journal of Clinical and Experimental Neuropsychology, 15*, 170–182.

Binder, L. M., & Rohling, M. L. (1996). Money matters: A meta-analytic review of the effects of financial incentives on recovery after closed-head injury. *American Journal of Psychiatry, 153*(1), 7–10.

Cartlidge, N. E. F., & Shaw, D. A. (1981). *Head injury*. Philadelphia: WB Saunders.

Cohen, J. (1994). The earth is round ($p < .05$). *American Psychologist, 49*, 997–1003.

Dean, R. S., & Reynolds, C. R. (in press). Cognitive processing and self-report of lateral preference. *Neuropsychology Review*.

de Armas, A. (1996). Detection of malingering in forensic psychological evaluations. *The Forensic Examiner, 5*, 26–28.

Denney, R. L. (1996). Symptom validity testing of remote memory in a criminal forensic setting. *Archives of Clinical Neuropsychology, 11*, 589–604.

Doty, L. (1995). *The Smell Identification Test administration manual*. (3rd ed.). Haddon Heights, NJ: Sensonics, Inc.

Fenton, G., McClelland, R., Montgomery, A., MacFlynn, G., & Rutherford, W. (1993). The postconcussional syndrome: Social antecedents and psychological sequelae. *British Journal of Psychiatry, 162*, 493–497.

Greiffenstein, M. E., Baker, W., & Gola, T. (1996). Comparison of multiple scoring methods for Rey's malingered amnesia measures. *Archives of Clinical Neuropsychology, 11*, 283–293.

Greiffenstein, M. F., Gola, T., & Baker, J. (1995). MMPI-2 validity scales versus domain specific measures in detection of factitious traumatic brain injury. *The Clinical Neuropsychologist, 9*, 230–240.

Hays, W. L. (1973). *Statistics for the social sciences*. New York: Holt, Rinehart & Winston.

Hickman, J. A., & Reynolds, C. R. (1994). Effects of false allegations of sexual assault on children and families. In B. Threatt (Ed.), *Evaluating children's allegations of sexual assault*. Austin: Texas Children's Legal Resource Center.

Jafek, B. W., Eller, P. M., Esses, B. A., & Moran, D. T. (1989). Post traumatic anosmia: Ultrastructural correlates. *Archives of Clinical Neuropsychology, 46*, 300–304.

Kaufman, A. S. (1979). *Intelligent testing with the WISC-R*. New York: Wiley–Interscience.

Kaufman, A. S. (1994). *Intelligent testing with the WISC-3*. New York: Wiley–Interscience.

Kleinmuntz, B. (1990). Why we still use our heads instead of the formulas: Toward an integrative approach. *Psychological Bulletin, 107*, 296–310.

Levinson, D. M., & Reeves, D. L. (1996). Monitoring recovery from traumatic brain injury using the automated neuropsychological assessment metrics (ANAM 1.0). *Archives of Clinical Neuropsychology, 11*, 419–420.

Malloy, P., Bihrle, A., Duffy, J., & Cimino, C. (1993). The orbitomedial frontal syndrome. *Archives of Clinical Neuropsychology, 8*, 185–201.

Matarazzo, J. (1990). Psychological assessment versus psychological testing: Validation from Binet to the school, clinic, and courtroom. *American Psychologist, 45*, 999–1017.

McKechnie, J. L. (Ed.). (1983). *Webster's new universal unabridged dictionary*. 2nd ed. New York: Simon & Schuster.

McLean, A., Dikmen, S. S., & Temkin, N. . (1993). Psychosocial recovery after head injury. *Archives of Physical Medicine and Rehabilitation, 74*, 1041–1046.

Meehl, P. E. (1954). *Clinical versus statistical prediction: A theoretical analysis and a review of the evidence*. Minneapolis: University of Minnesota Press.

Meehl, P. E. (1967). Theory testing in psychology and physics: A methodology paradox. *Philosophy of Science, 34*, 103–115.

Millis, S. (1992). The Recognition Memory Test in the detection of malingered and exaggerated memory deficits. *The Clinical Neuropsychologist*, *7*, 406–414.

Moore, R. E. (1996). Detecting guilty knowledge in violent crimes. *The Forensic Examiner*, *5*, 15–18.

Pankratz, L. (1979). Symptom validity testing and symptom retraining: Procedures for the assessment and treatment of functional sensory deficits. *Journal of Consulting and Clinical Psychology*, *47*, 409–410.

Pankratz, L., Fausti, S. A., & Peed, S. (1975). A forced-choice technique to evaluate deafness in the hysterical or malingering patient. *Journal of Consulting and Clinical Psychology*, *43*, 421–422.

Parzen, E. (1960). *Modern probability theory and its applications*. New York: Wiley.

Prigatano, G. P. (1990). Effective traumatic brain injury rehabilitation: Team/ patient interaction. In E. Bigler (Ed.), *Traumatic brain injury* (pp. 297–312), Austin, TX: PRO-ED.

Prigatano, G. P., & Amin, K. (1993). Digit Memory Test: Unequivocal cerebral dysfunction and suspected malingering. *Journal of Clinical and Experimental Neuropsychology*, *15*, 537–546.

Pritchard, D. A. (1997). Forensic neuropsychology. In M. Maruish & J. Moses (Eds.), *Clinical neuropsychology: Theoretical foundations for practioners* (pp. 81–118). Hillsdale, NJ: Erlbaum.

Reynolds, C. R. (1984). Critical issues in learning disabilities. *Journal of Special Education*, *18*, 451–476.

Reynolds, C. R. (1987a). Intelligent testing. In C. R. Reynolds & L. Mann (Eds.), *Encyclopedia of Special Education*, (pp. 855–857). New York: Wiley–Interscience.

Reynolds, C. R. (1987b). Raising intelligence: Clever Hans, Candide, and the miracle in Milwaukee. *Journal of School Psychology*, *25*, 309–312.

Reynolds, C. R. (1997). Measurement and statistical problems in neuropsychological assessment of children. In C. R. Reynolds & E. Fletcher-Janzen (Eds.), *Handbook of clinical child neuropsychology* (2nd ed., pp. 180–203). New York: Plenum.

Reynolds, C. R. (Ed.) (in press). Assessment of laterality. [Special issue]. *Neuropsychology Review*.

Reynolds, C. R., & Brown, R. T. (1984). Bias in mental testing: An introduction to the issues. In C. R. Reynolds & R. T. Brown (Eds.), *Perspectives on bias in mental testing*. (pp. 1–40). New York: Plenum Press.

Reynolds, C. R., & James, E. M. (1997). Development of neuropsychological measures. In M. Maruish & J. Moses (Eds.), *Clinical neuropsychology: Theoretical foundations for practitioners* (pp. 347–370). Hillsdale, NJ: Erlbaum.

Reynolds, C. R., & Kamphaus, R. W. (1992). *Behavior Assessment System for Children: Manual*. Circle Pines, MN: American Guidance Service.

Roget, P.M. (1962). *Roget's international thesaurus*. (3rd ed.). New York: Thomas Y. Crowell.

Shine, A. E., Morse, L. W., & Morse, D. T. (1996). A review of the neuropsychological symptoms endorsed by individuals reporting loss of consciousness. *Archives of Clinical Neuropsychology*, *11*, 448–449.

Tukey, J. W. (1962). The future of data analysis. *Annals of Mathematical Statistics*, *33*, 1–67.

Tukey, J. W. (1977). *Exploratory data analysis*. Reading MA: Addison Wesley.

Wesman, A. (1968). Intelligent testing. *American Psychologist*, *23*, 267–274.

Youngjohn, J. R., Burrows, L., & Erdal, K. (1995). Brain damage or compensation neurosis? The controversial post-concussion syndrome. *The Clinical Neuropsychologist*, *9*, 112–123.

Youssem, D. M., Geckle, R. J., Bilker, W. B., McKeown, D., & Doty, R. C. (in press). Post-traumatic olfactory dysfunction: MR evaluation. *Neurology*.

Index

ISBN 0-306-45655-9
90000
9 780306 456558